Treatment of Late-Life
INSOMNIA

TREATMENT OF LATE-LIFE
INSOMNIA

EDITORS

KENNETH L. LICHSTEIN
CHARLES M. MORIN

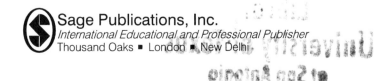
Sage Publications, Inc.
International Educational and Professional Publisher
Thousand Oaks ■ London ■ New Delhi

For information:

Sage Publications, Inc.
2455 Teller Road
Thousand Oaks, California 91320
E-mail: order@sagepub.com

Sage Publications Ltd.
6 Bonhill Street
London EC2A 4PU
United Kingdom

Sage Publications India Pvt. Ltd.
M-32 Market
Greater Kailash I
New Delhi 110 048 India

Printed in the United States of America

Library of Congress Cataloging-in-Publication Data

Treatment of late-life insomnia / edited by Kenneth L. Lichstein and
    Charles M. Morin.
      p. cm.
Includes bibliographical references and index.
ISBN 0-7619-1506-0 (cloth: acid-free paper)
ISBN 0-7619-1507-9 (pbk: acid-free paper)
    1. Insomnia. 2. Aged--Diseases. I. Lichstein, Kenneth L.
    II. Morin, Charles M.
    RC548 .T74 2000
    616.8'498--dc21   99-050603

This book is printed on acid-free paper.

00   01   02   03   04   05   06   7   6   5   4   3   2   1

Acquisition Editor:	Jim Brace-Thompson
Editorial Assistant:	Anna Howland
Production Editor:	Sanford Robinson
Editorial Assistant:	Cindy Bear
Typesetter/Designer:	Marion Warren
Indexer:	Molly Hall
Cover Designer:	Candice Harman

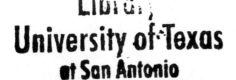

To Sarah, who taught me the importance
of a good night's sleep and other life's truths. (KLL)

To my parents. (CMM)

Contents

III. SPECIAL TREATMENT TOPICS

Foreword

Over 25 million Americans are 65 years of age or older, approximately 12% of the national population. Within 10 years this number will approach 30 million and probably exceed 20% of the population by 2020. One of the major changes that commonly accompanies the aging process is an often-profound disruption of an individual's daily sleep-wake cycle. Epidemiological studies have consistently shown that the prevalence of insomnia increases steadily with advancing age. As many as 40% of older individuals complain about sleep problems, including disturbed or "light" sleep, frequent awakenings, early morning awakenings, and undesired daytime sleepiness. Such disturbances can lead to impaired daytime function and seriously compromise quality of life.

It is within the context of this significant public health problem that Lichstein and Morin have produced this authoritative, comprehensive, and extremely useful book, *Treatment of Late-Life Insomnia*. The editors, nationally recognized experts in the field, have assembled an impressive group of authors, all of whom are themselves well-known scientist-practitioners, who have contributed significantly to our understanding of various aspects of insomnia and its treatment in the older population.

Treatment of Late-Life Insomnia provides the reader with a comprehensive overview of the major issues that the health care practitioner needs to appreciate in order to adequately address this major geriatric health concern. The text's opening chapters set the broad context for the more treatment-specific chapters to follow. These early chapters address such fundamental issues as definitions of insomnia; sleep and circadian rhythm changes with advancing age; causal factors of late-life insomnia; the complex relationship between "good" and "poor" sleep and insomnia complaints; assessment techniques, including the usefulness of sleep histories and diaries; issues of differential diagnosis; and finally, a general overview of treatment practice in this unique population.

The middle chapters provide clear, authoritative examinations of behavioral and cognitive treatment approaches to late-life insomnia. These approaches include sleep hygiene principles, sleep restriction therapy, stimulus control therapy, various relaxation techniques, and cognitive therapy. Each of these chapters offers much more than mere prescriptive information, but rather provides both a theoretical framework and a review of the supporting literature for each treatment approach. Where firm evidence for efficacy is lacking, as in the case of sleep hygiene, this lack is clearly recognized and a framework for what additional knowledge needs to be developed is offered.

The book's closing chapters focus on specialized areas of concern for treating late-life insomnia. The potential advantages and limitations of pharmacological treatment are thoughtfully examined. The rationale and treatment guidelines for discontinuation of sleep medications are discussed in the context of the questionable benefits of prolonged sleep medication use by the elderly. The issue of treatment of secondary insomnia, that is insomnia precipitated or aggravated by another disease, disorder, or substance, is explored. And finally, the difficult issue of treating insomnia in dementia patients and those in residential care facilities is examined.

In each of these chapters the authors have carefully evaluated the available scientific literature, in which their own works have often been seminal, to provide best practices models based on the most current and valid information available. All questions are certainly not answered here, and it is to the various authors' credit that they consistently recognize that much work still needs to be done. Rather than being a weakness, these caveats make the insights offered in *Treatment of Late-Life Insomnia* all the more valuable.

In sum, *Treatment of Late-Life Insomnia* is an extremely valuable, authoritative, and comprehensive resource not only for practitioners of sleep medicine but also for any health care practitioners who find themselves working with the elderly population.

Michael V. Vitiello, PhD
Professor of Psychiatry and Behavioral Sciences
University of Washington
Editor-in-Chief (for the Americas), Sleep Medicine Reviews

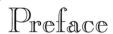

Preface

This book provides a comprehensive research/clinical accounting of insomnia treatment in older adults. We hope this book will serve a useful purpose in guiding practitioners in treating older adults with insomnia complaints and in stimulating additional research to refine our understanding of this condition.

The core of the book, the middle section titled "Intervention Strategies," reviews the clinical outcome research of the major treatments for late-life insomnia and teaches the clinical procedures in the style of a clinical handbook. The first section of the book, "Overview," describes typical normal and disturbed sleep patterns in older adults, demographics, and methods of evaluation and differential diagnosis. The final section, "Special Treatment Topics," explores cutting-edge research and methods of clinical management for pressing topics in late-life insomnia that have only recently attracted systematic investigation.

This book is geared toward students, scientists, and health practitioners engaged in the areas of geriatrics, sleep disorders, and behavioral medicine. These disciplines cut across a variety of professional groups whose members would find such a book useful, including practitioners in psychology, psychiatry, counseling, internal medicine, geriatric medicine, nursing, and social work.

About 12% of the population in this country is older than 65 years of age, and this rate is expected to climb to 20% over the next 20 years. Awareness of the special health needs of older adults is similarly rising, and the burgeoning area of sleep disorders research is rapidly expanding our knowledge of insomnia in this population. Insomnia occurs among older adults at a rate 25% to 50% higher than in younger age groups, and the consequences of insomnia in older adults are more severe than in younger age groups. Elders who exhibit a chronic pattern of insomnia dwell on their anticipation of a poor night's sleep. In many cases, this worry takes on an obsessive quality that degrades multiple aspects of the individual's life. Further, the impact of insomnia in older adults is partly mediated by their disproportionate high use of sleep medications and attendant rise in daytime sedation and cognitive confusion.

Insomnia and other sleep disorders motivate a high frequency of health complaints and utilization of health care services among the elderly. Perhaps half the older adult population is affected by some type of sleep disturbance. Often, there is an occult sleep disorder, such as sleep apnea or periodic limb movements, which mimics the presenting symptoms of insomnia and is prone to self- or professional misdiagnosis. Such misdiagnosis will lead to neglect of the underlying sleep disorder or the application of inappropriate treatments that may actually exacerbate the underlying condition. In either case, serious consequences may befall the individual. Within the health provider community, there is a great need to present effective treatments for the varieties of insomnia and to efficiently differentially diagnose related sleep disorders. This book will serve this dual purpose.

By the mid-1980s, psychological treatment of people with insomnia (PWI) had matured as a clinical science. Clinical interventions, methods of assessment, and strategies of research methodology were well developed and had secured a solid clinical reputation for this domain. By this time, however, the boundaries of refractory insomnia had been firmly established. Several subsets of PWI were judged to be poor candidates for psychological interventions and collectively may be said to have refractory insomnia. Among these groups were older adults with insomnia (OAWI), PWI dependent on sleep medications (hypnotics), and PWI secondary to a medical or psychiatric disorder. The large number of psychological studies on treating PWI consistently screened out people with refractory insomnia. This neglect prevailed even though these three subgroups—OAWI and people with secondary insomnia and hypnotic-dependent insomnia—constitute a majority of the population of PWI. Indeed, with respect to both prevalence and severity of impact, these subgroups of PWI are the most clinically needy.

Much progress has been made in the past decade with regard to psychological treatment of refractory insomnia. This book is devoted to OAWI, one type of refractory insomnia, and specific chapters focus on treating subsets of OAWI—those who are hypnotic dependent and those with insomnia secondary to a medical or psychiatric disorder.

The past 10 to 15 years have exploded myths about difficulties in treating OAWI, and more recently, substantial progress has been made in treating secondary insomnia and hypnotic-dependent insomnia as well. This book then gives testimony to the firm determination of science and celebrates the erosion of valued but misguided convictions.

—*Kenneth L. Lichstein*
—*Charles M. Morin*

PART I

Overview

1

Sleep and Aging

KEVIN MORGAN

With an elegance no longer characteristic of clinical writing, the impact and implications of chronic insomnia were summarized in *The Lancet* by Sigmond (1836) as follows:

> Obstinate sleeplessness is a malady that preys upon every system, disordering every function; during the darkness, the silence, and the solitude of night, all the causes of conflicting passion, of anxiety, and of corroding feeling, rise up with redoubled energy, and haunt the broken spirit. (p. 217)

Links between human aging and "obstinate sleeplessness" have long been recognized. Sigmond (1836), for example, suggested that "the duration of sleep should be, in manhood, about the fourth or the sixth of the 24 hours; children, the younger they are the more sleep they require; in advanced age there is more watchfulness" (p. 217). Similar conclusions are evident in the literature of that time, and associations between "watchfulness" (wakefulness) and advanced age did not escape the irony of Herman Melville. Disturbed by the repeated nocturnal pacing of Captain Ahab on the upper deck of the *Pequod*, Ishmael, the narrator of *Moby Dick*, reflects, "Old age is always wakeful; as if, the longer linked with life, the less man has to do with aught that looks like death" (Melville, 1851/1994, p. 132).

Developments in research methodology, particularly polysomnography, have since confirmed these changes in sleep structure that accompany advancing age (see Bliwise, 1993), while epidemiological studies have clearly described the age-related increase in complaints of insomnia (see Partininen, 1994). Sleep disorders in later life are now widely regarded as a significant policy issue (National Institutes of Health, 1991) and an important focus for clinical (Costa, Silva, Chase, Sartorius, & Roth, 1996) and economic (Leger, 1994, 1995) concern. Focusing mainly on the epidemiological literature and selected experimental studies, this chapter considers the causes and correlates of late-life insomnia in the context of age-related changes in sleep. Overall, the aim is to provide an overview of issues relevant to the assessment and management of sleep disturbance in later life. Because advances in sleep research have engendered an increasingly sophisticated taxonomy of sleep disorders, the issue of insomnia will first be considered in the context of diagnosis and classification.

Classification of Insomnia

Broadly, complaints of disturbed sleep may be divided into sleep onset problems (trouble getting to sleep), sleep maintenance problems (trouble staying asleep), and early morning awakening. These symptoms may occur singly or in combination, and may be transient or long term. Disturbed sleep may also present not as a complaint of sleeplessness but rather as a report of excessive daytime sleepiness (hypersomnia). Building on these rather straightforward subjective reports, insomnia is now explicitly defined in three diagnostic systems: the *ICD-10 Classification of Mental and Behavioral Disorders* (World Health Organization, 1993), the *Diagnostic and Statistical Manual of Mental Disorders* (*DSM-IV*; American Psychiatric Association, 1994), and the *International Classification of Sleep Disorders* (*ICSD*; American Sleep Disorders Association,

1990). Although all three classifications largely agree on the symptoms of insomnia, there are important differences in both terminology and emphasis.

Insomnia: ICD-10

The ICD-10 broadly divides sleep disorders into organic and nonorganic, with the latter category further subdivided into dyssomnias (disturbances of the amount, quality, or timing of sleep) and parasomnias (abnormal episodic events occurring during sleep, such as sleepwalking or nightmares). In this system, "nonorganic insomnia" is a dyssomnia characterized by persistent (i.e., at least three times a week for at least 1 month) difficulty in getting to sleep or staying asleep (or poor quality sleep) that causes the individual concern and markedly interferes with social or occupational functioning. The ICD-10 does not explicitly discriminate between primary insomnia (where the sleep disturbance may be the *only* presenting condition) and secondary insomnia (where the sleep disturbance accompanies other physical or mental disorders).

Insomnia: *DSM-IV*

The *DSM-IV* uses a broader classification that recognizes four main types of sleep disorder: sleep disorders related to another mental disorder, sleep disorders resulting from a general medical condition, substance-induced sleep disorders, and primary sleep disorders (i.e., those not associated with a psychiatric, medical, or pharmacological cause). *Primary sleep disorders* in *DSM-IV* are analogous to the *nonorganic sleep disorders* of ICD-10 and are similarly divided into dyssomnias and parasomnias, with insomnia (as "primary insomnia") again subsumed within the dyssomnias. In *DSM-IV*, the diagnostic features of primary insomnia are also similar to those described in the ICD-10 and include a persistent (i.e., for at least 1 month) complaint of difficulty initiating or maintaining sleep (or of nonrestorative sleep) that causes the individual "significant" distress and is associated with impaired social or occupational functioning. Unlike the ICD-10, however, *DSM-IV* taxonomically separates primary in-

somnia from those secondary insomnias associated with other disorders. Nevertheless, the system does recognize that, under some
circumstances, distinguishing *primary insomnia* from *insomnia related to
another mental disorder* can be especially difficult and that sleep disorders
resulting from general medical conditions are characterized by symptoms similar to those in primary sleep disorders.

Insomnia: *ICSD*

The most detailed classification of sleep disorders is that provided by
the *ICSD*, which defines 12 subtypes of "insomnia disorder" (i.e., disorders of initiating or maintaining sleep) and more than 50 different insomnia syndromes. Because many of these diagnoses require specialized instrumental monitoring (often laboratory-based polysomnography), the
value of the *ICSD* in everyday practice is probably limited. The most
common forms of insomnia recognized by this classification (and those
closest to the "nonorganic" and "primary" insomnias of the ICD-10 and
DSM-IV) include *psychophysiological insomnia* (characterized by psychosomatic arousal, excessive concern about sleep adequacy, and somatized
tension), *inadequate sleep hygiene* (where the sleep problem appears to be
caused or maintained by maladaptive practices), and so-called *sleep-state
misperception* (where the chronic complaint of insomnia is not "corroborated" by polysomnographic findings). The *ICSD* diagnosis of *idiopathic insomnia* (a near-lifelong constitutional predisposition to poor
quality sleep), though relatively rare, may also be regarded as a "classic"
insomnia.

Overall, then, the ICD-10, *DSM-IV*, and *ICSD* show widespread consensus as to what constitutes an insomnia, with many apparent differences being terminological rather than fundamental (in each system, for
example, the same clinical presentation could attract the diagnosis of
"organic insomnia," "primary insomnia," or "psychophysiological insomnia," respectively). In clinical field studies where all three systems
have been used, diagnoses have been found to logically interrelate
(Buysse et al., 1994). Nevertheless, there remain important areas of dis-
agreement. Trinder (1988), for example, described the *ICSD* label of *sleep
state misperception* (subjectively reported insomnia without objective
findings) as a judgmental and unhelpful pseudodiagnosis.

Insomnia and Aging

Although formal diagnostic classification is increasingly being used in epidemiological studies of insomnia (Foley et al., 1995; Ford & Kamerow, 1989; Ohayon, 1996), such categorization remains, at present, the exception. Nevertheless, since the seminal studies of McGhie and Russell (1962) in the United Kingdom and Karacan et al. (1976) in the United States, community surveys have been remarkably consistent in describing the prevalence and natural history of poor sleep quality.

Epidemiology

The prevalence of insomnia increases steadily with age (Gislason & Almqvist, 1987; Karacan et al., 1976; McGhie & Russell, 1962; Mellinger, Balter, & Uhlenhuth, 1985; Ohayon, 1996; Weyerer & Dilling, 1991), with estimates rising from approximately 5% among those aged 18 to 30 to more than 30% among those aged 65 and older (Foley et al., 1995; Gislason & Almqvist, 1987; Mellinger et al., 1985; Ohayon, 1996) (see Table 1.1.). Epidemiological studies also have consistently shown that dissatisfaction with sleep is more common among elderly women than among elderly men (Foley et al., 1995; Ford & Kamerow, 1989; Maggi et al., 1998; Morgan, Dallosso, Ebrahim, Arie, & Fentem, 1988; Newman, Enright, Manolio, Haponik, & Wahl, 1997; Ohayon, 1996) (see Table 1.2) and is higher among lower income and lower educational attainment groups (Blazer, Hays, & Foley, 1995; Ford & Kamerow, 1989; Geroldi, Frisoni, Rozzini, De Leo, & Trabucchi, 1996; Habte-Gabr et al., 1991; Ohayon, 1996). Evidence from the United States also shows clear racial differences in levels of insomnia, with older African Americans reporting significantly fewer sleep complaints than their white contemporaries (Blazer et al., 1995). Whether these latter findings reflect differences in the propensity to express complaints or fundamental differences in the sleep experience remains unclear.

In contrast to the abundance of prevalence data, information on the *incidence* of insomnia (i.e., the rate at which new cases come into existence) is scarce. A clear, though modest, age gradient in the 1-year incidence of insomnia was reported by Ford and Kamerow (1989), with incident complaints rising from 5.7% among those aged 18-25 to 7.3% among those

(Text continued on page 12)

Table 1.1 Age-Specific and Gender-Specific Prevalence Rates (in rounded percentages) of Insomnia From Community Studies, 1976-1996

Study	Gender	Overall Prevalence	Age-Specific Prevalence (range in years)					
Karacan, Thornby, Anch, et al. (1976)[a]	Women	15	9 (20-29)	15 (30-39)	16 (40-49)	17 (50-59)	23 (60-69)	29 (70+)
	Men	11	8 (20-29)	5 (30-39)	11 (40-49)	16 (50-59)	18 (60-69)	20 (70+)
Bixler, Kales, Soldatos, Kales, & Healey (1979)[b]	Total*	32	23 (18-30)	37 (31-50)	40 (51+)			
Mellinger, Balter, & Uhlenhuth (1985)[c]	Total*	17	14 (18-34)	15 (35-49)	20 (50-64)	25 (65-79)		
Ford & Kamerow (1989)[d]	Women	12						
	Men	8						
	Total*		11 (18-25)	9 (26-44)	11 (45-64)	12 (65+)		
Jacquinet-Salord, Lang, Fouriaud, Nicoulet, & Bingham (1993)[e]	Women	26	15 (< 25)	19 (25-34)	26 (35-44)	36 (45-54)	43 (55+)	
	Men	16	10 (< 25)	12 (25-34)	17 (35-44)	19 (45-54)	23 (55+)	

Ohayon (1996)[f]							
Women	24	15 (15-24)	16 (25-34)	22 (35-44)	26 (45-54)	30 (55-64)	37 (65+)
Men	16	10 (15-24)	11 (25-34)	12 (35-44)	19 (45-54)	18 (55-64)	29 (65+)

*Combined figures for women/men only.

a. Insomnia defined as trouble sleeping "often/all the time."

b. Insomnia defined as current difficulty falling or staying asleep, or waking too early.

c. Insomnia defined as "had trouble and was bothered a lot" by "trouble falling asleep or staying asleep."

d. Insomnia defined as "had trouble falling asleep, staying asleep, or waking too early" for a period of 2 weeks or more, *and* consulted a professional about it, took medication for it, or stated that it interfered with life a lot, *and* "if it was not always the result of physical illness."

e. Insomnia defined as self-perceived sleeping difficulties without sleeping tablets.

f. Insomnia defined as unsatisfied with sleep or taking medication for sleep difficulties or (taking medication for) anxieties about sleep difficulties.

Table 1.2 Prevalence of Insomnia (variously defined) Among Older People Living in the Community

Study	Location	Age	Number of Older Respondents	Prevalence (%) Overall	Women	Men
Karacan et al. (1976)	Florida	60-69	NR	20.9[a]	22.6	18.3
		70+	NR	25.9[a]	29.4	20.0
Mellinger, Balter, & Uhlenhuth (1985)	National sample, United States	65-79	798	25.0[b]	NR	NR
Morgan, Dallosso, Ebrahim, Arie, & Fentem (1988)	Nottingham, United Kingdom	65+	1,023	22.5[c]	27.7	14.6
				16.0[d]	19.0	11.6
Ford & Kamerow (1989)	NIMH catchment, United States	65+	1,801	12.0[e]	NR	NR
Jacquinet-Salord, Lang, Fouriaud, Nicoulet, & Bingham (1993)	Paris, France	55+	758	31.0[f]	42.5	22.5
Hohagen et al. (1994)	Mannheim, Germany	66-92	330	23.0[g]	29.1	7.9
				17.0[h]	17.5	16.9
Foley et al. (1995)	East Boston, Massachusetts	65+	3,537	33.7[i]	36.4	29.4
	New Haven, Connecticut	65+	2,717	27.5[i]	31.1	21.2
	Iowa	65+	3,028	23.2[i]	25.4	19.5

Study	Location	Age	N			
Ohayon (1996)	National sample, France	65+	NR	NR	37.3[j]	28.7[j]
Newman, Enright, Manolio, Haponik, & Wahl (1997)	4 U.S. states	65+	5,201	NR	30.0[k]	14.0[k]
	4 U.S. states	65+	5,201	NR	65.0[l]	65.0[l]
Maggi, et al. (1998)	Veneto, Italy	65+	2,398	NR	54.0[m]	35.6[m]

NR = data not reported.

a. Insomnia defined as trouble sleeping "often/all the time."
b. Insomnia defined as "had trouble and was bothered a lot" by "trouble falling asleep or staying asleep."
c. Insomnia defined as problems sleeping "often/all the time."
d. Insomnia defined as problems sleeping "sometimes."
e. Insomnia defined as "had trouble falling asleep, staying asleep, or waking too early" for a period of 2 weeks or more, *and* consulted a professional about it, took medication for it, or stated that it interfered with life a lot, *and* "if it was not always the result of physical illness."
f. Insomnia defined as reported "sleep disturbances."
g. Insomnia defined by DSM-III-R criteria for severe insomnia.
h. Insomnia defined by DSM-III-R criteria for severe insomnia but *without* daytime impairment.
i. Insomnia defined as "trouble falling asleep and/or waking up too early and not being able to fall asleep again most of the time."
j. Insomnia defined as "unsatisfied with sleep *or* taking medication for sleeping difficulties or anxiety with sleeping difficulties."
k. Insomnia defined as sleep onset insomnia, "difficulty falling asleep."
l. Insomnia defined as sleep maintenance insomnia, "frequent awakenings."
m. Insomnia defined as compound sleep disturbance index.

aged 65 and older. Lower estimates of incidence for the age group 65 years and older are reported by Morgan and Clarke (1997a), who nevertheless found that incidence continued to show a clear age gradient after 65 years. For each year at risk in a 4-year follow up, these researchers found incidence rates of 2.8%, 3.2%, and 3.5% for the age groups 65-69, 70-74, and 75-79, respectively.

Increasing age is also associated with changes in both the nature and the duration of sleep complaints. Problems in *getting* to sleep (sleep onset problems) tend to predominate in younger insomniacs, whereas problems *staying* asleep (sleep maintenance problems) become increasingly common in later life (Foley et al., 1995; Gislason & Almqvist, 1987; Maggi et al., 1998). Complaints of early morning awakening (EMA) also increase with age (see Morgan, 1996) but remain less common than sleep maintenance problems in elderly populations (see Maggi et al., 1998). Several epidemiological studies report data which indicate that symptoms of disturbed sleep are more likely to become chronic in older age groups (Hohagen et al., 1994; Mellinger et al., 1985). When asked to quantify the severity of insomnia, for example, older respondents are more likely to report that the problem occurs "often or all the time" (Karacan et al., 1976) or "a lot" (Mellinger et al., 1985). Recent longitudinal data (Morgan & Clarke, 1997a) show high levels of chronicity among prevalent cases of insomnia, with more than 36% of older adults with insomnia (OAWI) continuing to report severe symptoms 4 years later.

The extent to which reported dissatisfaction with sleep among elderly people (as measured in community surveys) translates into complaints of poor sleep (usually in primary care settings) has only recently attracted research attention. The evidence clearly shows, however, that insomnia among older adults remains both widely reported (Hohagen et al., 1994; Weyerer & Dilling, 1991) and widely treated (Hohagen et al., 1994; Pharoah & Melzer, 1995; Weyerer & Dilling, 1991) in general practice settings.

Structural Changes in Sleep

Since the discovery of rapid eye movement sleep (Aserinsky & Kleitman, 1953), the electroencephalogram (EEG), combined with recordings of eye movements (the electro-oculogram or EOG) and chin muscle tone (the electromyogram or EMG), has provided the standard

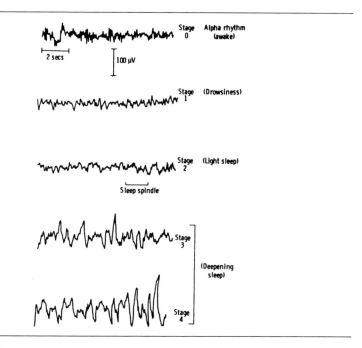

Figure 1.1. Electroencephalogram (EEG) Tracings of Sleep Stages Recorded From a Young Adult

tool for exploring the structure of human sleep. In 1968, internationally agreed criteria for interpreting the polysomnogram (i.e., the EEG, EOG, and EMG recordings made during sleep) were published (Rechtschaffen & Kales, 1968), identifying five "stages" of human sleep (see Figure 1.1).

When a person is relaxed (but with the eyes closed), his or her EEG is characterized by alpha waves, mixed voltage activity with a frequency of 8-13 cycles per second. Stage 1 sleep, drowsiness, is accompanied by lower voltage mixed frequency activity that may appear haphazard or "desynchronized" or may be regular and "synchronized" at about 4-6 cycles per second. The onset of light sleep is determined by the appearance of Stage 2, mixed voltage activity of the alpha type showing clear episodes ("sleep spindles") of 12-14 cycles per second. Stages 3 and 4 accompany "deep sleep" and are frequently subsumed within the single term "slow wave sleep" or SWS. These slow waves are of high voltage, with a frequency of between 1 and 4 cycles per second, the slower and more uniformly high voltage pattern being characteristic of Stage 4. The EEG of rapid eye movement or REM sleep is similar to that of Stage 1; however, unlike any other sleep stage, REM sleep is accompanied by episodic rapid eye movements and profound relaxation of the muscles that maintain posture (the so-called antigravity muscles of the limbs and trunk), both being events clearly visible on the EOG and EMG traces. (It is for this reason that REM sleep earned the epithet "paradoxical sleep," because the EEG shows arousal whereas the EOG and EMG show relaxation.) REM sleep is also accompanied by phases of quite intense physiological activity: the pulse rate quickens, blood pressure rises, respiration rates increase, and oxygen consumption is higher than at any other time during sleep. Finally, the REM stage is closely linked to dreaming. In experimental studies with young adults, more than 80% of REM awakenings are associated with the recall of vivid, narrative dreams. Non-REM awakenings, on the other hand, are associated with lower levels of dream recall or no dream recall at all (Dement & Kleitman, 1957).

A convenient way of graphically representing the EEG structure of a single sleep period (the hypnogram) is shown in Figure 1.2. The time spent in each stage is represented by horizontal lines, whereas the vertical lines indicate a shift from one stage to another. The five sleep stages follow each other in a cyclical fashion. Having progressed through Stages 1 through 4 (often referred to as the non-REM or NREM stages), an individual may then return, stepwise, to Stage 2 before the first REM period begins, after which the same cycle starts again. Although people of the same age may show wide individual differences in the characteristics of their normal sleep, one of the most influential factors determining the EEG structure of adult sleep is age. With increasing age, from early adulthood to later life, sleep becomes more fragmented, shorter, and lighter. Each of these changes has profound implications for subjective sleep quality as reported in population surveys, and each will be considered in turn.

Continuity of Sleep

Relative to that of the young, the sleep of elderly people is characterized by more frequent "shifts" from one sleep stage to another and more frequent intrasleep arousals (Figure 1.2; see also Bosselli, Parrino, Smerieri, & Terzano, 1998). Both events result in sleep that is more bro-

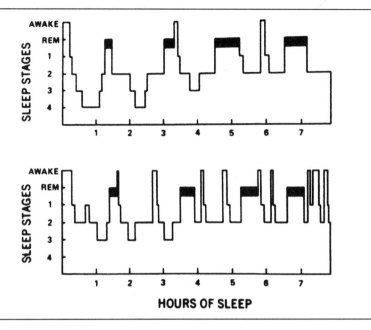

Figure 1.2. Typical Hypnograms for Younger (top) and Older (bottom) Adults
NOTE: Horizontal lines represent time spent in each stage of sleep and vertical lines indicate transitions between sleep stages.

ken and, at least in clinical trials, more likely to be rated as poor in quality (Oswald, 1980). Brief periods of EEG wakefulness (alpha activity) during the sleep period are normal at any age but tend to become both more frequent (e.g., Reynolds et al., 1985; Webb, 1982) and longer in duration in later life. Both changes are evident in the hypnograms shown in Figure 1.2. Throughout adult life, these "spontaneous" nocturnal awakenings tend to be more common among men, a finding possibly related to the disturbing effects of nocturnal penile tumescence (NPT), which occurs quite mechanically during REM sleep in sexually nondysfunctional men of all ages (see Gheorghiu, Mulligan, & Veldhuis, 1995; Karacan, Williams, Thornby, & Salis, 1975; Schiavi & Schreiner-Engel, 1988).

In addition to the more conventionally recorded EEG awakenings (which can last for several minutes), "transient arousals" (2- to 15-second bursts of alpha activity) also have been observed in the sleeping

EEG of elderly subjects (Carskadon, Brown, & Dement, 1982). Although unrelated to behavioral awakenings, these brief episodes of alpha activity, indicative of sleep fragmentation, are positively related to daytime sleepiness (as measured by the Multiple Sleep Latency Test; Carskadon et al., 1982).

Duration of Sleep

The total time spent asleep declines steadily throughout adulthood as a result of a progressive decrease in the sleep period itself (i.e., the time from sleep onset to final awakening) together with increases in the frequency and duration of intersleep arousals. Indeed, as shown by the data aggregated in Figure 1.3, the duration of human sleep shows a steady decline whether we are growing up or growing old. As a result, sleep efficiency (time spent asleep divided by time spent in bed) also tends to decrease (see Bliwise, 1993). Within the sleep period, the structure of sleep also changes, with some reports showing a progressive reduction in the proportion of REM sleep across the life span (see Figure 1.3). Not all studies agree, however, on the extent to which, or even whether, REM sleep percentage declines with age (see Bliwise, 1993). One of the most consistently reported age-related structural changes within NREM sleep is the progressive reduction in EEG slow waves (those associated with Stages 3 and 4 or slow wave sleep; e.g., Prinz, Peskind, et al., 1982). Many people experience a virtual disappearance of Stage 4 altogether.

Depth of Sleep

With advancing age, depth of sleep appears to be affected both quantitatively and qualitatively. Changes in the architecture of sleep so far considered (see Figure 1.2) show in a diminution of deeper slow wave sleep (SWS) and a reciprocal increase in Stages 2 (light sleep) and 1 (drowsiness). Older sleep is therefore *structurally* lighter. Such changes have direct clinical significance. Recent evidence suggests that among OAWI, variations in sleep depth (and sleep latency) are better predictors of subjective sleep quality than other polysomnographic variables (Riedel & Lichstein, 1998).

In addition to *structural* depth, studies of auditory awakening thresholds (the minimum amount of noise required to wake a sleeping person)

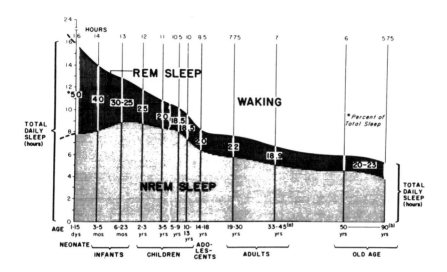

Figure 1.3. Sharp Diminution of REM Sleep in the Early Years

NOTE: REM sleep falls from 8 hours at birth to less than 1 hour in old age. The amount of non-REM (NREM) sleep throughout life remains more constant, falling from 8 hours to 5 five hours. In contrast to the steep decline of REM sleep, the quantity of NREM sleep is undiminished for many years. Although total daily REM sleep falls steadily during life, the percentage rises slightly in adolescence and early adulthood. This rise does not reflect an increase in amount; it is due to the fact that REM sleep does not diminish as quickly as total sleep.
SOURCE: Adapted by the original authors from "Ontogenetic Development of the Human Sleep-Dream Cycle," Roffwarg, Muzio, & Dement. © Copyright 1966 by the American Association for the Advancement of Science. Reprinted with permission.

show qualitative changes in the depth of individual sleep stages. It has been shown, for example, that during Stages 2 and 4 and during REM sleep, older people are more easily awakened by noise (i.e., have lower auditory awakening thresholds) than are younger people, despite reductions in the hearing sensitivity of older subjects (Zepelin, McDonald, & Zammit, 1984). Age-related differences in auditory awakening thresholds have also been observed in comparisons of pre- and postadolescent males, with older subjects again showing lower awakening thresholds (Busby, Mercier, & Pivik, 1994). Taken together, the evidence suggests a near-lifelong modification of processes underlying arousal from sleep. It is relevant to note, however, that *outside* the laboratory, auditory awakening thresholds may not be the best predictor of a given individual's response to nocturnal sound. In an extensive field study of the effects of aircraft noise on the sleep of people living near Heathrow Airport, London, Horne, Pankhurst, Reyner, Hume, and Diamond (1994) found that sleep disturbances did not increase with age. The behavior of bed partners and others living in the household appeared to be a more influential factor than aging in determining intrasleep arousals.

Gender Differences

Collectively, these structural changes in sleep are broadly consistent with the subjective reports from community surveys. It is interesting to note, however, that although epidemiological studies tend to show that women are more likely to report sleep difficulties in old age, the EEG studies (e.g., Reynolds et al., 1985) indicate that it is men who experience the greater deterioration in their sleep architecture. The reasons for this discrepancy are not clearly understood but possibly reflect cultural influences on the willingness of men and women to disclose symptoms and problems (for a discussion of these issues, see Rediehs, Reis, & Creason, 1990).

The Aging Circadian Rhythm

In addition to changes in the architecture and depth of (usually nighttime) sleep, the circadian rhythm itself also shows evidence of age-related decay, with sleep becoming desynchronized and more likely to encroach on daytime activities. Disturbances of the sleep-wake cycle, such as those that result from transmeridian travel (e.g., Dement, Seidel, Cohen, Bliwise, & Carskadon, 1986), shift work (see Monk, 1994), or sleep deprivation (e.g., Webb, 1981), are also less well tolerated by older people.

Evidence that the strength of the circadian rhythm is strongly influenced by age-related changes in melatonin secretion has accumulated in recent years (Garfinkel, Laudon, Nof, & Zisapel, 1995; Haimov et al., 1994). In clinical trials among elderly people, it has been shown that controlled-release melatonin replacement therapy can significantly improve both sleep efficiency (Garfinkel et al., 1995; Haimov et al., 1994) and sleep onset (Haimov et al., 1994), though the hormone appears to have little value in the treatment of psychophysiological insomnia unrelated to deficiency (Ellis, Lemmens, & Parkes, 1996). Nevertheless, psychological contributions to circadian synchronization, such as the ability to perceive and respond to social zeitgebers (time cues), and the importance of maintaining regular social habits should not be overlooked (Minors, Rabbitt, & Worthington, 1989; Monk, Reynolds, Machen, & Kupfer, 1992).

Structural Changes in Sleep: Normal or Abnormal?

Although contemporary sleep research has yielded several well-argued and scientifically profitable "global" theories (e.g., Adam & Oswald, 1983; Horne, 1988), there exists no overall consensus regarding either the functions of sleep or the specific relevance of age-related change in sleep architecture. Recent debate, however, has increasingly focused on whether such change is normal or pathological (Bliwise, 1993, 1994). It has long been assumed that many of the age-related structural changes recorded in EEG laboratories, ostensibly measured in healthy subjects, reflected aspects of normal ontogenetic change. The possibility has now arisen, however, that some of these apparently normal changes may be related to sleep-related respiratory disturbance (SRRD) or period leg movements (PLM), awareness of which has grown rapidly in the past 15 years. Both SRRD and PLM are extremely prevalent in later life (Ancoli-Israel et al., 1991a, 1991b; Mosko et al., 1988) and are known to be disruptive of sleep continuity and quality. Whether, and to what extent, these conditions have "contaminated" earlier normative studies of human sleep, or whether structural changes in sleep predispose the individual to SRRD and PLM (or vice versa), remains unknown. Issues relating to SRRD are more fully discussed below.

The Origins of Late-Life Insomnia

Given that, in old age, structural changes in sleep are experienced by the majority, and complaints of unsatisfactory sleep quality are expressed by the minority, it is reasonable to conclude that age-related change per se is not a sufficient condition for the development of insomnia. Rather, the experimental and epidemiological evidence clearly points to the existence of health, situational, and psychological factors that are strongly associated with the onset and/or the maintenance of disturbed sleep. Because these factors may occur in combination and are often superimposed upon sleep already compromised by ontogenetic change, it follows that sleep problems in later life are frequently multifactorial in origin. Factors known to influence sleep quality in later life can be clustered usefully into health, situational, and personal categories. Examples of each will be provided below.

Mental and Physical Health Status

As a correlate of psychological well-being, insomnia continues to be regarded as a useful indicant of mental ill health, appearing as a prominent diagnostic feature in both the ICD-10 (World Health Organization, 1993) and *DSM-IV* (1994). The symptom of disturbed sleep is also included in most of the available schedules for assessing the mental health of elderly people, including the Geriatric Mental State Schedule (GMS) (Copeland et al., 1976), the Cambridge Mental Disorders of the Elderly Examination (CAMDEX) (Roth et al., 1986), and the Comprehensive Assessment and Referral Evaluation (CARE) (Golden, Teresi, & Gurland, 1984). It is likely, however, that the specificity of insomnia as a symptom of mental ill health is lowest in later life. Thus, while complaints of insomnia steadily increase from early adulthood to at least the sixth or seventh decade of life (Gislason & Almqvist, 1987; Jacquinet-Salord, Lang, Fouriaud, Nicoulet, & Bingham, 1993; Maggi et al., 1998; Mellinger et al., 1985; Ohayon, 1996; Weyerer & Dilling, 1991), the prevalence of those mental health problems most closely associated with insomnia, depression and anxiety, appears to peak in earlier adulthood and decline thereafter (Blazer, Hughes, & George, 1987; Kay, 1988; Myers et al., 1984; Robins et al., 1984).

The relative contributions of mental and physical health factors to late-life insomnia can be more directly assessed from the existing literature. Comparing the performance of various CARE indicator scales, Golden et al. (1984) found high correlations not only between the sleep disorder and depression scales ($r = .55$) but also between sleep disorders and somatic symptoms ($r = .47$), arthritis ($r = .36$), and leg swelling ($r =

.36) scales. Similar associations are reported by Habte-Gabr et al. (1991) for 3,097 elderly people living in rural Iowa. In this extensive survey of health and disturbed sleep, recent hospitalization, limitations of physical function, self-perceptions of health, joint pain and stiffness, emphysema, a history of stroke or heart disease, and depressive symptoms were all significantly associated with poor-quality, unrefreshing sleep.

Similarly, Gislason and Almqvist (1987), in their extensive postal survey among a random sample of Swedish men of all ages, conclude, "Complaints of DMS [difficulty maintaining sleep] increased with increasing age . . . multiple regression clarified that the increase was related to reporting of somatic diseases and overweight" (p. 479). The same study also found that sleep complaints "were almost twice as common among men attending regular medical check-ups for somatic diseases" (p. 479). Mental health problems (particularly depression and anxiety) are, nevertheless, prevalent among OAWI, and in a recent review of community studies were found to be associated with more than 30% of later-life sleep complaints within random samples (Morgan, 1996). It is likely, however, that much higher levels of psychiatric comorbidity would be found among clinic populations and general practice attenders (e.g., Schramm, Hohagen, Käppler, Grasshoff, & Berger, 1994). Levels of psychiatric and somatic comorbidity among both people with insomnia (PWI) and OAWI, as indicated by prevalence studies, are shown in Tables 1.3 and 1.4, respectively. Although it is possible that, to some extent, somatic and psychiatric morbidity are confounded in epidemiological studies, it is interesting to note that, in both cross-sectional (Maggi et al., 1998; Newman et al., 1997) and longitudinal (Morgan & Clarke, 1997b) analyses, depressive symptoms and physical ill health have been shown to be independent predictors of late-life insomnia.

Although somatic disorders (as indexed in Table 1.4) form a heterogeneous category of symptoms and conditions, considerable attention has, in recent years, been paid to three specific health issues (sleep-related respiratory disturbance, periodic leg movements, and dementia) that appear to have far-reaching implications for understanding sleep quality in later life. Each will be considered briefly here.

Sleep-Related Respiratory Disturbance (SRRD)

Classified within the *ICSD* (American Sleep Disorders Association, 1990) as a dyssomnia giving rise either to insomnia disorders or to disor-

Table 1.3 Levels of Psychiatric Morbidity Associated With Insomnia in Community Samples

| Study | Location | Age | Proportion of People With Insomnia Diagnostically Categorized | |
			Depression (%)	Other (%)
Mellinger, Balter, & Uhlenhuth (1985)	United States	18-79	21.0[a]	42.0[b]
Bixler, Kales, Soldatos, Kales, & Healey (1979)	United States	18-80	19.4[c]	29.2[d]
Morgan (1996)	United Kingdom	65+	NR	27.5[e]
Ford & Kamerow (1989)	United States	18-65+	14.0[f]	40.4[g]
Livingston et al.	United Kingdom	60+ (women) 65+ (men)	35.6[h]	NR
Mallon & Hetta (1997)	Sweden	65-79	29.8[i]	48.7[j]

NOTE: Recent studies have tended to report insomnia-health associations as odds ratios rather than proportions (see Newman, Enright, Manolio, Haponik, & Wahl, 1997 and Maggi et al., 1998). NR = data not reported.
a. "Symptoms resembling major depression" (DSM-III criteria).
b. "Generalized anxiety" (DSM-III criteria).
c. Undefined.
d. "Tension" (undefined).
e. "Significant emotional disturbance" (frequency and severity of symptoms of anxiety/depression).
f. Major depression (DSM-III criteria).
g. "Any psychiatric disorder" (defined by the Diagnostic Interview Schedule).
h. As defined by the SHORT-CARE depression scale (calculated from reported data).
i. "Possible depression."
j. "Possible anxiety disorder."

ders of excessive sleepiness, SRRD refers to episodes of apnea (a temporary cessation of breathing) and hypopnea (shallow, rapid breathing) that, in affected individuals, suppress the deeper stages of sleep. Al-

Table 1.4 Levels of Physical Ill Health Associated With Insomnia in Community Samples

Study	Location	Age	Percentage of People With Insomnia Reporting Physical Health Problems
Bixler, Kales, Soldatos, Kales, & Healey (1979)	United States	18-80	53.0[a]
Mellinger, Balter, & Uhlenhuth (1985)	United States	18-79	53.0[b]
Morgan et al. (1988)	United Kingdom	65+	30.6[c]
			42.8[d]
Ford & Kamerow (1989)	United States	18-65+	68.8[e]

NOTE: Recent studies have tended to report insomnia-health associations as odds ratios rather than proportions (see Newman, Enright, Manolio, Haponik, & Wahl, 1997 and Maggi et al., 1998).
a. Ill health defined as "recurring health problem present."
b. Ill health defined as having "2 or more health problems."
c. Ill health defined as rating health "below average."
d. Ill health defined as contact with general practitioner in previous month.
e. Ill health defined as utilization in past 6 months of medical services "with no mental health component."

though criteria and terminology used to describe SRRD varied considerably in earlier studies (Berry & Phillips, 1988), the use of the respiratory disturbance index (RDI) has now been widely adopted for clinical and research purposes. Defined as the average number of apneic + hypopneic episodes per hour of sleep, an RDI ≥ 5 was originally considered pathognomonic of sleep apnea (Guilleminault, van den Hoed, & Mitler, 1979). In recent years, however, higher RDI levels (e.g., RDI ≥ 15) have been found to offer a more realistic criterion for sleep apnea (Gould et al., 1988).

SRRD increases significantly with age (Ancoli-Israel & Coy, 1994), with additional risk factors including being male, snoring, and obesity (Bliwise et al., 1987). Indeed, associations with daytime sleepiness and snoring have proved so robust that these two factors have been described as the "cardinal symptoms" of sleep apnea (Bliwise, 1993). The clinical relevance of SRRD in the absence of daytime symptoms, however, remains unclear. Community-based studies have shown that low levels of SRRD (RDI $\geq$ 5) are relatively common among noncomplaining older people, affecting approximately 24% of asymptomatic Americans aged 65 and older (Ancoli-Israel, Kripke, Mason, Gabriel, & Kaplan, 1986). In studies that have found similar levels of SRRD among healthy elderly volunteers, no relationships were found between SRRD and measures of daytime sleepiness (Berry et al., 1987; Carskadon et al., 1982), sleep-wake complaints (Mosko et al., 1988), cognitive performance, personality, or health status (Berry et al., 1987).

Although high in populations of healthy elderly people, levels of SRRD appear to be even higher among older people with dementia (Erkinjuntti et al., 1987), particularly older women with dementia (Frommlet, Prinz, Vitiello, Ries, & Williams, 1986). Within small groups of women selected from an Australian retirement village, for example, 72% of people with dementia, compared with 46% of controls, were found to have RDIs $\geq$ 5 (Mant et al., 1988). Again, the precise clinical relevance of these events is uncertain. It seems reasonable to assume that respiratory disturbances that can be accompanied by prolonged oxygen desaturation and hypoxemia may further compromise neuropsychological functioning in dementing illness. In mildly and moderately demented people, however, Hoch et al. (1989) found no consistent correlations between RDIs, apneic events/hour, lowest oxyhemoglobin desaturation, and psychometric test performance.

Periodic Leg Movements (PLM)

Also classified within the *ICSD* (American Sleep Disorders Association, 1990) as a cause of both insomnia and excessive daytime sleepiness, PLM is characterized by involuntary limb movements that can occur in all stages of sleep but tend to predominate in the lighter stages (Stages 1 and 2; Montplaisir, Godbout, Pelletier, & Warnes, 1994). Although movement and positional changes occur throughout normal sleep, four or more consecutive limb movements lasting 0.5-5 seconds (with an intermovement interval of 4-90 seconds) are regarded as PLM episodes, with five such episodes per night considered pathological (Coleman, 1982). As does SRRD, PLM increases with age, with an estimated prevalence among elderly people living at home of about 45% (Ancoli-Israel et al., 1991a). Once again, however, not all those showing signs of PLM experience disturbed sleep. Thus, although PLM undoubtedly is a cause of disturbed sleep in later life, many of the links between PLM and sleep complaints remain to be explored.

Dementia

Dementia presents a special area of concern in late-life sleep disturbance because many of the polygraphic sleep changes seen in normal older individuals, and described above, are amplified in dementing illness. Relative to age-matched controls, older people with dementia take longer to get to sleep (Allen, Seiler, Stähelen, & Speigel, 1987), wake up more frequently during the night (Allen et al., 1987; Prinz, Vitaliano, et al., 1982), stay awake longer when disturbed (Prinz, Vitaliano, et al., 1982), tend to be more active during periods of wakefulness (Allen et al., 1987), and in one study were found to be up to 20 times as likely to fall asleep during the day (Prinz, Vitaliano, et al., 1982). Changes in the circadian organization of *total* sleep also have been reported. In a detailed comparison of demented and nondemented inpatients, Allen et al. (1987) found not only that patients with dementia slept more during the day but also that some (10%) actually slept more during the day than during the night (so-called day-night reversal).

These changes in the architecture and circadian timing of sleep, often accompanied by episodes of nighttime agitation and wandering (or "sundowning"; see Bliwise, 1993), contribute substantially to the demands of caring and are among the most frequently cited reasons for the breakdown of caregiving in the community (Gilhooly, 1984; Gilleard, 1986; Pollak & Perlick, 1991). Evidence linking the severity of cognitive impairment, as indexed by psychometric ratings, with the degree of sleep disturbance (Prinz, Vitaliano, et al., 1982) highlights the role of neuronal degeneration in explaining dementia-related sleep disorders; however, the existence of wide individual differences in the degree of sleep disturbance among similarly impaired individuals (e.g., Regestein & Morris, 1987) and the failure of sleep disturbance indicators to discriminate reliably between mildly demented patients and nondemented controls (Meguro et al., 1995) suggest that etiologic factors are not alone in determining sleep disruptions in dementia. This conclusion is supported by Meguro et al. (1995), who report that dementia severity (as indexed by the extent of white-matter lesions) and lowered activity levels (as measured by "activities of daily living" scores) interact to increase sleep fragmentation.

Whatever the organic origin, it is likely that the disruption of sleep in dementia is exacerbated by behavioral factors. The research evidence clearly indicates that regularizing daytime and nighttime activities, optimizing daytime stimulation, minimizing daytime naps, and maximizing the psychological association between the bedroom and sleep all make significant contributions to the maintenance of satisfactory sleep-wake cycles in nondemented insomniacs. In dementing illness, however, the influence of these and other factors may be greatly diminished or lost. For example, a demented patient with severely disturbed nighttime sleep may be left to nap ad lib during the day by an exhausted relative. As a result, the patient may be less tired and less likely to sleep during the night, which in turn can lead to sleepiness and excess napping the following day, and so on. Support for the general proposition that behavioral factors exacerbate sleep fragmentation in dementia can be found in the clinical literature. Hinchcliffe, Hyman, Blizard, and Livingston (1991), for example, describe the successful management of dementia-related nighttime sleeplessness and wandering through stimulating daytime "distractions" that prevented excessive napping.

Institutionalization

Relationships between institutionalization and disturbed sleep are strongly suggested by the high levels of hypnotic drug consumption that consistently have been found in hospitals and rest, residential, and nursing homes (e.g., Alessi, Schnelle, Traub, & Ouslander, 1995; Buck, 1988; Middelkoop, Kerkhof, Smilde-Van Den Doel, Ligthart, & Kamphuisen, 1994; Schmidt, Claesson, Westerholm, Nilsson, & Svarstad, 1998; Seppala, Rajala, & Sourander, 1993; Snowdon, Vaughan, Miller, Burgess, & Tremlett, 1995). Within each of these settings, sleep disturbance can be related to the act of admission itself, the personal circumstances necessitating admission, or the institutional environment. It is well recognized in contemporary sleep research, for example, that environmental novelty (such as the first night in the EEG laboratory) results in sleep that is shorter, lighter, and more broken, a phenomenon originally described as the "first night effect" (Agnew, Webb, & Williams, 1966; Scharf, Kales, & Bixler, 1975) and observed in laboratory studies of older subjects

(Reynolds et al., 1985). After a brief period of adaptation (say, 1-2 nights), however, sleep returns to its more "normal" structure (Reynolds et al., 1985). There is no reason to suppose that such phenomena do not accompany institutional admissions and may sometimes be inappropriately treated with hypnotic drugs.

In addition, institutionalization is often accompanied by events that in themselves can be expected to disturb sleep—anxiety, discomfort, pain, bereavement, and so forth. In hospital settings, it is also becoming increasingly apparent that many surgical and medical procedures have a quite detrimental effect on sleep continuity (Aureff & Elmqvist, 1985; Meyer et al., 1994; Southwell & Wistow, 1995). One of the most significant environmental factors that has been shown to influence sleep quality in institutional settings is noise (Grumet, 1993; Yinnon, Ilan, Tadmor, Altarescu, & Hershko, 1992). Thus, institutionalization remains both a high-probability event for older people and a major cause of insomnia.

The research evidence also suggests that institutional regimes can adversely affect sleep quality in old age. Again, although days lacking in structure and stimulation can disturb sleep at almost any age, elderly people do appear to be most at risk. In nursing home residents, for example, disturbed nighttime sleep has been associated with excessive periods in bed. Using wrist actigraphy (see Sadeh, Hauri, Kripke, & Lavie, 1995) to monitor sleep and waking, Ancoli-Israel, Parker, Sinaee, Fell, and Kripke (1989) recorded up to 5 episodes of sleep during the day and up to 32 episodes of wakefulness during the night in nursing home residents. These investigators concluded that residents had very little sustained wakefulness and very little sustained sleep. Physical activity levels also have been implicated as a factor contributing to poor sleep in nursing home residents, though the evidence cautions against a simple cause-effect explanation. Thus, although lower activity levels have been significantly associated with sleep fragmentation in elderly nursing home residents (Meguro et al., 1995), structured activity programs appear to have little impact on the sleep quality of elderly people who are similarly institutionalized (Alessi, Schnelle, MacRae, et al., 1995).

Lifestyle

In recent years, the clinical and research literature has established clear links between aspects of lifestyle (e.g., diet, exercise, sleeping habits) and sleep quality. Degraded sleep quality in later life has been associated with tea consumption (Morgan, Healey, & Healey, 1989), excessive daytime napping and excessive time spent in bed (Ancoli-Israel et al., 1989), unaccustomed nighttime food drinks (Adam, 1980), and low levels of physical activity (Morgan & Clarke, 1997b). Regularizing daytime and nighttime activities, optimizing daytime stimulation, minimizing daytime naps, and maximizing the psychological association between the bedroom and sleep can all make a significant contribution to the maintenance of satisfactory sleep-wake cycles in both older (e.g., Morin & Azrin, 1988) and younger adults (Lacks & Morin, 1992) with insomnia.

Individual Differences

Studies comparing the personality profiles of otherwise healthy good and poor sleepers have found consistent differences in young (Monroe, 1967), middle-aged (Adam, Tomeny, & Oswald, 1986), and elderly (Morgan et al., 1989) subjects. In all cases, poor sleepers have shown significantly elevated levels of anxiety and neuroticism as measured by the Minnesota Multiphasic Personality Inventory (Monroe, 1967), the Taylor Manifest Anxiety Inventory (Adam et al., 1986), the Spielberger State-Trait Anxiety Inventory, and the Eysenck Personality Questionnaire (Morgan et al., 1989). Similar relationships between insomnia and anxiety/neuroticism have been found in sleep clinic patients (Kales, Caldwell, Soldatos, Bixler, & Kales, 1983) and representative survey populations (Hyyppa, Kronholm, & Mattlar, 1991). Personality factors are also strongly related to *components* of insomnia. In a factor-analytic study of Espie, Lindsay, Brooks, Hood, and Turvey's (1989) Sleep Disturbance Questionnaire, Coyle and Watts (1991) found neuroticism (as measured by the EPI) to be significantly correlated with both the first (concern about the aftereffects of insomnia) and third (mental activity) principal components. Given that many of these personality assessments reflect what are presumed to be enduring traits, it is possible that such characteristics may act as risk factors for insomnia either directly, by contributing to levels of emotional arousal, or perhaps indirectly by lowering the threshold at which sleep is perceived to be a problem. That sleep quality is significantly influenced by constitutional factors is also strongly supported by evidence on hereditary predispositions. In a study of more than 10,000 elderly people in Sweden, levels of insomnia were found to be significantly higher among people both of whose parents were also poor sleepers (Asplund, 1995).

Conclusions

In addition to senescent changes that directly influence the structure and quality of sleep, advancing age is also associated with an increasing number of events that can influence and disturb sleep indirectly. As a result, later-life insomnia is both prevalent and complex. Sleep research has, in recent years, made considerable progress in identifying and clarifying some of the specific causes and correlates of disturbed sleep in older people. Clinically, this improved understanding of the nature and the origins of late-life insomnia is, perhaps, of particular relevance in the *assessment* of the presenting sleep disorder. Based on the information outlined in this chapter, such assessment (which should form the basis of all treatment programs) should recognize at least three important principles. First, for most older people (with or without insomnia), the continuity, duration, and depth of sleep are reduced in later life. It is incumbent upon the clinician, therefore, to distinguish treatable causes of insomnia from apparently normal ontogenetic change. Second, late-life insomnias are frequently multifactorial in origin, with specific risk factors interacting with one another and with sleep patterns already compromised by the aging process. An important aim of assessment in the present context, therefore, is to identify the most appropriate targets for psychological intervention. Third, it is important to remember that insomnias that *present* in later life do not necessarily *originate* in later life, and that many younger PWI will grow old with their sleep disorder. This latter point clearly emphasizes the need to base both therapy and, ultimately, client expectations on a carefully taken sleep history.

References

Adam, K. (1980). Dietary habits and sleep after bedtime food drinks. *Sleep, 3,* 47-58.

Adam, K., & Oswald, I. (1983). Protein synthesis, bodily renewal and the sleep-wake cycle. *Clinical Science, 65,* 561-567.

Adam, K., Tomeny, M., & Oswald, I. (1986). Physiological and psychological differences between good and poor sleepers. *Journal of Psychiatric Research, 20,* 301-316.

Agnew, H. W., Webb, W. B., & Williams, R. L. (1966). The first night effect: An EEG study of sleep. *Psychophysiology, 12,* 412-415.

Alessi, C. A., Schnelle, J. F., MacRae, P. G., Ouslander, J. G., Al-Samarrai, N., Simmons, S. F., & Traub, S. (1995). Does physical activity improve sleep in impaired nursing home residents? *Journal of the American Geriatrics Society, 43,* 1098-1102.

Alessi, C. A., Schnelle, J. F., Traub, S., & Ouslander, J. G. (1995). Psychotropic medications in incontinent nursing home residents: Association with sleep and bed mobility. *Journal of the American Geriatrics Society, 43,* 789-792.

Allen, S. R., Seiler, W. O., Stähelen, H. B., & Speigel, R. (1987). Seventy-two hour polygraphic and behavioral recordings of wakefulness and sleep in a hospital geriatric unit: Comparison between demented and nondemented patients. *Sleep, 10,* 143-159.

American Psychiatric Association. (1994). *Diagnostic and statistical manual of mental disorders.* Washington, DC: Author.

American Sleep Disorders Association. (1990). *The International Classification of Sleep Disorders: Diagnostic and coding manual.* Rochester, MN: Author.

Ancoli-Israel, S., & Coy, T. (1994). Are breathing disturbances in elderly equivalent to sleep apnea syndrome? *Sleep, 17,* 77-83.

Ancoli-Israel, S., Kripke, D. F., Klauber, M. R., Mason, W. J., Fell, R., & Kaplan, O. (1991a). Periodic limb movements in sleep in community dwelling elderly. *Sleep, 14,* 496-500.

Ancoli-Israel, S., Kripke, D. F., Klauber, M. R., Mason, W. J., Fell, R., & Kaplan, O. (1991b). Sleep disordered breathing in community dwelling elderly. *Sleep, 14,* 486-495.

Ancoli-Israel, S., Kripke, D. F., Mason, W. J., Gabriel, S., & Kaplan, D. (1986). Sleep apnea and PMS in a randomly selected elderly population: Final prevalence results [Abstract]. *Sleep Research, 15,* 101.

Ancoli-Israel, S., Parker, L., Sinaee, R., Fell, R. L., & Kripke, D. F. (1989). Sleep fragmentation in patients from a nursing home. *Journal of Gerontology: Medical Sciences, 44,* M18-M21.

Aserinsky, E., & Kleitman, N. (1953). Regularly occurring periods of eye motility, and concomitant phenomena during sleep. *Science, 118,* 273-274.

Asplund, R. (1995). Are sleep disorders hereditary? A questionnaire survey of persons about themselves and their parents. *Archives of Gerontology and Geriatrics, 21,* 231.

Aureff, J., & Elmqvist, D. (1985). Sleep in the surgical intensive care unit: Continuous polygraphic recording of sleep in nine patients receiving postoperative care. *British Medical Journal, 290,* 1029-1032.

Berry, D.T.R., & Phillips, B. A. (1988). Sleep disordered breathing in the elderly: Review and methodological comment. *Clinical Psychology Review, 8,* 101-120.

Berry, D.T.R., Phillips, B. A., Cook, Y. R., Schmitt, F. A., Gilmore, R. L., Patel, R., Keener, T. M., & Tyre, E. (1987). Sleep-disordered breathing in healthy aged persons: Possible daytime sequelae. *Journal of Gerontology, 42,* 620-626.

Bixler, E. O., Kales, A., Soldatos, C. R., Kales, J. D., & Healey, S. (1979). Prevalence of sleep disorders in the Los Angeles metropolitan area. *American Journal of Psychiatry, 10,* 1257-1262.

Blazer, D. G., Hays, J. C., & Foley, D. J. (1995). Sleep complaints in older adults: A racial comparison. *Journal of Gerontology, 50A,* M280-M284.

Blazer, D., Hughes, D. C., & George, L. K. (1987). The epidemiology of depression in an elderly community population. *Gerontologist, 27,* 281-287.

Bliwise, D. (1993). Sleep in normal aging and dementia. *Sleep, 16,* 40-81.

Bliwise, D. L. (1994). Normal aging. In M. H. Kryger, T. Roth, & W. C. Dement (Eds.), *Principles and practice of sleep medicine* (2nd ed., pp. 26-39). Philadelphia: W. B. Saunders.

Bliwise, D. L., Feldman, D. E., Bliwise, N. G., Carskadon, M. A., Kraemer, H., North, C. S., Petta, D. F., Seidel, W. F., & Dement, W. C. (1987). Risk factors for sleep disordered breathing in heterogeneous geriatric populations. *Journal of the American Geriatric Society, 35*, 132-141.

Bosselli, M., Parrino, L., Smerieri, A., & Terzano, M. G. (1998). Effects of age on EEG arousals in normal sleep. *Sleep, 21*, 351-357.

Buck, J. A. (1988). Psychotropic drug practice in nursing homes. *Journal of the American Geriatric Society, 36*, 409-418.

Busby, K. A., Mercier, L., & Pivik, R. T. (1994). Ontogenic variations in auditory arousal threshold during sleep. *Psychophysiology, 31*, 182-188.

Buysse, D. J., Reynolds, C. F., Kupfer, D. J., Thorpy, J. T., Bixler, E., Manfredi, R., Kales, A., Vgontzas, A., Stepanski, E., Roth, T., Hauri, P., & Mesiano, D. (1994). Clinical diagnoses in 216 insomnia patients using the International Classification of Sleep Disorders (ICSD), DSM-IV and ICD-10 categories: A report from the APA/NIMH DSM-IV field trial. *Sleep, 17*, 630-637.

Carskadon, M. A., Brown, E. D., & Dement, W. C. (1982). Sleep fragmentation in the elderly: Relationship to daytime sleep tendency. *Neurobiology of Aging, 3*, 321-327.

Coleman, R. M. (1982). Periodic movements in sleep (nocturnal myoclonus) and restless legs syndrome. In C. Guilleminault (Ed.), *Sleeping and waking disorders: Indications and techniques* (pp. 265-295). Menlo Park, CA: Addison-Wesley.

Copeland, J.R.M., Kelleher, M. J., Kellett, J. M., Gourlay, A. J., Gurland, B. J., Fleiss, J. L., & Sharpe, L. (1976). A semi-structured clinical interview for the assessment of diagnosis and mental state in the elderly. The Geriatric Mental State Schedule. 1. Development and reliability. *Psychological Medicine, 6*, 439-449.

Costa, E., Silva, J. A., Chase, M., Sartorius, N., & Roth, T. (1996). Special report from a symposium held by the World Health Organization and the World Federation of Sleep Research Societies: An overview of insomnias and related disorders: Recognition, epidemiology and rational management. *Sleep, 19*, 412-416.

Coyle, K., & Watts, F. N. (1991). The factorial structure of sleep dissatisfaction. *Behaviour Research and Therapy, 29*, 513-520.

Dement, W., & Kleitman, N. (1957). The relation of eye movements during sleep to dream activity: An objective method for the study of dreaming. *Journal of Experimental Psychology, 53*, 339-346.

Dement, W. C., Seidel, W. F., Cohen, S. A., Bliwise, N. G., & Carskadon, M. A. (1986). Sleep and wakefulness in aircrew before and after transoceanic flights. *Aviation Space and Environmental Medicine* (Suppl. 12), B14-B28.

Ellis, C. M., Lemmens, G., & Parkes, J. D. (1996). Melatonin and insomnia. *Journal of Sleep Research, 5*, 61-65.

Erkinjuntti, T., Partinen, M., Sulkava, R., Telakivi, T., Salmi, T., & Tilvis, R. (1987). Sleep apnea in multi-infarct dementia and Alzheimer's disease. *Sleep, 10*, 419-425.

Espie, C. A., Lindsay, W. R., Brooks, D. N., Hood, E. M., & Turvey, T. (1989). A controlled comparative investigation of psychological treatments for chronic sleep-onset insomnia. *Behaviour Research and Therapy, 27*, 79-88.

Foley, D. J., Monjan, A. A., Brown, S. L., Simonsick, E. M., Wallace, R. B., & Blazer, D. G. (1995). Sleep complaints among elderly persons: An epidemiologic study of three communities. *Sleep, 18*, 425-432.

Ford, D. E., & Kamerow, D. B. (1989). Epidemiologic study of sleep disturbances and psychiatric disorders. *Journal of the American Medical Association, 262*, 1479-1484.

Frommlet, M., Prinz, P., Vitiello, M. V., Ries, R., & Williams, D. (1986). Sleep hypoxemia and apnea are elevated in females with mild Alzheimer's disease [Abstract]. *Sleep Research, 15*, 189.

Garfinkel, D., Laudon, M., Nof, D., & Zisapel, N. (1995). Improvement of sleep quality in elderly people by controlled-release melatonin. *The Lancet, 346*, 541-544.

Geroldi, C., Frisoni, G. B., Rozzini, R., De Leo, D., & Trabucchi, M. (1996). Principal lifetime occupation and sleep quality in the elderly. *Gerontology, 42*, 163-169.

Gheorghiu, S., Mulligan, T., & Veldhuis, J. D. (1995). Lack of temporal association among REM sleep, LH secretion, testosterone secretion, and nocturnal penile tumescence (NPT) in healthy aged men. *Journal of the American Geriatric Society, 43*, SA81.

Gilhooly, M. (1984). The social dimensions of senile dementia. In I. Hanley & J. Hodge (Eds.), *Psychological approaches to the care of the elderly* (pp. 88-135). London: Croom Helm.

Gilleard, C. J. (1986). *Living with dementia*. London: Croom Helm.

Gislason, T., & Almqvist, M. (1987). Somatic diseases and sleep complaints. *Acta Medica Scandinavica, 221*, 475-481.

Golden, R. R., Teresi, J. A., & Gurland, B. J. (1984). Development of indicator scales for the Comprehensive Assessment and Referral Evaluation (CARE) interview schedule. *Journal of Gerontology, 39*, 138-146.

Gould, G. A., Whyte, K. F., Rhind, G. B., Airlie, M.A.A., Catterall, J. R., Shapiro, C. M, & Douglas N. J. (1988). The sleep hypopnea syndrome. *American Review of Respiratory Diseases, 137*, 895-898.

Grumet, G. W. (1993). Pandemonium in the modern hospital. *New England Journal of Medicine, 328*(6), 433-437.

Guilleminault, C., van den Hoed, J., & Mitler, M. (1979). Clinical overview of the sleep apnea syndromes. In C. Guilleminault & W. Dement (Eds.), *Sleep apnea syndromes* (pp. 1-11). New York: Alan R. Liss.

Habte-Gabr, E., Wallace, R. B., Colsher, P. L., Hulbert, J. R., White, L. R., & Smith, I. M. (1991). Sleep patterns in rural elders: Demographic, health, and psychobehavioral correlates. *Journal of Clinical Epidemiology, 44*, 5-13.

Haimov, I., Laudon, M., Zisapel, N., Souroujon, M., Nof, D., Shlitner, A., Herer, P., Tzischinsky, O., & Lavie, P. (1994). Sleep disorders and melatonin rhythms in elderly people. *British Medical Journal, 309*, 167.

Hinchcliffe, A. C., Hyman, I., Blizard, B., & Livingston, G. (1991). The impact on carers of behavioural difficulties in dementia: A pilot study on management. *International Journal of Geriatric Psychiatry, 7*, 579-583.

Hoch, C. C., Reynolds, C. F., III, Nebes, R. D., Kupfer, D. J., Berman, S. R., & Campbell, D. (1989). Clinical significance of sleep-disordered breathing in Alzheimer's disease: Preliminary data. *Journal of the American Geriatric Society, 37*, 138-144.

Hohagen, F., Käppler, C., Schramm, E., Rink, K., Weyerer, S., Riemann, D., & Berger, M. (1994). Prevalence of insomnia in general practice attenders and the current treatment modalities. *Acta Psychiatrica Scandinavica, 90*, 102-108.

Horne, J. (1988). *Why we sleep: The functions of sleep in humans and other mammals*. Oxford, UK: Oxford University Press.

Horne, J. A., Pankhurst, F. L., Reyner, L. A., Hume, K., & Diamond, I. D. (1994). A field study of sleep disturbance: Effects of aircraft noise and other factors on 5,742 nights of actimetrically monitored sleep in a large subject sample. *Sleep, 17*, 146-159.

Hyyppa, M. T., Kronholm, E., & Mattlar, C. E. (1991). Mental well-being of good sleepers in a random population sample. *British Journal of Medical Psychology, 64*, 25-34.

Jacquinet-Salord, M. C., Lang, T., Fouriaud, C., Nicoulet, I., & Bingham, A. (1993). Sleeping tablet consumption, self reported quality of sleep, and working conditions. *Journal of Epidemiology and Community Health, 47*, 64-68.

Kales, A., Caldwell, A. B., Soldatos, C. R., Bixler, E. O., & Kales, J. D. (1983). Biopsychobehavioral correlates of insomnia II: Pattern specificity and consistency with MMPI. *Psychosomatic Medicine, 45*, 341-356.

Karacan, I., Thornby, J. I., Anch, H., Holzer, C. E., Warheit, G. J., Schwab, J. J., & Williams, R. L. (1976). The prevalence of sleep disturbance in a primarily urban Florida county. *Social Science and Medicine, 10*, 239-244.

Karacan, I., Williams, R. L., Thornby, J. I., & Salis, P. J. (1975). Sleep-related tumescence as a function of age. *American Journal of Psychiatry, 132*, 932-937.

Kay, D.W.K. (1988). Anxiety in the elderly. In R. Noyes, M. Roth, & G. D. Burrows (Eds.), *Handbook of anxiety: Vol. 2. Classification, etiological factors and associated disturbances* (pp. 289-310). Amsterdam: Elsevier Science.

Lacks, P., & Morin, C. M. (1992). Recent advances in the assessment and treatment of insomnia. *Journal of Consulting and Clinical Psychology, 60*, 586-594.

Leger, D. (1994). The cost of sleep related road accidents: A report for the National Commission on Sleep Disorders Research. *Sleep, 17*, 84-93.

Leger, D. (1995). The cost of sleepiness: A response to comments. *Sleep, 18*, 281-284.

Livingston, G., Hawkins, A., Graham, N., Blizard, B., & Mann, A. (1990). The Gospel Oak study: Prevalence rates of dementia, depression and activity limitation among elderly residents in Inner London. *Psychological Medicine, 20*, 137-146.

Maggi, S., Langlois, J. A., Minicuci, N., Grigoletto, F., Pavan, M., Foley, D. J., & Enzi, G. (1998). Sleep complaints in community-dwelling older persons: Prevalence, associated factors, and reported causes. *Journal of the American Geriatrics Society, 46*, 161-168.

Mallon, L., & Hetta, J. (1997). A survey of sleep habits and sleeping difficulties in an elderly Swedish population. *Uppsala Journal of Medical Sciences, 102*, 185-197.

Mant, A., Saunders, N. A., Eyland, A. E., Pond, C. D., Chancellor, A. H., & Webster, I. W. (1988). Sleep-related respiratory disturbance and dementia in elderly females. *Journals of Gerontology (Medical Science), 43*(5), M140-M144.

McGhie, A., & Russell, S. M. (1962). The subjective assessment of normal sleep patterns. *Journal of Mental Science, 108*, 642-654.

Meguro, K., Ueda, M., Kobayashi, I., Yamaguchi, S., Yamazaki, H., Oikawa, Y., Kikuchi, Y., & Sasaki, H. (1995). Sleep disturbance in elderly patients with cognitive impairment, decreased daily activity and periventricular white matter lesions. *Sleep, 18*, 109-114.

Mellinger, G. D., Balter, M. B., & Uhlenhuth, E. H. (1985). Insomnia and its treatment. *Archives of General Psychiatry, 42*, 225-232.

Melville, H. (1994). *Moby Dick*. London: Penguin. (Original work published 1851)

Meyer, T. J., Eveloff, S. E., Bauer, M. S., Schwartz, W. A., Hill, N. S., & Millman, R. P. (1994). Adverse environmental conditions in the respiratory and medical ICU settings. *Chest, 105*, 1211-1216.

Middelkoop, H.A.M., Kerkhof, G. A., Smilde-Van Den Doel, D. A., Ligthart, G. J., & Kamphuisen, H.A.C. (1994). Sleep and ageing: The effects of institutionalisation on subjective and objective characteristics of sleep. *Age and Ageing, 23*, 411-417.

Minors, D. S., Rabbitt, P.M.A., & Worthington, H. (1989). Variation in meals and sleep-activity patterns in aged subjects—its relevance to circadian rhythm studies. *Chronobiology International, 6*, 139-146.

Monk, T. H. (1994). Shift work. In M. H. Kryger, T. Roth, & W. C. Dement (Eds.), *Principles and practice of sleep medicine* (pp. 321-330). Philadelphia: W. B. Saunders.

Monk, T. H., Reynolds, C. F., Machen, M. A., & Kupfer, D. J. (1992). Daily social rhythms in the elderly and their relationship to objectively recorded sleep. *Sleep, 15*, 322-329.

Monroe, L. J. (1967). Psychological and physiological differences between good and poor sleepers. *Journal of Abnormal Psychology, 72*, 255-264.

Montplaisir, J., Godbout, R., Pelletier, G., & Warnes, H. (1994). Restless legs syndrome and periodic movements during sleep. In M. H. Kryger, T. Roth, & W. C. Dement (Eds.), *Principles and practice of sleep medicine* (pp. 589-597). Philadelphia: W. B. Saunders.

Morgan, K. (1996). Mental health factors in late-life insomnia. *Reviews in Clinical Gerontology, 6*, 75-83.

Morgan, K., & Clarke, D. (1997a). Longitudinal trends in late-life insomnia: Implications for prescribing. *Age and Ageing, 26*, 179-184.

Morgan, K., & Clarke, D. (1997b). Risk factors for late-life insomnia in a representative general practice sample. *British Journal of General Practice, 47*, 166-169.

Morgan, K., Dallosso, H., Ebrahim, S., Arie, T., & Fentem, P. (1988). Characteristics of subjective insomnia among the elderly living at home. *Age and Ageing, 17*, 1-7.

Morgan, K., Healey, D. W., & Healey, P. J. (1989). Factors influencing persistent subjective insomnia in old age: A follow-up study of good and poor sleepers aged 65-74. *Age and Ageing, 18*, 117-122.

Morin, C. M., & Azrin, N. H. (1988). Behavioral and cognitive treatments of geriatric insomnia. *Journal of Consulting and Clinical Psychology, 56*, 748-753.

Mosko, S. S., Dickel, M. J., Paul, T., LaTour, T., Dhillon, S., Ghanim, A., & Sassin, J. F. (1988). Sleep apnea and sleep-related periodic leg movements in community resident seniors. *Journal of the American Geriatric Society, 36*, 502-508.

Myers, J. K., Weissman, M. M., Tischler, G. L., Holzer, C. E., Leaf, P. J., Orvaschel, H., Anthony, J. C., Boyd, J. H., Burke, J. D., Kramer, M., & Stolzman, R. (1984). Six-month prevalence of psychiatric disorders in three communities: 1980-1982. *Archives of General Psychiatry, 41*, 959-967.

National Institutes of Health. (1991). Consensus development conference statement: The treatment of sleep disorders of older people. *Sleep, 14*, 169-177.

Newman, A. B., Enright, P. L., Manolio, T. A., Haponik, E. F., & Wahl, P. W. (1997). Sleep disturbance, psychosocial correlates, and cardiovascular disease in 5201 older adults: The cardiovascular health study. *Journal of the American Geriatrics Society, 45*, 1-7.

Ohayon, M. (1996). Epidemiologic study on insomnia in the general population. *Sleep, 19*, S7-S15.

Oswald, I. (1980). Sleep studies in clinical pharmacology. *British Journal of Clinical Pharmacology, 10*, 317-326.

Partininen, M. (1994). Epidemiology of sleep disorders. In M. H. Kryger, T. Roth & W. C. Dement (Eds.), *Principles and practice of sleep medicine* (pp. 437-452). Philadelphia: W. C. Saunders.

Pharoah, P.D.P., & Melzer, D. (1995). Variations in prescribing of hypnotics, anxiolytics and antidepressants between 61 general practices. *British Journal of General Practice, 45*, 595-599.

Pollak, C. P., & Perlick, D. (1991). Sleep problems and institutionalization of the elderly. *Journal of Geriatric Psychiatry and Neurology, 15*, 123-135.

Prinz, P. N., Peskind, E. R., Vitaliano, P. P., Raskind, M. A., Eisdorfer, C., Zemcuznikov, N., & Gerber, C. J. (1982). Changes in the sleep and waking EEGs of nondemented and demented elderly subjects. *Journal of the American Geriatric Society, 30*, 86-93.

Prinz, P. N., Vitaliano, P. P., Vitiello, M. V., Bokan, J., Raskind, M., Peskind, E., & Gerber, C. (1982). Sleep, EEG and mental function changes in senile dementia of the Alzheimer's type. *Neurobiology of Aging, 3*, 361-370.

Rechtschaffen, A., & Kales, A. (1968). *A manual of standardized terminology, techniques, and scoring system for sleep stages of human subjects* (National Institute of Health Publication No. 24). Washington, DC: Government Printing Office.

Rediehs, M. H., Reis, J. S., & Creason, N. S. (1990). Sleep in old age: Focus on gender differences. *Sleep, 13*, 410-424.

Regestein, Q. R., & Morris, J. (1987). Daily sleep patterns observed among institutionalized elderly residents. *Journal of the American Geriatric Society, 35*, 767-772.

Reynolds, C. F., Kupfer, D. J., Taska, L. S., Hoch, C. C., Sewitch, D. E., & Spiker, D. G. (1985). Sleep of healthy seniors: A revisit. *Sleep, 8*, 20-29.

Riedel, B. W., & Lichstein, K. L. (1998). Objective sleep measures and subjective sleep satisfaction: How do older adults with insomnia define a good night's sleep? *Psychology and Aging, 13*, 159-163.

Robins, L. N., Helzer, J. E., Weissman, M. M., Orvaschel, H., Gruenberg, E., Burke, J. D., & Regier, D. A. (1984). Lifetime prevalence of specific psychiatric disorders in three sites. *Archives of General Psychiatry, 41*, 949-958.

Roffwarg, H. P., Muzio, J. N., & Dement, W. C. (1966). Ontogenetic development of the human sleep-dream cycle. *Science, 152*, 604-619.

Roth, M., Tym, E., Mountjoy, C. Q., Huppert, F. A., Hendrie, H., Verma, S., & Goddard, R. (1986). CAMDEX: A standardised instrument for the diagnosis of mental disorder in the elderly with special reference to the early detection of dementia. *British Journal of Psychiatry, 149*, 698-709.

Sadeh, A., Hauri, P., Kripke, D. F., & Lavie, P. (1995). The role of actigraphy in the evaluation of sleep disorders. *Sleep, 18*, 288-302.

Scharf, M. B., Kales, A., & Bixler, E. O. (1975). Readaptation to the sleep laboratory in insomniac subjects. *Psychophysiology, 12*, 412-415.

Schiavi, R. C., & Schreiner-Engel, P. (1988). Nocturnal penile tumescence in healthy aging men. *Journals of Gerontology (Medical Science), 43*, M146-M150.

Schmidt, I., Claesson, C. B., Westerholm, B., Nilsson, L. G., & Svarstad, B. L. (1998). The impact of regular multidisciplinary team interventions on psychotropic prescribing in Swedish nursing homes. *Journal of the American Geriatrics Society, 46*, 77-82.

Schramm, E., Hohagen, F., Käppler, C., Grasshoff, U., & Berger, M. (1994). Mental comorbidity of chronic insomnia in general practice attenders using DMS-III-R. *Acta Psychiatrica Scandinavica, 91*, 10-17.

Seppala, M., Rajala, T., & Sourander, L. (1993). Subjective evaluation of sleep and the use of hypnotics in nursing-homes. *Aging—Clinical and Experimental Research, 5*, 199-205.

Sigmond, G. G. (1836). Lectures on materia medica and therapeutics. *The Lancet, 37*(1), 214-220.

Snowdon, J., Vaughan, R., Miller, R., Burgess, E. E., & Tremlett, P. (1995). Psychotropic-drug use in Sydney nursing-homes. *Medical Journal of Australia, 163*, 70-72.

Southwell, M. T., & Wistow, G. (1995). Sleep in hospitals at night: Are patients' needs being met? *Journal of Advanced Nursing, 21*, 1101-1109.

Trinder, J. (1988). Subjective insomnia without objective findings: A pseudodiagnostic classification? *Psychological Bulletin, 103*, 87-94.

Webb, W. B. (1981). Sleep stage responses of older and younger subjects after sleep deprivation. *Electroencephalography and Clinical Neurophysiology, 52*, 368-371.

Webb, W. B. (1982). Sleep in older persons: Sleep structures in 50- to 60-year-old men and women. *Journal of Gerontology, 52*, 368-371.

Weyerer, S., & Dilling, H. (1991). Prevalence and treatment of insomnia in the community—results from the upper Bavarian field-study. *Sleep, 14*, 392-398.

World Health Organization. (1993). *The ICD-10 classification of mental and behavioural disorders*. Geneva: World Health Organization.

Yinnon, A. M., Ilan, Y., Tadmor, B., Altarescu, G., & Hershko, C. (1992). Quality of sleep in the medical department. *British Journal of Clinical Practice, 46*, 88-91.

Zepelin, H., McDonald, C. S., & Zammit, G. K. (1984). Effects of age on auditory awakening thresholds. *Journal of Gerontology, 39*, 294-300.

2

Characteristics of Older Adults With Insomnia

CATHERINE S. FICHTEN
EVA LIBMAN
SALLY BAILES
IRIS ALAPIN

Purpose

The goals of this chapter are (a) to describe the characteristics of three groups of healthy, independent, community dwelling older adults: good sleepers and poor sleepers with and without insomnia complaints; (b) to present a working operational definition of insomnia that is based on both sleep/wake parameters and distress experienced; and (c) to explore the multifaceted nature of the insomnia complaint in older adults. In particular, we will show that at least the following aspects of the insomnia experience must be taken into consideration both when conceptualizing insomnia and during assessment and treatment:

1. Nocturnal sleep/wake experiences such as total sleep and wake times
2. Nocturnal cognitive arousal, activity, and tension
3. Psychologically laden sleep variables such as sleep-related distress

4. Aspects of daytime psychological adjustment, such as low levels of anxiety and depression
5. Self-reported as well as objective aspects of daytime functioning and performance (e.g., fatigue, sleepiness)

To arrive at an operational definition of insomnia in older adults, we will discuss what is meant by "older adults" and will briefly examine how existing classificatory systems deal with definitions of insomnia. We will then evaluate the daytime and nocturnal components of the insomnia complaint, examine characteristics of older adults with and without insomnia, and explore how insomnia and related complaints are measured and evaluated.

Methodological and Conceptual Problems in Determining Whether Increasing Age Causes Insomnia

Studies show age-related changes in sleep architecture and in the prevalence of insomnia (Dement et al., 1985; Kales, 1975; Miles & Dement, 1980; Morin, 1993; Morin & Gramling, 1989; Prinz, Vitiello, Raskind, & Thorpy, 1990; Williams, Karacan, & Hursch, 1974). Does this mean that increasing age causes insomnia? Not necessarily. There are five major confounds in the literature that prevent definitive statements: Much of the data reflect prevalence rather than incidence, the effects of illness and medications are often not taken into account, studies are cross-sectional rather than longitudinal, age ranges of older adults studied vary widely, and diverse and sometimes inconsistent definitions of poor sleep and insomnia are used.

Prevalence Rather Than Incidence and the Effects of Illness and Medications

The bulk of the findings reflect the prevalence of insomnia (e.g., "do you have" or "have you ever had") rather than its incidence (e.g., "did you develop during the past year") (see Morgan, Chapter 1, this volume, for an extended discussion of this topic). Thus, the available data concerning age and insomnia may reflect the chronicity of sleep complaints rather than the rate at which new sleep problems develop.

A variety of other changes occur with age, and factors such as deteriorating physical health, the adverse effects of many prescription and over-the-counter drugs on sleep, and high rates of sleep apnea and restless legs syndrome/periodic limb movements in sleep (RLS/PLMS) all contribute to confounding the findings (e.g., Ancoli-Israel & Coy, 1994; Edinger et al., 1989; Jacobs, Reynolds, Kupfer, Lovin, & Ehrenpreis, 1988; Libman, Creti, Levy, Brender, & Fichten, 1997; Reynolds et al., 1980).

Cross-Sectional Rather Than Longitudinal Investigations

The widely held assumption that aging causes insomnia may not be supported by the available evidence on older healthy adults. For example, although increases in sleep disturbances with increasing age have been found in non-elderly samples (Janson et al., 1995; McGhie & Russell, 1962; Weyerer & Dilling, 1991), a reexamination of studies from the 1960s as well as more recent investigations suggests that rather than accelerating after age 65, insomnia problems appear to peak considerably earlier—in the 50 to 60 age group (Hammond, 1964; McGhie & Russell, 1962; Mellinger, Balter, & Uhlenhuth, 1985). In addition, epidemiological studies of older individuals have demonstrated that when health problems were controlled for or when studies were longitudinal, insomnia complaints generally showed no age-related increases (Bliwise, King, Harris, & Haskell, 1992; Foley et al., 1995; Hoch et al., 1994; Monjan & Foley, 1995). Moreover, both cross-sectional and longitudinal studies that examined healthy, well-functioning seniors have demonstrated exceptionally low levels of sleep complaints (Kronholm & Hyyppa, 1985; Morgan, Healey, & Healey, 1989). Some studies of sleep patterns in aging populations have found that when older individuals were divided into "young old" and "old old" categories, sleep quality did not decline with age (Frisoni et al., 1993; Gislason, Reynisdottir, Kristbjarnarson, & Benediktsdottir, 1993; Kronholm & Hyyppa, 1985; Libman et al., 1998; Schmitt, Phillips, Cook, Berry, & Wekstein, 1996). Similar results are reported by Hoch et al. (1994), who used both physiological and self-report assessment. When older subjects are divided into good and poor sleepers, some longitudinal studies have even suggested that sleep quality can improve over time (Libman et al., 1998; Mellinger et al., 1985; Mendelson, 1995; Monjan & Foley, 1995; Morgan et al., 1989). Such findings suggest that insomnia does not necessarily develop as a consequence of increasing age, per se, in older adults.

Age Ranges Vary Widely

An additional confound relates to "older adults" having been defined in a variety of ways in the literature. The lower limit may be 55, 60, or 65 years of age. The upper limit is usually not specified, but frequently there are 90-year-old participants, as is the case in our research. Thus, it is entirely possible that findings on "older adults" reflect data on individuals aged 55 to well over 90. Not only does this age range span 35 or more years, but it also involves two generations—two distinct cohorts— of older adults. This vast age range, along with comorbidities such as illness and iatrogenic effects of medications, may contribute to findings of large numbers of older adults with insomnia. To further knowledge in this realm, we must be clear whom we are talking about.

Most studies of insomnia exclude individuals age 55 and over. This is due, in part, to differences between younger adults, on one hand, and middle-aged and older adults on the other, both in sleep architecture and in the nature of insomnia complaints. Whereas younger individuals generally have problems falling asleep (sleep onset insomnia), older adults are also likely to have problems maintaining sleep (sleep maintenance insomnia) (e.g., Gislason & Almqvist, 1987). As noted earlier, studies of older adults often use age 65 as the cutoff. Thus, data on the fastest growing segment of North American society—people aged 55 to 65—are especially scarce. Future research should target this group for evaluation. Studies should be longitudinal, if possible, and evaluate both the prevalence and the incidence of poor sleep and insomnia.

Varied Definitions

Another confound relates to the diagnostic criteria for insomnia. There are three popular classificatory systems for sleep disorders: the *Di-*

agnostic and Statistical Manual of Mental Disorders (*DSM-IV*; American Psychiatric Association, 1994), the International Classification of Sleep Disorders or *ICSD* (American Sleep Disorders Association, 1990), and the International Classification of Diseases (*ICD-10*; World Health Organization, 1992). These are described in detail by Morgan (Chapter 1, this volume). When it comes to defining insomnia, each classificatory system has important weaknesses, leading to considerable confusion about the definition of poor sleep and insomnia in both the clinical and research literatures. These classification systems not only differ in the categories they use but also utilize different diagnostic criteria to define insomnia (Edinger et al., 1996). For example, whereas the *ICD-10* provides both a frequency criterion (at least 3 nights per week) and a duration criterion (at least 1 month), the *DSM-IV* contains only a duration requirement (at least 1 month), and the *ICSD* contains neither.

All three systems are consistent in that a diagnosis of primary insomnia is made only after excluding insomnia associated with (a) a mental disorder (e.g., major depressive disorder, generalized anxiety disorder), (b) a general medical condition (e.g., hyperthyroidism), (c) another sleep disorder (e.g., narcolepsy), or (d) the physiological effects of substance abuse or medication. All three nosologies include criteria for daytime "consequences" of poor sleep and require the presence of a complaint of insomnia, rather than merely poor sleep. In fact, the *DSM-IV* and *ICD-10* both include a "clinical significance" criterion of distress related to the sleep problem as a central feature of primary insomnia. Unfortunately, none of the classificatory systems has operationalized how to evaluate or measure "distress" or "complaint."

Research definitions of insomnia also use the exclusion criteria noted above. Because the existing nosologies are not entirely consistent with one another and because some criteria are only loosely operationalized, however, variations in definitions abound. This problem has been especially serious in epidemiological investigations, where sleep-related questions formulated by non–sleep specialists are frequently used.

The most popular research definition involves 30 minutes of undesired awake time at least 3 nights per week with a problem duration at least 6 months. The distress criterion usually is not formally included, in part because there is no generally acceptable measure for the construct. Often, research relies on self-selection—if someone volunteers for an insomnia study or is referred to a sleep laboratory and meets the other selection criteria, he or she is assumed to have insomnia rather than merely poor sleep.

We contend that the failure to use a uniform definition across studies and the universal lack of research attention to the distress component of insomnia have allowed a false picture to emerge about poor sleep and the complaint of insomnia in older adults. Younger adults who do not have insomnia frequently experience uninterrupted sleep during the night. Most older adults, including those who report sleeping well, experience at least one awakening during the night (Libman, Creti, Amsel, Brender, & Fichten, 1997). Therefore, whereas older adults may indeed experience disrupted sleep with lengthy nocturnal awake times, the individual may not find this experience especially distressing and thus may not be *suffering* from insomnia. As one research participant told us, "Yes, I stay up for a while. But it is really quiet, and I can get many things done. I do my best baking in the middle of the night."

High- and Low-Distress: Poor Sleepers

Reports such as this, coupled with the difficulties with definitions of insomnia noted above, forced us to identify and distinguish two groups of older poor sleepers whose sleep parameters were very similar: poor sleepers who were highly distressed about their sleep and those who were minimally distressed about it (Fichten et al., 1995; Libman, Creti, Amsel, et al., 1997). There had already been hints in the literature that some "insomniacs" fail to experience high levels of anxiety, tension, or arousal (Chambers & Kim, 1993; Seidel et al., 1984; Stepanski et al., 1989), and others have discussed noncomplaining poor sleepers (Dorsey & Bootzin, 1997; Lavidor et al., 1996; Mellinger et al., 1985; Mendelson, Garnett, Gillin, & Weingartner, 1984; Ohayon, Caulet, & Guilleminault, 1997).

We clearly identified, categorized, and described these two types of poor sleepers—those who are highly distressed by their sleep problem and those who have similarly serious sleep disturbance but are minimally distressed about it. The "low-distress poor sleeper" group consists of people who are relatively untroubled by the psychophysiological changes in sleep architecture that accompany aging. This group is critical to understanding successful coping with age-related changes in sleep. For example, comparisons of good sleepers with high- and low-distress poor sleepers show that where quantitative sleep parameters are concerned, such as total sleep time, total wake time, and sleep efficiency, high- and low-distress poor sleepers are fairly similar to each other and very different from good sleepers. On measures of distress related to sleep disruption, however, there is greater similarity between good sleepers and low-distress poor sleepers than there is between the two poor sleeper groups. This finding mirrors the pattern of results obtained on personality and psychological adjustment (Fichten et al., 1995; Lavidor et al., 1996).

Contributors to the Insomnia Complaint

The requirement that insomnia be defined not merely through sleep and wake parameters, such as total sleep and wake times or sleep efficiency, but also through presumed daytime consequences poses additional difficulties both for assessment and for treatment.

Presumed Daytime Consequences: Impaired Daytime Performance

People who complain of difficulty falling asleep or staying asleep during the night often complain of being impaired in their ability to function during the day. For example, they report feeling unrefreshed, sleepy, and tired, and they report problems with memory and concentration (Alapin et al., 2000; Hauri & Fisher, 1986; Zammit, 1988). Most cite fatigue (tiredness, lethargy) as a greater problem than drowsiness (feeling sleepy, struggling to stay awake) (Chambers & Keller, 1993; Stepanski, Zorick, Sicklesteel, Young, & Roth, 1986).

Despite the ubiquity of self-reported complaints about daytime functioning in individuals with insomnia, studies generally have failed to find significant differences between people with insomnia and normal controls on behavioral measures of daytime performance and functioning (e.g., Alapin, 1996; Lichstein, Wilson, Noe, Aguillard, & Bellur, 1994; Mendelson et al., 1984; Seidel et al., 1984).

Correlations between self-reports of feeling sleepy or fatigued and behavioral measures of the same constructs are generally small and nonsignificant (cf. Alapin et al., 2000; Johnson, Freeman, Spinweber, & Gomez, 1991; Seidel et al., 1984). This lack of consistency between subjective and behavioral measures of daytime "consequences" have played a key role in conceptualizations of the nature and meaning of insomnia as well as of the role of sleep deprivation in the "secondary" symptoms of insomnia such as sleepiness and fatigue (cf. Chambers & Keller, 1993). Indeed, some investigators have gone as far as to posit "that the secondary symptoms reported by patients with primary insomnia are probably not related to their poor sleep per se" (Bonnet & Arand, 1998, p. 359). By contrast, self-reports of poor daytime functioning are related to distress about insomnia as well as to poor scores on measures of psychological adjustment (Fichten, Libman, et al., 1998a, 2000b). This suggests that subjectively experienced daytime performance and the behavioral or biological expressions of these aspects of daytime functioning may not be fully controlled by the same physiological mechanisms. Indeed, it has been suggested that central nervous system (CNS) hyperarousal may provide the mediational link between distress about one's insomnia and self-perceived poor performance during the day (Bonnet & Arand, 1998). To explore this possibility, research is needed that includes both daytime and nocturnal polysomnography (PSG) as well as self-reported and behavioral measures of daytime sleepiness, fatigue, and difficulty concentrating. In such investigations, poor sleepers reporting both high and low levels of distress concerning their sleep difficulty should be studied.

Presumed Daytime Causes: Myths About Lifestyle Factors

The ubiquity of chronic sleep complaints, even in the "well elderly," has prompted a variety of plausible but unsubstantiated causal explanations related to lifestyle factors: irregular schedules permitted by retirement, napping, early bedtimes, overly long periods spent in bed, unrealistic expectations about sleep needs, erroneous beliefs about how well comparable age peers sleep, and major life stresses such as death or illness of a loved one. Given the pervasiveness of such beliefs, there has been a surprising lack of confirmatory data. Our own work (Fichten et al., 1995) as well as studies by others (e.g., Monk, Reynolds, Machen, & Kupfer, 1992) demonstrates that as far as daytime activities and lifestyle are concerned, older individuals with no insomnia complaints lead neither more regular nor less stressful lives than their poor sleeper counterparts.

Sleep Expectations

It has been suggested that older individuals complaining of insomnia have unrealistic beliefs and expectations about sleep that, when not met, increase anxiety and distress, thereby perpetuating and aggravating the sleep problem (Morin & Gramling, 1989). Our data do not support the hypothesis that older poor sleepers have unreasonable expectations about sleep (Fichten et al., 1995). Poor sleepers in our study were surprisingly optimistic about how their sleep experience compared to that of others; this was true both for poor sleepers who were highly distressed about their sleep problem (highly distressed poor sleepers) and for poor sleepers who were not troubled by their poor sleep (minimally distressed poor sleepers). For example, approximately 50% of both highly and minimally distressed poor sleepers indicated that their sleep was much the same as that of others their age. Good sleepers and highly distressed poor sleepers also wanted similar amounts of sleep—approximately 7 hours—the amount actually obtained by our good sleepers. Minimally distressed poor sleepers wanted somewhat less (6.25 hours).

Sleep Lifestyle Practices

The literature contains suggestions and assertions that poor sleep in older individuals is associated with maladaptive sleep lifestyle practices and poor "sleep hygiene," such as spending excessive amounts of time in bed, going to bed too early, taking frequent naps, and having erratic bedtimes and arising times (e.g., Hoelscher & Edinger, 1988; Marchini, Coates, Magistad, & Waldum, 1983). Our data show that good sleepers and highly distressed as well as minimally distressed poor sleepers were all very similar on these dimensions (Fichten et al., 1995). First, they experienced similarly regular lifestyles; they did not differ on variability in mealtimes or in the times they went to bed or got up in the morning. In addition, all three groups spent similar amounts of time in bed—approximately 8 hours. They also had similar bedtimes (around 11 p.m.) and arising times (around 7 a.m.), and they napped equally frequently—almost twice per week. Our findings indicate no significant differences in either coffee or alcohol consumption between good and poor sleepers while they are trying to fall asleep or during noctural wake times (Libman, Creti, Amsel, et al., 1997); this is similar to others' findings (e.g., Adam, Tomeny, & Oswald, 1986; Gourash-Bliwise, 1992; Morgan et al., 1989), although Morgan and his colleagues did find a difference in daytime tea, but not coffee, consumption.

Another area of presumed difference between good sleepers and poor sleepers with insomnia revolves around the ease with which they fall asleep outside their bedrooms. Contrary to popular beliefs and clinical lore, which state that poor sleepers fall asleep more easily in locations other than their bedrooms, our data show that only about 20% of both highly and minimally distressed poor sleepers—as well as of good sleepers—indicated that they found it easier to fall asleep in places other than their bedrooms.

Demographics and Daytime Aspects of Lifestyle

Equally important are our consistently negative findings on demographic factors. These show that good sleepers, poor sleepers who are highly distressed about their insomnia, and poor sleepers who are minimally distressed closely resemble each other on all variables examined in our research (Fichten et al., 1995). For example, there were no differences in the diversity of activities engaged in or in perceptions about how fully one's time was occupied. Nor did the three groups in our study—good sleepers and highly and minimally distressed poor sleepers—differ on education or on either income level or its perceived adequacy. Our findings support reports by other investigators who have shown economic dissatisfaction to be unrelated to sleep quality in older individuals (Frisoni et al., 1993). Epidemiological surveys have found that people with low incomes were considerably more likely to experience poor sleep than people with higher incomes (e.g., Tait, 1992). Here, however, other health and psychosocial variables related to poverty must be taken into consideration.

Life Events

Exposure to stressful life events (such as the death of a loved one) was also similar in our three groups (Fichten et al., 1995). Consistent with our results, others also have shown that older good and poor sleepers did not differ on life stress (e.g., Friedman, Brooks, Bliwise, Yesavage, & Wicks,

1995). Although major negative life events have been implicated in the onset of insomnia (Healey et al., 1981; Kales et al., 1984), it seems that large but infrequent stressors are not involved in the maintenance of chronic sleep problems.

Summary of Lifestyle Factors

Our results (Fichten et al., 1995) add to the growing body of evidence (e.g., Gourash-Bliwise, 1992); Morin & Gramling, 1989) that highlights the absence of differences in lifestyle in older individuals with and without insomnia. Evidence on the effectiveness of lifestyle changes in alleviating sleep complaints (e.g., Edinger, Hoelscher, Marsh, Lipper, & Ionescu-Pioggia, 1992) should not be used to justify the assumption that older poor sleepers' maladaptive sleep hygiene and lifestyle practices cause either poor sleep or the complaint of insomnia, just as the efficacy of aspirin in alleviating headaches is never used to infer that lack of aspirin causes headaches.

Personality and Daytime Psychological Adjustment

Of course, diagnosable psychiatric conditions, such as major depression and anxiety disorders, are well known to be associated with insomnia (e.g., Ford & Kamerow, 1989; Henderson et al., 1995; Kales, Caldwell, Preston, Healy, & Kales, 1976; Morgan & Clarke, 1997; Reynolds, Kupfer, Burpse, Cable, & Yeager, 1991; Schramm, Hohagen, Kappler, Grasshoff, & Berger, 1995). Other psychological factors also have been found to be important. For example, numerous studies have shown that healthy older individuals with no psychiatric diagnosis who complain of insomnia experience more negative affect and have poorer scores on a large variety of measures of daytime psychological adjustment than do good sleepers (e.g., Frisoni et al., 1993; Gourash-Bliwise, 1992; Monk et al., 1992; Morin & Gramling, 1989; Morgan, Dallosso, Ebrahim, Arie, & Fentem, 1988; Morgan et al., 1989). Our own work (Fichten et al., 1995; Fichten, Libman, et al., 1998a) also indicates that psychological adjustment (e.g., an anxious worrying "neurotic" personality style and low, subclinical levels of depression) is poorer in healthy older adults with insomnia than in those who sleep well.

As noted earlier, an interesting finding to emerge from our studies has been the identification of substantial numbers of older individuals who, in spite of sleeping badly, are only minimally distressed by their poor sleep. This group of poor sleepers differs relatively little from highly distressed poor sleepers with respect to severity of problematic sleep. These two groups are more easily distinguished by the absence of poor psychological adjustment and negative affect in the minimally distressed poor sleeper group and by the presence of maladjustment and emotional turmoil in the other.

Why are people who are somewhat anxious or depressed more likely to suffer from insomnia than those who are less so? How do personality and daytime psychological adjustment influence nocturnal sleep experiences? Our research suggests that thoughts during the day and during the night may pose a mediational link between personality and psychological adjustment, on one hand, and distress about insomnia on the other (Fichten, Libman, et al., 1998a, 2000). Of course, it is also possible that the underlying root cause is central nervous system (CNS) hyperarousal (Bonnet & Arand, 1998; Lamarche & Ogilvie, 1997; Perlis, Giles, Mendelson, Bootzin, & Wyatt, 1997). Even if this is so, it is still necessary to explain how CNS hyperarousal translates into distress about insomnia. Thus, the CNS hyperarousal formulation is entirely consistent with our view that negative thoughts and experienced cognitive arousal mediate various aspects of the insomnia complaint. This position—that aversive cognitions, including negative thoughts, worry, a poor balance between positive and negative thinking, and high levels of mental "tension" are related both to poor sleep and to distress about one's sleep problem—is developed in subsequent sections of this chapter.

Problems Related
to How Relevant
Constructs Are Measured

Sleep/Wake Parameters:
All ParametersAre Not Created Equal

The most common sleep parameters evaluated are total sleep time (TST), sleep onset latency (SOL), wake time after sleep onset (WASO), sleep efficiency (TST/time spent in bed), and frequency of nocturnal awakenings (FNA).

TST, SOL, and WASO

Total nocturnal sleep time (TST) is, we believe, the best single indicator of sleep status, in spite of large discrepancies between individual sleep needs (e.g., Hicks, Marical, & Conti, 1991; Hicks & Youmans, 1989; Kripke, Simons, Garfinkel, & Hammond, 1979; Rutter & Waring-Paynter, 1992). TST is easily reported by most individuals, and TST scores are more closely related than are SOL or WASO to a variety of other measures of sleep and wake as well as to psychologically laden sleep variables (cf. Alapin et al., 2000). Moreover, unpublished data show that of all sleep/wake parameters evaluated in our research, the correlation between scores measured via retrospective questionnaire and via daily sleep diary was highest for TST (Libman et al., 1999).

Measures of nocturnal wake times tend to be problematic. For example, sleep onset latency (SOL), generally defined as the interval between lights out and sleep onset, has long been known to be overestimated by poor sleepers (compared to objective evaluation using polysomnography) and underestimated by good sleepers (e.g., Carskadon et al., 1976; Coursey, Frankel, Gaardner, & Mott, 1980; Frankel, Coursey, Buchbinder, & Snyder, 1976; Knab & Engle, 1988; Morin, Kowatch, Barry, & Walton, 1993). But when does one turn the lights out? Some people turn lights out based on a regular sleep schedule, whereas others keep lights on and read, watch TV, or work until they feel sleepy. This can be very late at night. There is a confound because some people keep lights on late into the night precisely because they cannot fall asleep, but this interval is not included in the definition of SOL. Waking after sleep onset (WASO) is even more problematic to evaluate, especially when it is based on self-reports. For example, people may experience several separate nocturnal awake intervals as a single long period of wakefulness. Alternately, people are expected to "sum" several wake periods to come up with a total. The issue of what to do about waking too early compounds the problem, regardless of whether WASO is measured through objective or subjective means. For example, if someone's final awakening occurred at 5 a.m. and that person got out of bed at 8, should the 3 hours spent in bed be considered wake time? What if the individual fell asleep for 10 minutes just before 8 a.m. or if the 3 hours spent in bed occurred between 8 a.m. and 11 a.m.? In addition, contrary to findings on SOL, where poor sleepers *over*estimate how long it takes them to fall asleep, data indicate that older poor sleepers tend to *under*estimate WASO compared to objective measures (Coates et al., 1983; Libman, Creti, Levy, et al., 1997; Lichstein & Johnson, 1991; Morin, Colecchi, Stone, Brink, & Sood, 1994).

Sleep Efficiency

Sleep efficiency is a ratio calculated by dividing TST by the total time spent in bed (arising time minus bedtime). Although at first glance this appears to be an ideal measure, as it seems to reflect both sleep and wake times, this is not the case. First, there is lack of agreement about what is meant by bedtime and by arising time. If one watches TV, knits, and reads in bed before lights out, is the time spent doing these activities counted? Of course, there is a similar problem defining arising time. What does one do with people who enjoy an hour in bed after awakening before getting out of bed as part of their regular sleep experience?

Perhaps more important, sleep efficiency is a ratio and, as such, is affected by changes in both the numerator and the denominator. Thus, one may achieve a sleep efficiency of 80%—a score widely used as a cutoff for good and poor sleep—by spending 8 hours asleep and 10 hours in bed, as well as by sleeping 2 hours out of $2\frac{1}{2}$. The fact that the score is a ratio poses serious limitations on its use as the single best measure of good and poor sleep (cf. Amsel & Fichten, 1990, 1998).

Frequency of Nocturnal Awakenings (FNA)

Evaluation of FNA is meaningful in younger adults. In older populations, however, where nocturnal arousals are fairly common, FNA scores are problematic. There are problems both with what scores mean and with measurement modality. For example, one may obtain a low score on FNA by waking up only once but staying awake for 3 hours as well as by waking up once and returning to sleep almost immediately. Indeed, higher scores may reflect better sleep—that is, longer rather than shorter sleep. Another problem relates to how FNA is measured. Self-reports of

FNA by both good and poor sleepers generally are substantially lower than those indicated by polysomnographic (PSG) data (e.g., Carskadon et al., 1976; Knab & Engle, 1988; Morin et al., 1994). It has been suggested that this occurs because poor sleepers may not be aware of having slept (Knab & Engle, 1988). Of course, forgetting is another possibility, as reporting of nocturnal events has been related to retrograde and anterograde amnesia (Lichstein & Johnson, 1991; Wyatt, Bootzin, Anthony, & Bazant, 1994). Whatever the cause of the underreporting, self-reported FNA scores do not appear to be a good index of sleep/wake parameters in older adults.

Sleep/Wake Parameters: Variations in Technique

Sleep parameters such as TST, SOL, WASO, and sleep efficiency can be measured in various ways. There are two concepts to note here. One is the issue of objective measurement, for example polysomnography (PSG) (cf. Chesson et al., 1997), vs. self-report (interview, questionnaire, daily self-monitoring). The second revolves around how to best measure self-report: through retrospective questionnaires ("generally") vs. ongoing self-monitoring (sleep diaries).

Objective vs. Self-Report Measures

In the sleep literature, polysomnography (PSG) is considered the "gold standard" for assessment of sleep disorders. This is so in spite of a variety of data showing that although PSG may be vital in the diagnosis of sleep disorders such as sleep apnea and restless legs syndrome/periodic limb movements in sleep (RLS/PLMS), it may have little to add to self-report in the case of insomnia (Reite, Buysse, Reynolds, & Mendelson, 1995; Vgontzas, Kales, Bixler, Manfredi, & Vela-Bueno, 1995). Poor sleepers generally report shorter sleep times and longer sleep onset than comparable PSG data (e.g., Carskadon et al., 1976; Coursey et al., 1980; Frankel et al., 1976; Knab & Engle, 1988; Kryger, Siteljes, Pouliot, Neufeld, & Odgnoki, 1991; Lichstein & Johnson, 1991; Morin et al., 1994; Morin et al., 1993). Nevertheless, correlations between self-reports and PSG are high (e.g., Frankel et al., 1976; Hoch et al., 1987; Knab & Engle, 1988; Kryger et al., 1991; Morin et al., 1993). Whereas the findings suggest that poor sleepers exaggerate the extent of their sleep problem, paradoxically, poor sleepers have also been shown to underestimate nocturnal wake times compared to objective measures (Coates et al., 1983, Libman, Creti, Levy, et al., 1997; Lichstein & Johnson, 1991; Morin et al., 1994), suggesting a role for information processing rather than motivational factors and bringing into question the exaggeration hypothesis.

Most self-reported poor sleepers differ from good sleepers on PSG-scored sleep parameters (e.g., Morin et al., 1993). Yet a substantial number of self-reported poor sleepers do not have "objective findings" on PSG—a diagnostic entity currently called sleep state misperception (American Sleep Disorders Association, 1990) but referred to by various other names throughout the years, including subjective insomnia, pseudo-insomnia, and normal sleeping insomniacs. Self-reports of poor sleepers with and without "objective findings" tend to be very similar on most sleep-related variables in spite of substantial differences on PSG. For example, the data show little if any difference between the symptoms, prognostic indicators, daytime complaints, or personality factors of self-reported poor sleepers with and without PSG-documented objective findings (Dorsey & Bootzin, 1997; Lichstein et al., 1994; Mendelson, 1995; Mendelson et al., 1984; Salin-Pascual, Roehrs, Merlotti, Zorick, & Roth, 1992; Seidel et al., 1984; Trinder, 1988). For all practical purposes, then, the contribution of PSG in this realm is also negligible.

Moreover, polysomnography, as it is currently practiced in many sleep laboratories, may be altogether inappropriate for the evaluation of insomnia. As an example, in one of our studies we sent some of the participants for the customary 2 nights of testing to our collaborating, research-minded sleep laboratory (Libman, Creti, Levy, et al., 1997) and encountered a variety of problems. First, some subjects never completed testing—they found the atmosphere austere and somewhat intimidating. In addition, they found themselves in a small, sparsely furnished room that had little in common with their bedroom. Certainly, the conditions for sleep in the lab were not typical of participants' natural environments. Such environmental factors can result in first night effects (and reverse first night effects)—that is, people may sleep either worse or better in locales other than their homes (e.g., Edinger et al., 1997; Hauri, 1983; Randazzo & Schweitzer, 1995). Perhaps more important, even 2 nights of PSG may not be representative of highly variable sleep experiences (cf.

Babkoff, Weller, & Lavidor, 1995; Bootzin et al., 1995; Coates et al., 1983; Edinger, Marsh, McCall, Erwin, & Lininger, 1991).

In addition, sleep laboratories may not accommodate insomnia patients. In the case of our collaborating lab, lights were always turned out around midnight, regardless of whether the subject was ready to sleep or not. Similarly, subjects were asked to get out of bed at 6 a.m., again regardless of whether they were ready to get up. Needless to say, this does not give a realistic picture of SOL, WASO, TST, or sleep efficiency. The laboratory experience lacked external validity. Doubtless, the lab's protocol was fine for what typically was studied there: sleep apnea and RLS/PLMS. For the assessment of insomnia, however, such a protocol was clearly inappropriate.

There are suggestions in the literature that the EEG data of people complaining of insomnia show higher levels of cortical arousal (cf. Bonnet & Arand, 1998; Perlis et al., 1997). Most PSG evaluations, however, do not routinely score such criteria. Nor are the etiological or treatment implications of such findings clear at this time.

Although PSG is clearly more "objective" than self-report, it should be noted that the criteria used to define sleep and wake are, to some extent, arbitrary. For example, Hauri and Olmstead (1989) postulated that the traditional PSG-assessed measure of sleep onset (i.e., first epoch scored as Stage 2 sleep) is inappropriate for people with insomnia because of demonstrated random alpha rhythm activity in all sleep stages.

For all the reasons cited above, we concur with the Standards of Practice Committee of the American Sleep Disorders Association (1995) and believe that self-report is a more valid means than PSG of evaluating the complaint of insomnia. People *complain* of insomnia. This is not an asymptomatic or hidden disease entity, like hypertension, which requires indirect tests for verification. Indeed, it is the complaint that is of interest. Minimally distressed poor sleepers do not seek out treatment and, according to virtually all diagnostic nosologies, would not be classified as having insomnia. It is thus a corollary that self-reports of sleep parameters and distress about insomnia are legitimate ways of evaluating the extent and import of insomnia in an individual's life.

That having been said, do we recommend PSG for older adults with insomnia? The answer, in spite of the foregoing, is a firm "Yes." We recommend PSG not to verify the insomnia complaint but to rule out sleep apnea and RLS/PLMS, which are known to be extremely common in older adults (e.g., Ancoli-Israel & Coy, 1994; Edinger et al., 1989; Jacobs et al., 1988; Libman, Creti, Levy, et al., 1997; Reynolds et al., 1980). These medically treatable sleep disorders are very difficult to detect based on clinical interviews (cf. Libman, Creti, Levy, et al., 1997; McCall & Edinger, 1991).

Retrospective Questionnaire vs. Ongoing Self-Monitoring (Daily Sleep Diary)

When conducting assessment, it is more convenient to administer a single questionnaire about a typical week's sleep than to ask individuals to self-monitor by completing daily sleep diaries for up to 2 weeks. In most clinical evaluations and in much sleep and insomnia research, however, daily sleep diaries are used to evaluate insomnia. Data are reduced by averaging the daily scores. In some studies, only 1 to 3 nights are evaluated, although recent clinical outcome studies often report up to 1 or 2 weeks.

Generally, sleep parameter scores on daily sleep diaries and retrospective questionnaires are highly correlated, with longer administrations of sleep diary yielding higher correlations (Babkoff et al., 1995). For example, in an unpublished study on 156 community-dwelling older adults, we found significant and reasonably high correlations between corresponding scores on a retrospective sleep questionnaire and on 7 days of self-monitoring on a daily sleep diary (Total Sleep Time, $r = .83$; Total Wake Time, $r = .72$; Sleep Efficiency, $r = .77$) (Libman et al., 1999).

When there are discrepancies between a daily sleep diary and retrospective questionnaire scores, it is usually assumed that the daily sleep diaries provide more accurate information. We contend that this is not necessarily the case. For example, self-monitoring may involve an atypical period in the individual's life; this is important because it is well documented that there is significant night-to-night variability in sleep parameters of people diagnosed with insomnia (Bootzin et al., 1995; Edinger et al., 1991). Perhaps more important, it has long been known that self-monitoring can be a reactive process in a variety of contexts and that it may cause either improvement or deterioration (Fichten et al., 1991; Mahoney, 1977; Nelson, 1977), thereby affecting the very variables it is meant to assess.

We believe that retrospective questionnaires provide a useful "snap-shot" of the extent of an insomnia problem and that they can be used profitably for research as well as for screening and assessment. Daily sleep diary scores, however, can pinpoint variations in night-to-night sleep experience, shed light on sequences of events, and monitor progress in therapy. Therefore, when undertaking treatment or obtaining a baseline, daily sleep diaries should be used.

Distress Related to Poor Sleep and Insomnia

One of the problems encountered in diagnosing insomnia is difficulty operationalizing distress. As we noted earlier, even though classificatory systems include distress in the criteria for insomnia, there are no well-accepted techniques for operationalizing the construct. In particular, it should be noted that the severity of the sleep problem, as measured by examination of sleep parameters such as TST, WASO, and sleep efficiency, is only moderately related to distress experienced about the sleep problem in older adults (Fichten et al., 1995).

In many insomnia research projects, it is assumed that the people who volunteer for the study must have an insomnia problem if they meet the sleep parameter criteria for a diagnosis of insomnia. This is not the case. For example, in our own research, we were interested in both good and poor sleep; therefore, we accepted all volunteers who fit our nonsleep-related selection criteria. We then offered a brief analog treatment to all individuals who met the criteria for poor sleeper status (i.e., 30 minutes of undesired awake time at least 3 nights per week, problem duration at least 6 months). To our surprise, almost one quarter of poor sleepers who completed our intensive 6-week treatment program were only minimally distressed by their poor sleep (Creti, 1996). This type of finding underscores the need to develop a distress criterion to be used in making a diagnosis of insomnia.

Operationalizing the Distress Criterion of Insomnia

To operationalize the construct for our own studies, we developed two ways of measuring distress related to poor sleep. We asked a single question using a 10-point Likert-type scale, "How distressed are you about an insomnia problem?" (1 = *not at all*, 10 = *very much*). We also asked a series of three 7-point questions concerning the frequency of experiencing distress related to a sleep problem and summed the scores. Participants were asked, "During a typical week, how many days per week does difficulty falling asleep distress you?" (also difficulty getting back to sleep during the night and difficulty getting back to sleep again after waking up too early). The maximum score was 21, with higher scores indicating more frequent distress episodes experienced during the week. Correlations between the composite frequency of distress score and the single 10-point item evaluating level of distress ranged from .75 to .84; temporal stability data for the single item showed acceptable reliability, with *r* values ranging from .66 to .73. These psychometric properties suggest that the single item inquiring about one's level of distress may be used in research to quantify the distress criterion.

The Multidimensional Components of Insomnia

The foregoing analysis, based on data both from our own research (Alapin et al., 2000; Fichten, Libman, et al., 1998a) and from that of others (cf. Bonnet & Arand, 1998; Chambers & Keller, 1993; Lichstein et al., 1994), suggests that more or less sleep or wake time does not fully explain either the severity of the insomnia complaint or the accompanying daytime fatigue and impairment that typically are reported. Thus, the question "If sleep deprivation is not the main culprit, what is?" We propose that insomnia complaints in older individuals are multidimensional in nature and have both physiological and psychological components.

Central Nervous System Hyperarousal

The view that insomnia complaints as well as some "secondary symptoms" of insomnia, such as poorer daytime psychological adjustment and functioning, are due to central nervous system (CNS) hyperarousal has recently been gaining ground (Lamarche & Ogilvie, 1997). For example, CNS hyperarousal has been invoked as an explanation not only of poor sleep but also of difficulties related to personality and adjustment, negative affect and thoughts, self-reports of poor daytime functioning and performance, and biased time estimation (e.g., Bonnet & Arand, 1998). In addition, a physiological predisposition for certain personality characteristics has been suggested, and high-frequency EEG activity has been linked to cognitive hyperarousal during the sleep onset latency period (cf. Perlis et al., 1997). Indeed, Perlis and his colleagues have implicated both neurological processes (i.e., high-frequency EEG activity at sleep onset) and information and memory processing both in sleep state misperception and in the overestimation of sleep onset latency—phenomena that are both typically observed in people complaining of insomnia.

Personality and Psychological Adjustment

The literature indicates that people who do not have a diagnosable psychiatric disorder and who complain of insomnia generally tend to be more anxious, worrying, "neurotic," and depressed than either those who sleep well or those with poor sleep who are not distressed about their sleep disruption (e.g., Fichten et al., 1995; Fichten, Libman, et al., 1998a; Gourash-Bliwise, 1992; Libman, Creti, Amsel, et al., 1997; Morgan et al., 1989; Morin & Gramling, 1989). Moreover, individuals from nonclinical populations who score higher on measures of anxiety and worry experience poorer sleep on PSG than their non-anxious counterparts (Fuller, Waters, Binks, & Anderson, 1995).

Affect

Sleep disruption itself may have a physical basis in older adults. The observation that a sizable percentage of older adults experience extensive sleep disruption but minimal or no accompanying distress (cf. Dorsey & Bootzin, 1997; Fichten et al., 1995; Henderson et al., 1995; Kales et al., 1976; Lavidor et al., 1996; Mellinger et al., 1985; Mendelson et al., 1984; Morgan et al., 1988; Morgan et al., 1989; Ohayon et al., 1997) illustrates the important contribution of affect to the insomnia complaint in older adults.

Time Estimation

People who complain of insomnia consistently overestimate sleep on-set latency compared with polysomnographic data (cf. Borkovec, 1982; Frankel et al., 1976); good sleepers do not do this (Hauri & Olmstead, 1989). Although it is often assumed that poor sleepers are merely exag-gerating the extent of their sleep problem, there are also two information processing explanations for this discrepancy: (a) people with insomnia subjectively experience being awake during EEG-recorded Stage 2 sleep, whereas good sleepers do not (Borkovec, Lane, & Van Oot, 1981; Hauri & Olmstead, 1989), and (b) subjective time passes slowly during distress-ing and unpleasant bedtime experiences (Frankel et al., 1976). We pro-pose that lengthy "empty" time intervals, such as those experienced by poor sleepers, when filled with negative cognitive activity, can make the nocturnal experience aversive. Lengthy wake times can also seem longer than they actually are, and time can be felt to be passing slowly. For ex-ample, analog data from our laboratory show that people generally over-estimate the duration of "empty" blocks of time and that they perceive empty time as "dragging" (Fichten et al., 1992).

Behaviors

With the exception of our own studies, we know of no systematic eval-uation of behaviors engaged in by older individuals during periods of nocturnal wakefulness. To learn about how such behaviors relate to the insomnia complaint, we developed and validated a measure of what people do during the night when they are awake—the Sleep Behaviors Scale: 60+ (Libman, Creti, Amsel, et al., 1997). The study of sleep behav-iors suggests that maladaptive and adaptive nighttime behaviors also play a role in the insomnia experience.

Our findings indicate that although good sleepers engage less fre-quently in virtually all nocturnal behaviors than poor sleepers—be-cause they obviously spend less time awake during the night—they still manifest a similar range of behaviors in a similar rank ordering of frequency. When they find themselves awake during the night, how-ever, good sleepers are most likely to lie in bed quietly or rest and relax. Poor sleepers, on the other hand, most frequently toss and turn and go to the toilet.

Daytime Performance
and Functioning

Highly distressed poor sleepers report more daytime fatigue, sleepiness, and difficulty concentrating than do minimally distressed poor sleepers or good sleepers (Alapin, 1996; Alapin et al., 2000; Fichten et al., 1995). This suggests that perceived poor daytime functioning is related to distress about poor sleep (i.e., insomnia) rather than to simple sleep disruption (Chambers & Kim, 1993). With some exceptions (e.g., Hauri, 1997; Hart, Morin, & Best, 1995), scores on behavioral aspects of daytime impairment, such as falling asleep in inappropriate contexts, however, generally fail to distinguish poor sleepers from good sleepers (cf. Alapin, 1996; Nau, 1997; Stone, Morin, Hart, Remsberg, & Mercer, 1994). Perhaps the factors that impede sleep during the night, such as cognitive or physiological arousal, interfere with falling asleep during the day as well; this topic needs further investigation.

Cognitive Arousal and Tension

Sleep researchers and clinicians have increasingly implicated cognitive factors, such as cognitive hyperarousal and distressing and intrusive thoughts, in the etiology and maintenance of insomnia (Borkovec et al., 1981; Coates et al., 1983; Coyle & Watts, 1991; Kuisk, Bertelson, & Walsh, 1989; Lichstein & Fanning, 1990; Lichstein & Rosenthal, 1980; Lundh, Lunqvist, Broman, & Hetta, 1991; Marchini et al., 1983; Morin, 1993; Nicassio, Mendlowitz, Fussell, & Petras, 1985; Perlis et al., 1997; Van Egeren, Haynes, Franzen, & Hamilton, 1983; Waters, Adams, Binks, & Varnado, 1993). Indeed, some have argued that a common mediating mechanism—interruption of negative and intrusive cognitive activity—can best explain the demonstrated effectiveness of a wide variety of cognitive-behavioral interventions in treating sleep problems (cf. Borkovec, 1982; Lacks, 1987; Lichstein & Fischer, 1985). We posit that negative cognitive activity and high levels of mental "tension" during periods of wakefulness contribute to poor sleep experiences and may act as mediators between personality factors and negative affect, on one hand, and self-reported poor daytime functioning and insomnia complaints on the other.

To facilitate exploration of the notion that cognitive factors are involved in the complaint of insomnia, we recently developed and validated three measures that relate to nocturnal tension and to thinking and behavior during periods of nocturnal wakefulness.

Tension Thermometer

An easy-to-use, reliable, and valid single-item measure evaluates how much tension is experienced during nocturnal wake times: the Tension Thermometer ("When you are lying in bed trying to fall asleep, how tense do you generally feel?"). Responses are made on an 11-point scale: 0 = *not at all tense*, 100 = *very tense*, with ratings made at 10-point intervals. Our data indicate reasonable temporal stability for this item ($r = .67$), and the pattern of correlations between scores on this measure and relevant sleep variables shows logical, highly significant relationships (Fichten et al., 1995; Fichten, Libman, et al., 1998a).

Sleep Self-Statement Test: 60+ (SST: 60+)

Our research has also explored both the nature and the valence of thoughts experienced during periods of nocturnal wakefulness by older adults who are good sleepers as well as those who sleep poorly and are either minimally or highly distressed about this (Fichten et al., 1995; Fichten, Libman, et al., 1998a, 2000). At first we used open-ended thought listing; this helped identify the content areas and provided the impetus to develop an easy-to-use inventory measure: the Sleep Self-Statement Test: 60+ (SST: 60+) (Fichten, Libman, et al., 1998a). The measure contains two valenced subscales—generalized positive thinking and generalized negative thinking—as well as Schwartz and Garamoni's (1986) States-of-Mind (SOM) ratio [Positive/(Positive + Negative)] (for a discussion of SOMs and insomnia, see Amsel & Fichten, 1990, 1998). Our data using this measure indicate that negative thoughts are strongly and significantly related to sleep measures with an appreciable psychological loading (e.g., sleep self-efficacy expectations, distress concerning one's sleep problem). Measures of personality and psychological adjustment were also related to these variables. It is notable, however, that unlike personality and psychological adjustment measures, which were generally unrelated to sleep parameters, negative thoughts were also highly and significantly related to the more "quantitative" aspects of sleep (i.e., total sleep and wake times and sleep efficiency).

Sleep Behaviors Scale: 60+

This measure, which evaluates what people do during periods of sleeplessness, also provides data to support the assumption that cognitive arousal, negative thoughts, and nocturnal tension are important aspects of the insomnia experience (Libman, Creti, Amsel, et al., 1997). For example, when minimally distressed and highly distressed poor sleepers and good sleepers were compared on this measure, the two poor sleeper groups resembled each other on most variables, both differing from good sleepers. This was to be expected, as poor sleepers spend longer periods awake than good sleepers. One exception to this pattern was on the Cognitive Arousal subscale, where the highly distressed poor sleepers had substantially higher scores than minimally distressed poor sleepers, suggesting that items on this subscale are associated with the distress related to insomnia, not merely with the presence of disrupted sleep. Scores on the Cognitive Arousal subscale were also shown to be related to both poor daytime and nighttime adjustment. This is consistent with findings that (a) minimally distressed poor sleepers manifest significantly less psychological maladjustment and negative affect than highly distressed poor sleepers (Fichten et al., 1995; Lavidor et al., 1996), and (b) a higher frequency of cognitive activity, negative activity in particular, characterizes people who complain of insomnia (e.g., Fichten & Libman, 1991; Fichten, Libman, et al., 1998a, 2000; Kales et al., 1984).

A Theoretical View: The Cognitive Model of Insomnia

Multidimensional and interactive aspects of the insomnia complaint are summarized in our Cognitive Model of Insomnia (Fichten & Libman, 1991; Fichten, Libman, et al., 1998a, 2000). This model provides a description of a mediational mechanism by which personality and daytime psychological "adjustment" can influence nocturnal distress (i.e., through negative thoughts and self-statements). It pro-

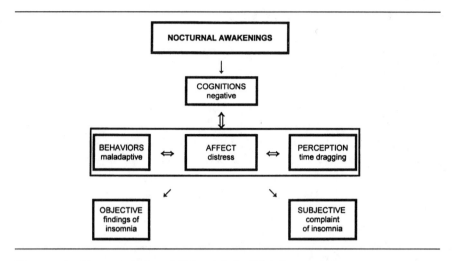

Figure 2.1. Characteristics of Older Adults With Insomnia
SOURCE: From "What Do Older Good and Poor Sleepers Do During Periods of Nocturnal Wakefulness? The Sleep Behaviors Scale: 60+," *Psychology and Aging*, Libman, Creti, Amsel, Brender, and Fichten, © Copyright 1997 by the American Psychological Association. Reprinted with permission.

poses that negative cognitive activity—primarily negative, worrying, and anxious thoughts and self-statements during periods of nocturnal wakefulness—is likely to be an important mediator of insomnia complaints.

Our model begins with the recognition that nocturnal awakenings will occur in most older individuals. It then proposes that negative cognitive activity, such as concerns about the day's events and worry about miscellaneous matters, including the consequences of not getting enough sleep, is associated with other maladaptive nocturnal events that, in turn, both magnify the sleep complaint and contribute to the negative cognitive experiences that interfere with falling asleep or returning to sleep. The model predicts that minimizing negative thoughts is likely to be effective because this targets cognitive activities that may (a) prevent sleep, (b) cause negative affect, (c) result in maladaptive sleep-related behaviors, and (d) contribute to distorted perceptions of the passage of time.

Findings from our studies provide support for heuristic, descriptive aspects of our Cognitive Model of Insomnia and also provide some support for the mediational role of negative thoughts in insomnia-related distress (Fichten, Libman, et al., 2000). For example, the data show that perceived severity of the sleep problem and negative thoughts both make significant and independent contributions to the variability in distress about poor sleep. Indeed, the data show that aversive cognitions, including negative thoughts, a poor balance between positive and negative thinking, and high levels of mental "tension" are all strongly and clearly related both to poor sleep and to distress about one's sleep problem. These cognitive aspects were more closely related to the various components of the insomnia experience than *any* of the state or trait measures of anxiety and adjustment explored in our study, suggesting a specific mediational role for negative thinking during nocturnal awake times. The possibility of CNS hyperarousal (cf. Bonnet & Arand, 1998; Lamarche & Ogilvie, 1997; Perlis et al., 1997) is consistent with this formulation, as are findings showing that when good sleepers are "yoked" (i.e., awakened at the same time as a matched insomnia sufferer) to insomnia patients for 7 days, they do not come to resemble insomnia patients on variables such as mood, daytime metabolic rate, or behavioral performance (Bonnet & Arand, 1996). Nevertheless, the issue of causality in our model needs further research attention; much of the evidence supporting the model has, to date, been correlational in nature.

Whatever the source, the powerful impact of negative thinking on affect and behavior has been amply demonstrated in the vast cognitive therapy literature. Because effective techniques for altering negative thoughts are readily available, our findings have a variety of applied implications for the treatment of insomnia.

Using the Model to Conceptualize
Where and How to Intervene

The therapeutic approach clearly suggested by our model and our data is to reduce negative thoughts, worry, and "tension" during nocturnal awakenings. This may be accomplished in a variety of ways. First, individuals may be taught to replace negative thoughts with neutral, "defusing," or positive thoughts and images. Second, people may be instructed to refocus attention away from internal information processing toward externally generated content (cf. Mathews & Milroy,

1994) by, for example, watching TV, reading, or listening to the radio or to audiotapes with verbal content (Creti, Libman, & Fichten, 2000). Third, it is possible to interrupt negative thoughts by engaging in incompatible activities either in bed (e.g., relaxation exercises) or out of bed, as prescribed in Bootzin's popular stimulus control insomnia treatment (Bootzin, Epstein, & Wood, 1991). Finally, our data also implicate daytime contributors to insomnia in otherwise healthy older adults, including subclinical levels of anxiety, tension, and depression and an anxious, worrying personality style. This suggests that an effective therapeutic intervention for insomnia might address the broader goal of modifying maladaptive daytime thoughts and feelings as well by treating subclinical anxiety or depression when these are evident.

Research Issues

An Operational Definition of Insomnia for People With Disrupted Sleep

As sleep researchers, we have been much troubled by the lack of consistency in defining insomnia. As noted earlier, existing classificatory systems do not specify operationalizable criteria. To remedy this problem, we propose an operational definition below.

Exclusion Criteria

This definition assumes that insomnia secondary to other problems such as those noted in the *DSM-IV* (1994) has been excluded: (a) a mental disorder (e.g., major depressive disorder, generalized anxiety disorder), (b) a general medical condition (e.g., hyperthyroidism), (c) the physiological effects of a substance (e.g., medication, abuse of drugs), or (d) another sleep disorder (e.g., sleep apnea, RLS/PLMS, narcolepsy). In older populations, it may be necessary to use polysomnographic evaluation to rule out sleep apnea and RLS/PLMS.

Inclusion Criteria

To diagnose insomnia, we propose that two requirements must be met: individuals must experience poor sleep for at least 1 month (i.e., have Difficulty Initiating or Maintaining Sleep [DIMS]) and must be distressed about their poor sleep.

Poor sleep: Determining the presence or absence of Difficulty Initiating or Maintaining Sleep (DIMS). To designate poor sleeper status, *the individual must self-report at least 30 minutes of undesired wakefulness at sleep onset or during nocturnal awakenings at least 3 nights per week, with a problem duration of at least 1 month.* We do not believe that PSG findings are suitable to meet this criterion, because this would require at least 1 week of polysomnographic (PSG) evaluation either in the sleep laboratory or at home. Sleep during this period would need to be typical of naturalistic circumstances, and the sleep evaluation would have to follow the participant's usual sleep schedule.

Our data show high correlations between scores based on self-monitoring for 7 days and scores on a retrospective questionnaire based on the past typical month. Thus, the constructs related to DIMS may be *evaluated either through 1 to 2 weeks of self-monitoring or through a single retrospective questionnaire based on the last typical month.*

Daily sleep diary. To establish the presence or absence of DIMS, we recommend using the following items on a daily basis for a minimum of 7 consecutive days during a "typical" week:

1	How long did it take you to fall asleep last night?	___hours	___minutes	
2	After you had fallen asleep for the first time, when you woke up during the night, approximately how long were you awake? (If you were awake more than once, write the total amount of time that you were awake.)	___hours	___minutes	___did not wake up
3	Did you have difficulty falling asleep or getting back to sleep?	___yes	___no	

4	(The following item needs to be asked only once:) How long have you had a problem with falling asleep or getting back to sleep? (Indicate duration in weeks, months, or years.)	___weeks ___months ___years ___I do not have a problem.

Although not required to establish the presence or absence of DIMS, we also recommend obtaining estimates of time slept, bedtime, out of bed time, and time of last awakening. This information is useful for reporting total sleep time (TST) and sleep efficiency [TST/(time spent in bed)] as well as for determining the existence of a problem with waking up too early in the morning (early morning or terminal insomnia). We recommend the following items:

5	Approximately how many hours did you sleep last night?	___hours ___minutes
6	What time did you go to bed last night?	___
7	What time did you wake up this morning (for the last time)?	___
8	What time did you get out of bed this morning?	___

Retrospective questionnaire. An alternative to using a daily sleep diary is to use a retrospective questionnaire that is administered only once. To establish the presence or absence of DIMS, we recommend using the following items. Unless stated otherwise, respondents are instructed to refer to the last typical month.

1	At bedtime, how long does it usually take you to fall asleep?	___hours ___minutes
2	After you have fallen asleep for the first time, when you wake up during the night, approximately how long are you usually awake? (If you wake more than once, write the total amount of time that you are usually awake.)	___hours ___minutes ___Do not usually wake up.

3	During a typical week, how often do you have difficulty falling asleep or getting back to sleep?	___nights per week
4	How long have you had a problem with falling asleep or getting back to sleep? (Indicate duration in weeks, months or years)	___weeks ___months ___years ___I do not have a problem.

As was the case for the daily sleep diary, here, too, we recommend that estimates of total sleep time, bedtime, out of bed time, and time of last awakening be obtained. We recommend the following items:

5	How many hours do you usually sleep per night?	___hours ___minutes
6	What is the usual time you go to bed?	___
7	What is the usual time you wake up in the morning (for the last time)?	___
8	What is the usual time you get out of bed?	___

Scoring. To classify individuals as having DIMS, they have to report, at a minimum:

a. One of the following: 3 nights of sleep onset latency (SOL) equal to or greater than 30 minutes (Question 1), *or* 3 nights of waking after sleep onset (WASO) equal to or greater than 30 minutes (Question 2), *or* 1 night of SOL and 2 nights of WASO equal to or greater than 30 minutes, *or* 2 nights of SOL and 1 night of WASO equal to or greater than 30 minutes, and

b. 3 nights of difficulty falling or staying asleep (Question 3), and

c. Problem duration (Question 4) of at least 1 month—if respondent states two durations, one for sleep onset and one for sleep maintenance, use the longer of the two intervals.

Distress: A necessary criterion for diagnosing insomnia. The definition of insomnia is based on both sleep/wake parameters and experienced distress. We propose that to diagnose insomnia, the individual must meet the criteria for DIMS specified above and must also score above the midpoint (i.e., score equal to or greater than 6) on the following distress item, which has been validated in our laboratory. Again, respondents complete this item only once and base their answers on the last typical month.

| 9 | How distressed are you by an insomnia problem? | 10-point scale, with 1 = not at all and 10 = very much |

Better Sample Specification

When conducting research, we must do a better job of specifying and describing our samples; this refers to age categories as well as to defining comparison groups.

Age

For now, we propose the following possibilities. If the sample is large enough, decade intervals should be used. If possible, data should be obtained for the understudied but fast-growing age group of those aged 50 to 60. Otherwise, researchers should not only specify means, standard deviations, and ranges but also divide the sample, if possible, into "young old" and "old old" groups. "Young old" samples may start as young as age 55. Age 75 and over is a typical age for the "old old" cutoff.

The Comparison Group: Good Sleepers or "Non-Poor Sleepers"?

In our research, we made a concerted effort to have two very different groups—poor sleepers who met the criteria for DIMS proposed above and good sleepers who not only failed to meet the criteria for DIMS but also showed evidence of excellent sleep on a variety of other measures as well. This resulted in two very dissimilar contrast groups; however, we also lost about one-third of our sample because some subjects were neither good nor poor sleepers. Deemed "medium quality" sleepers, these subjects had elements of both good and poor sleep.

Of course, selection criteria for such "good sleeper" status is arbitrary, especially in older adults. We therefore propose that, as is the case in other clinical areas (e.g., depressed and nondepressed, anxious and non-anxious), the comparison group be defined in future research not in terms of utopia, population means, or an ideal, but in terms of the absence of pathology.

Selection criteria for "non-poor sleepers." We propose the following. For an individual to be designated as a non-poor sleeper, he or she *must (a) fail to meet the criteria for DIMS and (b) if he or she takes sleep medication, it must be no more than twice a week.* Of course, one does not want to include poor sleepers who are "non-poor" only by dint of their sleep medications. This is especially important because hypnotics and other drugs used to induce sleep can have effects on aspects other than sleep, such as psychological adjustment and daytime functioning. The rationale for a maximum of 2 nights per week of sleep medication use is as follows. Everyone occasionally has a bad night, and some people cope by taking medication on these occasions to help them sleep. If medications are taken more frequently, for example 3 times per week, then those 3 nights may mask the 3 bad nights necessary to classify individuals as poor sleepers.

More Precise and Targeted Measurement

It is also necessary to select the right instrument for the right question. For example, instead of lamenting the observed discrepancies between subjective and behavioral measures of the same aspects of daytime functioning, such as sleepiness or fatigue, we should be administering both sets of measures and exploring the reasons for similarities and inconsistencies. Similarly, we should not simply follow typical usage in the literature but should recognize and make use of the strengths and weaknesses of evaluating sleep parameters through retrospective self-reports, daily sleep diaries, and polysomnography (PSG).

Implications for Research and Evaluation

Problems plaguing the literature clearly need to be circumvented. First, more data on incidence rather than prevalence are needed. This is especially important for the "midlife" years, as this seems to be an important time for sleep problems to develop. Samples also need to be better defined. This means that older adults must be separated into more finely grained age groups. Also, standards and criteria for health and illness as well as for medications that affect sleep need to be elaborated. More longitudinal studies are needed to better understand the factors that predispose, cause, and help maintain sleep problems, as well as factors that help improve or eliminate existing problems. To make findings more comparable across studies, a set of operationally defined definitions must be agreed upon for poor sleep, for the distress component of insomnia, and for "non-poor sleep." In this chapter, we propose such a set of definitions. In addition, future research needs to evaluate the role of cortical arousal and needs to pay more careful attention to the meaning of discrepancies in the daytime "consequences" of insomnia.

Conclusions

Summary of Characteristics of Older Adults Who Sleep Well and Those Who Sleep Poorly

Older adults who sleep poorly may or may not be distressed about their poor sleep. Although their sleep is substantially poorer than that of good sleepers, poor sleepers who are minimally distressed tend to sleep slightly better than their highly distressed counterparts. Older adults who are distressed about their sleep problem are likely to be somewhat more anxious, tense, worrying, and "neurotic" than their minimally distressed poor sleeper counterparts. They are also more likely to manifest subclinical levels of depression. In addition, they are more likely to have negative thoughts during nocturnal awake times and to toss and turn and engage in a variety of maladaptive sleep-related behaviors during the night. Recent research also suggests that these highly distressed individuals may have higher cortical arousal, both during the day and during the night. Although unselected poor sleepers are likely to report impaired daytime performance, such as fatigue, sleepiness, and difficulty concentrating, poor sleepers who are distressed about their sleep problem are likely to report more serious problems in these domains. Such deficits, however, are generally not likely to be evident on behavioral tests of these constructs.

Older adults' lifestyles are often blamed for their insomnia. This is generally unjustified and is the result of a variety of widely held but incorrect assumptions about how good and poor older sleepers differ. Variables that fail to distinguish between good sleepers and highly and minimally distressed poor sleepers include self-reported frequency of nocturnal awakenings, lifestyle practices, demographics, life events, and sleep expectations. For example, there are no differences between groups on usual bedtimes, arising times, naps, ease of falling asleep outside the bedroom, or the variability of nocturnal or daytime (e.g., mealtime) schedules. Nor do they differ in age; demographics such as education, income, and income adequacy (within middle-class populations); diversity of daytime activities; perceptions of how fully one's time is occupied during the day; and life stressors such as illness or death of friends or family members.

Assessment and Treatment

Factors to attend to during the clinical management of insomnia. It is evident from the foregoing that the insomnia complaint is multifaceted and that clinicians need to take the following aspects of the insomnia experience into consideration during evaluation, assessment, and treatment:

- ⇨ Nocturnal sleep-wake experiences (e.g., self-reports of total sleep times, sleep onset latency, waking after sleep onset, sleep efficiency, frequency of difficulty initiating or maintaining sleep, problem duration, time of last awakening in the morning)—self-reports may be obtained using daily sleep diary or retrospective questionnaire, depending on whether assessment is conducted once or whether it is ongoing throughout therapy.
- ⇨ Medically based sleep disorders that are common in older adults and are difficult to detect via interview (e.g., sleep apnea, RLS/PLMS) should be evaluated in a sleep laboratory.
- ⇨ Psychologically laden aspects of sleep and nocturnal wakefulness should be evaluated through paper-and-pencil measures (e.g., distress about sleep, sleep self-efficacy beliefs).
- ⇨ Aspects of daytime psychological adjustment should be evaluated using standardized measures of anxiety (e.g., Spielberger, Gorsuch, Lushene, Vagg, and Jacobs's [1983] State-Trait Anxiety Inventory), neuroticism (e.g., Eysenck and Eysenck's [1991] measure), and depression (e.g., Beck, Steer, and Brown's [1996] revised edition of the Beck Depression Inventory).

↺ Negative thinking and cognitive activity during nocturnal wake times should be assessed (e.g., Self-Statement Test: 60+, Tension Thermometer [cf. Fichten, Libman, et al., 1998a]); an EEG-based measure of cortical arousal may also be of interest.

↺ Subjective and behavioral aspects of daytime functioning should be evaluated (e.g., self-reports and behavioral measures of fatigue, sleepiness, difficulty concentrating).

↺ Sleep-related behaviors during periods of nocturnal wakefulness could shed light on behaviors and practices that promote or interfere with sleep (e.g., Sleep Behaviors Scale: 60+ [cf. Libman, Creti, Amsel, et al., 1997]).

Paying attention to these aspects is likely to yield more accurate identification of the problem and will permit more targeted therapeutic interventions. In addition, evaluation of these aspects allows the clinician to construct a profile of the older client with insomnia that will indicate the appropriate therapeutic avenue.

We must stress that it is entirely possible that the so-called "consequences" or "secondary symptoms" of insomnia (e.g., daytime fatigue, difficulty concentrating, depression, anxiety) are, in fact, its causes. If this turns out to be the case, then insomnia associated with chronic fatigue syndrome or with low levels of depression or anxiety, for example, may best be dealt with by addressing these problems directly, rather than by targeting sleep parameters.

References

Adam, K., Tomeny, M., & Oswald, I. (1986). Physiological and psychological differences between good and poor sleepers. *Journal of Psychiatric Research, 20*, 301-316.

Alapin, I. (1996). *Daytime functioning among older good and poor sleepers.* Unpublished undergraduate thesis, McGill University, Montréal, Québec, Canada.

Alapin, I., Fichten, C. S., Libman, E., Creti, L., Bailes, S., & Wright, J. (2000). *Sleepiness, fatigue, and concentration problems: Are these due to sleep loss?* Unpublished manuscript, Jewish General Hospital, Montréal, Québec, Canada.

American Psychiatric Association. (1994). *Diagnostic and Statistical Manual of Mental Disorders (DSM-IV).* Washington, DC: Author.

American Sleep Disorders Association. (1990). *The International Classification of Sleep Disorders: Diagnostic and coding manual.* Rochester, MN: Author.

Amsel, R., & Fichten, C. S. (1990). Ratios versus frequency scores: Focus of attention and the balance between positive and negative thoughts. *Cognitive Therapy and Research, 14*, 257-277.

Amsel, R., & Fichten, C. S. (1998). Recommendations for self-statement inventories: Use of valence, endpoints, frequency and relative frequency. *Cognitive Therapy and Research, 22*(3), 255-277.

Ancoli-Israel, S., & Coy, T. (1994). Are breathing disturbances in elderly equivalent to sleep apnea syndrome? *Sleep, 17*, 77-83.

Babkoff, H., Weller, A., & Lavidor, M. (1995). A comparison of prospective and retrospective assessments of sleep. *Journal of Clinical Epidemiology, 48*, 1-9.

Beck, A., Steer, R., & Brown, G. (1996). *BDI-II: Beck Depression Inventory manual—Second edition.* San Antonio, TX: The Psychological Corporation, Harcourt Brace & Company.

Bliwise, D. L., King, A. C., Harris, R. B., & Haskell, W. L. (1992). Prevalence of self reported poor sleep in a healthy population aged 50-65. *Social Science and Medicine, 34*, 49-55.

Bonnet, M. H., & Arand, D. L. (1996). The consequences of a week of insomnia. *Sleep, 19*, 453-461.

Bonnet, M. H., & Arand, D. L. (1998). The consequences of a week of insomnia II: Patients with insomnia. *Sleep, 21*, 359-370.

Bootzin, R. R., Bell, I. R., Habisch, R., Kuo, T., Wyatt, J. K., Roder, S. P., & Manber, R. (1995). Night-to-night variability in measures of sleep and sleep disorders: A six night PSG study. *Proceedings: 9th Annual Meeting of the APSS.* Rochester, MN: Association of the Professional Sleep Societies.

Bootzin, R. R., Epstein, D., & Wood, J. M. (1991). Stimulus control instructions. In P. J. Hauri (Ed.), *Case studies in insomnia* (pp. 19-28). New York: Plenum.

Borkovec, T. D. (1982). Insomnia. *Journal of Consulting and Clinical Psychology, 50*, 880-895.

Borkovec, T. D., Lane, T. W., & Van Oot, P. H. (1981). Phenomenology of sleep among insomniacs and good sleepers: Wakefulness experience when cortically asleep. *Journal of Abnormal Psychology, 90*, 607-609.

Carskadon, M. A., Dement, W. C., Mitler, M. M., Guilleminault, C., Zarcone, V. P., & Spiegal, R. (1976). Self report versus sleep laboratory findings in 122 drug-free subjects with complaints of chronic insomnia. *American Journal of Psychiatry, 133*, 1382-1388.

Chambers, M. J., & Keller, B. (1993). Alert insomniacs: Are they really sleep deprived? *Clinical Psychology Review, 13*, 649-666.

Chambers, M. J., & Kim, J. Y. (1993). The role of state-trait anxiety in insomnia and daytime restedness. *Behavioral Medicine, 19*(1), 42-46.

Chesson, A. L., Ferber, R. A., Fry, J. M., Grigg-Damberger, M., Hartse, K. M., Hurwitz, T. D., Johnson, S., Kader, G. A., Littner, M., Rosen, G., Sangal, R. B., Schmidt-Nowara, W., & Sher, A. (1997). The indications for polysomnography and related procedures. *Sleep, 29*, 423-487.

Coates, T. J., Killen, J. D., Silverman, S., George, J., Marchini, E., Hamilton, S., & Thoresen, C. E. (1983). Cognitive activity, sleep disturbance, and stage specific differences between recorded and reported sleep. *Psychophysiology, 20*, 243-250.

Coursey, R. D., Frankel, B. L., Gaardner, K. R., & Mott, D. E. (1980). A comparison of relaxation techniques with electro-sleep therapy for chronic, sleep-onset insomnia: A sleep-EEG study. *Biofeedback Self Regulation, 33*, 615-623.

Coyle, K., & Watts, F. N. (1991). The factorial structure of sleep dissatisfaction. *Behavior Research and Therapy, 29*, 513-520.

Creti, L. (1996). *An evaluation of a new cognitive-behavioral technique for the treatment of insomnia in older adults.* Unpublished doctoral thesis, Concordia University, Montréal, Québec, Canada.

Creti, L., Libman, E., & Fichten, C. S. (2000). *Cognitive behavioral treatment effects in late-life insomnia: Can these really be attributed to therapy?* Unpublished manuscript, Jewish General Hospital, Montréal, Québec, Canada.

Dement, W. C., Richardson, G., Prinz, P., Carskadon, M., Kripke, O., & Czeisler, C. (1985). Changes of sleep and wakefulness with age. In C. Finch & E. L. Schneider (Eds.), *Handbook of the biology of aging* (2nd ed., pp. 692-717). New York: Van Nostrand Reinhold.

Dorsey, C. M., & Bootzin, R. R. (1997). Subjective and psychophysiologic insomnia: An examination of sleep tendency and personality. *Biological Psychiatry, 41,* 209-216.

Edinger, J. D., Fins, A. I., Goeke, J. M., McMillan, D. K., Gersh, T. L., Krystal, A. D., & McCall, W. V. (1996). The empirical identification of insomnia subtypes: A cluster analytic approach. *Sleep, 19,* 398-411.

Edinger, J. D., Fins, A. I., Sullivan, R. J., Jr., Marsh, G. R., Dailey, D. S., Hope, T. V., Young, M., Shaw, E., Carlson, D., & Vasilas, D. (1997). Do our methods lead to insomniacs' madness?: Daytime testing after laboratory and home-based polysomnographic studies. *Sleep, 20,* 1127-1134.

Edinger, J. D., Hoelscher, T. J., Marsh, G. R., Lipper, S., & Ionescu-Pioggia, M. (1992). A cognitive-behavioral therapy for sleep-maintenance insomnia in older adults. *Psychology and Aging, 7,* 282-289.

Edinger, J. D., Hoelscher, T. J., Webb, M. D., Marsh, G. R., Radtke, R. A., & Erwin, C. W. (1989). Polysomnographic assessment of DIMS: Empirical evaluation of its diagnostic value. *Sleep, 12,* 315-322.

Edinger, J. D., Marsh, G. R., McCall, W. V., Erwin, C. W., & Lininger, A. W. (1991). Sleep variability across consecutive nights of home monitoring in older mixed DIMS patients. *Sleep, 14,* 13-17.

Eysenck, H. J., & Eysenck, S.B.G. (1991). *Eysenck Personality Scales.* London: Hodder & Stoughton.

Fichten, C. S., Creti, L., Amsel, R., Brender, W., Weinstein, N., & Libman, E. (1995). Poor sleepers who do not complain of insomnia: Myths and realities about psychological and lifestyle characteristics of older good and poor sleepers. *Journal of Behavioral Medicine, 18*(2), 189-223.

Fichten, C. S., Creti, L., Bailes, S., Weinstein, N., Gay, A., Lennox, H., Tagalakis, V., Amsel, R., Brender, W., & Libman, E. (1992, July). *Time estimation in the experience of insomnia/L'évaluation du temps dans l'expérience de l'insomnie.* Paper presented at the 25th International Congress of Psychology, Brussels.

Fichten, C. S., & Libman, E. (1991). L'insomnie et son traitment chez les personnes âgées: une nouvelles approche. [A new look at the complaint of insomnia and its treatment in older adults]. *Santé Mentale au Québec, 16*(1), 99-116.

Fichten, C. S., Libman, E., Amsel, R., Creti, L., Weinstein, N., Rothenberg, P., Liederman, G., & Brender, W. (1991). Evaluation of the sexual consequences of surgery: Retrospective and prospective strategies. *Journal of Behavioral Medicine, 14*(3), 267-285.

Fichten, C. S., Libman, E., Creti, L., Amsel, R., Sabourin, S., & Brender, W. (2000). *Role of thoughts during nocturnal awake times in the insomnia experience of older adults.* Unpublished manuscript, Jewish General Hospital, Montréal, Québec, Canada.

Fichten, C. S., Libman, E., Creti, L., Amsel, R., Tagalakis, V., & Brender, W. (1998a). Thoughts during awake times in older good and poor sleepers: The Self-Statement Test: 60+. *Cognitive Therapy and Research, 22*(1), 1-20.

Foley, D. J., Monjan, A. A., Brown, S. L., Simonsick, E. M., Wallace, R. B., & Blazer, D. G. (1995). Sleep complaints among elderly persons: An epidemiological study of three communities. *Sleep, 18,* 425-432.

Ford, D. E., & Kamerow, D. B. (1989). Epidemiologic study of sleep disturbances and psychiatric disorders: An opportunity for prevention. *JAMA: Journal of the American Medical Association, 262,* 1479-1484.

Frankel, B. L., Coursey, R. D., Buchbinder, R., & Snyder, F. (1976). Recorded and reported sleep in chronic primary insomnia. *Archives of General Psychiatry, 33,* 615-623.

Friedman, L., Brooks, J. O., III, Bliwise, D. L., Yesavage, J. A., & Wicks, D. S. (1995). Perceptions of life stress and chronic insomnia in older adults. *Psychology and Aging, 10,* 352-357.

Frisoni, G. B., De Leo, D., Rozzini, R., Bernardini, M., Della Buono, M., & Trabucchi, M. (1993). Night sleep symptoms in an elderly population and their relation with age, gender, and education. *Clinical Gerontologist, 13,* 51-68.

Fuller, K. H., Waters, W. F., Binks, P. G., & Anderson, T. (1995). The impact of trait anxiety and worry on sleep architecture. *Proceedings: 9th Annual Meeting of the APSS* (p. 236). Rochester, MN: Association of the Professional Sleep Societies.

Gislason, T., & Almqvist, M. (1987). Somatic diseases and sleep complaints: An epidemiological study of 3201 Swedish men. *Acta Medica Scandinavica, 221,* 475-481.

Gislason, T., Reynisdottir, H., Kristbjarnarson, H., & Benediktsdottir, B. (1993). Sleep habits and sleep disturbances among the elderly—An epidemiological survey. *Journal of Internal Medicine, 234,* 31-39.

Gourash-Bliwise, N. (1992). Factors related to sleep quality in healthy elderly women. *Psychology and Aging, 7,* 83-88.

Hammond, E. (1964). Some preliminary findings on physical complaints from a prospective study of 1,604,004 men and women. *American Journal of Public Health, 54,* 11-23.

Hart, R. P., Morin, C. M., & Best, A. M. (1995). Neuropsychological performance in elderly insomnia patients. *Aging and Cognition, 2*(4), 268-278.

Hauri, P. J. (1983). A cluster analysis of insomnia. *Sleep, 6,* 326-328.

Hauri, P. J. (1997). Cognitive deficits in insomnia patients. *Acta Neurologica Belgica, 97,* 113-117.

Hauri, P., & Fisher, J. (1986). Persistent psychophysiologic insomnia. *Sleep, 9,* 38-53.

Hauri, P., & Olmstead, E. (1989). Reverse first night effect in insomnia. *Sleep, 12,* 97-105.

Healey, E. S., Kales, A., Monroe, L. J., Bixler, E. O., Chamberlain, K., & Soldatos, C. R. (1981). Onset of insomnia: Role of life-stress events. *Psychosomatic Medicine, 43,* 439-451.

Henderson, S., Jorm, A. F., Scott, L. R., Mackinnon, A. J., Christensen, H., & Korten, A. E. (1995). Insomnia in the elderly: Its prevalence and correlates in the general population. *Medical Journal of Australia, 162,* 22-24.

Hicks, R. A., Marical, C. M., & Conti, P. A. (1991). Coping with a major stressor: Differences between habitual short- and longer-sleepers. *Perceptual and Motor Skills, 72,* 631-636.

Hicks, R. A., & Youmans, K. (1989). The sleep-promoting behaviors of habitual short- and longer-sleeping adults. *Perceptual and Motor Skills, 69,* 145-146.

Hoch, C. C., Dew, M. A., Reynolds, C. F., III, Monk, T. H., Buysse, D. J., Houck, P. R., Machen, M. A., & Kupfer, D. J. (1994). A longitudinal study of laboratory and diary-based sleep measures in healthy "old old" and "young old" volunteers. *Sleep, 17,* 489-496.

Hoch, C. C., Reynolds, C. F., III, Kupfer, D. J., Berman, S. R., Houck, P. R., & Stack, J. A. (1987). Empirical note: Self report versus recorded sleep in healthy seniors. *Psychophysiology, 24,* 293-299.

Hoelscher, T. J., & Edinger, J. D. (1988). Treatment of sleep-maintenance insomnia in older adults: Sleep period reduction, sleep education and modified stimulus control. *Psychology and Aging, 3,* 258-263.

Jacobs, E. A., Reynolds, C. F., Kupfer, D. J., Lovin, B. A., & Ehrenpreis, A. B. (1988). The role of polysomnography in the differential diagnosis of chronic insomnia. *American Journal of Psychiatry, 145,* 346-349.

Janson, C., Gislason, T., DeBacker, W., Plashke, P., Bjornsson, E., Hetta, J., Kristbjarnason, H., Vermaire, P., & Boman, G. (1995). Prevalence of sleep disturbances among young adults in 3 European countries. *Sleep, 18,* 589-597.

Johnson, L. C., Freeman, C. R., Spinweber, C. L., & Gomez, S. A. (1991). Subjective and objective measures of sleepiness: Effects of benzodiazepine and caffeine on their relationship. *Psychophysiology, 28*, 65-71.

Kales, A., Caldwell, A. B., Preston, T. A., Healy, S., & Kales, J. D. (1976). Personality patterns in insomnia. *Archives of General Psychiatry, 33*, 1128-1134.

Kales, J. D. (1975). Aging and sleep. In R. Goldman & M. Rockstein (Eds.), *Symposium on the physiology and pathology of aging*. New York: Academic Press.

Kales, J. D., Kales, A., Bixler, E. O., Soldatos, C. R., Cadieux, R. J., Kashurba, G. J., & Vela-Bueno, A. (1984). Biopsychobehavioral correlates of insomnia V: Clinical characteristics and behavioral correlates. *American Journal of Psychiatry, 141*, 1371-1376.

Knab, B., & Engle, R. R. (1988). Perception of waking and sleeping: Possible implications for the evaluation of insomnia. *Sleep, 11*, 265-272.

Kripke, D. F., Simons, R. N., Garfinkel, L., & Hammond, C. (1979). Short and long sleep and sleeping pills: Is increased mortality associated? *Archives of General Psychiatry, 36*, 103-116.

Kronholm, E., & Hyyppa, M. T. (1985). Age-related sleep habits and retirement. *Annals of Clinical Research, 17*, 257-264.

Kryger, M. H., Siteljes, D., Pouliot, Z., Neufeld, H., & Odgnoki, T. (1991). Subjective versus objective evaluation of hypnotic efficacy: Experience with zolpidem. *Sleep, 14*, 399-407.

Kuisk, L. A., Bertelson, A. D., & Walsh, J. K. (1989). Presleep cognitive hyperarousal and affect as factors in objective and subjective insomnia. *Perceptual and Motor Skills, 68*, 1219-1225.

Lacks, P. (1987). *Behavioral treatment for persistent insomnia*. New York: Pergamon.

Lamarche, C. H., & Ogilvie, R. D. (1997). Electrophysiological changes during the sleep onset period of psychophysiological insomniacs, psychiatric insomniacs, and normal sleepers. *Sleep, 20*, 724-733.

Lavidor, M., Libman, E., Babkoff, H., Creti, L., Weller, A., Amsel, R., Brender, W., & Fichten, C. S. (1996, November). *Psychologically laden sleep parameters in aging*. Paper presented at the meeting of the Association for Advancement of Behavior Therapy, New York.

Libman, E., Fichten, C. S., Creti, L., Amsel, R., Bailes, S., Wright, J., Alapin, I., Brender, W., Baltzan, M., & Spector, I. (1999, November). *How should one measure sleep parameters: Retrospective questionnaire vs. ongoing self-monitoring (daily sleep diary)?* Presentation at the annual convention of the Association for advancement of Behavior Therapy (AABT), Toronto, Ontario.

Libman, E., Creti, L., Amsel, R., Brender, W., & Fichten, C. S. (1997). What do older good and poor sleepers do during periods of nocturnal wakefulness? The Sleep Behaviors Scale: 60+. *Psychology and Aging, 12*(1), 170-182.

Libman, E., Creti, L., Levy, R. D., Brender, W., & Fichten, C. S. (1997). A comparison of reported and recorded sleep in older poor sleepers. *Journal of Clinical Geropsychology, 3*(3), 199-211.

Libman, E., Fichten, C. S., Weinstein, N., Tagalakis, V., Amsel, R., Brender, W., & Creti, L. (1998). Improvement and deterioration in sleep status of "younger" and "older" seniors: A longitudinal study. *Journal of Mental Health and Aging, 4*(1), 183-192.

Lichstein, K. L., & Fanning, J. (1990). Cognitive anxiety in insomnia: An analogue test. *Stress Medicine, 6*, 47-51.

Lichstein, K. L., & Fischer, S. M. (1985). Insomnia. In M. Hersen & A. S. Bellack (Eds.), *Handbook of clinical behavior therapy with adults* (pp. 319-352). New York: Plenum.

Lichstein, K. L., & Johnson, R. S. (1991). Older adults' objective self recording of sleep in the home. *Behavior Therapy, 22*, 531-548.

Lichstein, K. L., & Rosenthal, T. L. (1980). Insomniacs' perceptions of cognitive vs. somatic determinants of sleep disturbance. *Journal of Abnormal Psychology, 89*, 105-107.

Lichstein, K. L., Wilson, N. M., Noe, S. L., Aguillard, R. N., & Bellur, S. N. (1994). Daytime sleepiness in insomnia: Behavioral, biological and subjective indices. *Sleep, 17*, 693-702.

Lundh, L. G., Lunqvist, K., Broman, J. E., & Hetta, J. (1991). Vicious cycles of sleeplessness, sleep phobia, and sleep-compatible behaviors in patients with persistent insomnia. *Scandinavian Journal of Behavior Therapy, 20*, 101-114.

Mahoney, M. J. (1977). Some applied issues in self monitoring. In J. D. Cone & R. P. Hawkins (Eds.), *Behavioral assessment: New directions in clinical psychology* (pp. 241-254). New York: Brunner/Mazel.

Marchini, E. J., Coates, T. J., Magistad, J. G., & Waldum, S. J. (1983). What do insomniacs do, think and feel during the day? A preliminary study. *Sleep, 6*, 147-155.

Mathews, A., & Milroy, R. (1994). Effects of priming and suppression of worry. *Behaviour Research & Therapy, 32*, 843-850.

McCall, W. V., & Edinger, J. D. (1991). Need for polysomnographic studies in research on initiating and maintaining sleep [Letter to the editor]. *American Journal of Psychiatry, 148*, 957-958.

McGhie, A., & Russell, S. M. (1962). The subjective assessment of normal sleep patterns. *The Journal of Mental Science, 108*, 642-654.

Mellinger, G. D., Balter, M. B., & Uhlenhuth, E. H. (1985). Insomnia and its treatment: Prevalence and correlates. *Archives of General Psychiatry, 42*, 225-232.

Mendelson, W. B. (1995). Long-term follow-up of chronic insomnia. *Sleep, 18*, 698-701.

Mendelson, W. B., Garnett, D., Gillin, J. C., & Weingartner, H. (1984). The experience of insomnia and daytime and nighttime functioning. *Psychiatry Research, 12*, 235-250.

Miles, L. E., & Dement, W. C. (1980). Sleep and aging. *Sleep, 3*, 119-230.

Monjan, A. A., & Foley, D. J. (1995). Longitudinal study of chronic insomnia in older people. *Proceedings: 9th Annual Meeting of the APSS*. Rochester, MN: Association of the Professional Sleep Societies.

Monk, T. H., Reynolds, C. F., Machen, M. A., & Kupfer, D. J. (1992). Daily social rhythms in the elderly and their relation to objectively recorded sleep. *Sleep, 15*, 322-329.

Morgan, K., & Clarke, D. (1997). Risk factors for late-life insomnia in a representative general practice sample. *British Journal of General Practice, 47*, 166-169.

Morgan, K., Dallosso, H., Ebrahim, S., Arie, T., & Fentem, P. H. (1988). Characteristics of subjective insomnia in the elderly living at home. *Age and Ageing, 17*, 1-7.

Morgan, K., Healey, D. W., & Healey, P. J. (1989). Factors influencing persistent subjective insomnia in old age: A follow-up study of good and poor sleepers age 65-74. *Age and Ageing, 18*, 117-122.

Morin, C. M. (1993). *Insomnia: Psychological assessment and management*. New York: Guilford.

Morin, C. M., Colecchi, C., Stone, J., Brink, D., & Sood, R. (1994). Cognitive-behavior therapy for insomnia. *Convention Proceedings for the 28th Annual AABT*, 65.

Morin, C. M., & Gramling, S. E. (1989). Sleep patterns and aging: Comparison of older adults with and without insomnia complaints. *Psychology and Aging, 4*, 290-294.

Morin, C. M., Kowatch, R. A., Barry, T., & Walton, E. (1993). Cognitive-behavior therapy for late-life insomnia. *Journal of Consulting and Clinical Psychology, 61*, 137-146.

Nau, S. D. (1997). The measurement of daytime sleepiness. In M. R. Pressman & W. C. Orr (Eds.), *Understanding sleep—The evaluation and treatment of sleep disorders* (pp. 209-225). Washington, DC: American Psychological Association.

Nelson, R. O. (1977). Methodological issues in assessment via self-monitoring. In J. D. Cone & R. P. Hawkins (Eds.), *Behavioral assessment*. New York: Brunner/Mazel.

Nicassio, P. M., Mendlowitz, D. R., Fussell, J. J., & Petras, L. (1985). The phenomenology of the presleep state: The development of the presleep arousal scale. *Behavior Research and Therapy, 23*, 263-271.

Ohayon, M. M., Caulet, M., & Guilleminault, C. (1997). How a general population perceives its sleep and how this relates to the complaint of insomnia. *Sleep, 20*, 715-723.

. Perlis, M. L., Giles, D. E., Mendelson, W. B., Bootzin, R. R., & Wyatt, J. K. (1997). Psychophysiological insomnia: The behavioral model and a neurocognitive perspective. *Journal of Sleep Research, 6*, 179-188.

Prinz, P. N., Vitiello, M. V., Raskind, M. R., & Thorpy, M. J. (1990). Geriatrics: Sleep disorders and aging. *New England Journal of Medicine, 323*, 520-526.

Randazzo, A. C., & Schweitzer, P. K. (1995). First night effect in elderly insomniacs. *Proceedings: 9th Annual Meeting of the APSS*. Rochester, MN: Association of the Professional Sleep Societies.

Reite, M., Buysse, D., Reynolds, C., & Mendelson, W. (1995). The use of polysomnography in the evaluation of insomnia. *Sleep, 18*, 58-70.

Reynolds, C. F., III, Coble, P. A., Black, R. S., Holzer, B., Carral, R., & Kupfer, D. J. (1980). Sleep disturbances in a series of elderly patients: Polysomnographic findings. *Journal of the American Geriatrics Society, 28*, 164-170.

Reynolds, C. F., III, Kupfer, D. J., Burpse, D. J., Cable, P. A., & Yeager, A. (1991). Subtyping DSM-III-R primary insomnia: A literature review by the DSM-IV work group on sleep disorders. *American Journal of Psychiatry, 148*, 432-438.

Rutter, S., & Waring-Paynter, K. (1992). Prebedtime activity and sleep satisfaction of short and long sleepers. *Perceptual and Motor Skills, 75*, 122.

Salin-Pascual, R. J., Roehrs, T. A., Merlotti, L. A., Zorick, F., & Roth, T. (1992). Long-term study of insomnia patients with sleep state misperception and other insomnia patients. *American Journal of Psychiatry, 149*, 904-908.

Schmitt, F. A., Phillips, B. A., Cook, Y. R., Berry, D.T.R., & Wekstein, D. R. (1996). Self report of sleep symptoms in older adults: Correlates of daytime sleepiness and health. *Sleep, 19*, 59-64.

Schramm, E., Hohagen, F., Kappler, C., Grasshoff, U., & Berger, M. (1995). Mental comorbidity of chronic insomnia in general attenders using DSM-III-R. *Acta Psychiatrica Scandinavica, 91*, 10-17.

Schwartz, R. M., & Garamoni, G. L. (1986). A structural model of positive and negative states of mind: Asymmetry in the internal dialogue. In P. C. Kendall (Ed.), *Advances in cognitive-behavioral research and therapy* (Vol. 5, pp. 1-62). New York: Academic Press.

Seidel, W. F., Ball, S., Cohen, S., Patterson, N., Yost, D., & Dement, W. C. (1984). Daytime alertness in relation to mood, performance, and nocturnal sleep in chronic insomniacs and noncomplaining sleepers. *Sleep, 7*, 230-238.

Spielberger, C. D., Gorsuch, R. L., Lushene, R., Vagg, P. R., & Jacobs, G. A. (1983). *Manual for the State-Trait Anxiety Inventory (Form Y)*. Palo Alto, CA: Consulting Psychologists Press.

Standards of Practice Committee of the American Sleep Disorders Association. (1995). Practice parameters for the use of polysomnography in the evaluation of insomnia. *Sleep, 18*, 55-57.

Stepanski, E., Koshorek, G., Zorick, F., Glinn, M., Roehrs, T., & Roth, T. (1989). Characteristics of individuals who do or do not seek treatment for chronic insomnia. *Psychosomatics, 30*, 421-424.

Stepanski, E., Zorick, F., Sicklesteel, J., Young, D., & Roth, T. (1986). Daytime alertness-sleepiness in patients with chronic insomnia. *Sleep Research, 15*, 174.

Stone, J., Morin, C. M., Hart, R. P., Remsberg, S., & Mercer, J. (1994). Neuropsychological functioning in older insomniacs with or without obstructive sleep apnea. *Psychology and Aging, 9*, 213-236.

Tait, H. (1992). Sleep problems: Whom do they affect? *Canadian Social Trends, 4*, 8-10.

Trinder, J. (1988). Subjective insomnia without objective findings: A pseudo diagnostic classification. *Psychological Bulletin, 103*, 87-94.

Van Egeren, L., Haynes, S. N., Franzen, M., & Hamilton, J. (1983). Presleep cognitions and attributions in sleep-onset insomnia. *Journal of Behavioral Medicine, 6*, 217-232.

Vgontzas, A. N., Kales, A., Bixler, E. O., Manfredi, R. L., & Vela-Bueno, A. (1995). Usefulness of polysomnographic studies in the differential diagnosis of insomnia. *International Journal of Neuroscience, 82*, 47-60.

Waters, W. F., Adams, S. G., Jr., Binks, P., & Varnado, P. (1993). Attention, stress and negative emotion in persistent sleep onset and sleep maintenance insomnia. *Sleep, 16*, 128-136.

Weyerer, S., & Dilling, H. (1991). Prevalence and treatment of insomnia in the community: Results from the Upper Bavarian Field Study. *Sleep, 14*, 392-398.

Williams, R. L., Karacan, I., & Hursch, C. J. (1974). *Electroencephalography (EEG) of human sleep: Clinical applications.* New York: John Wiley & Sons.

World Health Organization. (1992). *International classification of diseases (ICD-10).* Geneva: Author.

Wyatt, J. K., Bootzin, R. R., Anthony, J., & Bazant, S. (1994). Sleep onset is associated with retrograde and anterograde amnesia. *Sleep, 17*, 502-511.

Zammit, G. K. (1988). Subjective ratings of the characteristics and sequelae of good and poor sleep in normals. *Journal of Clinical Psychology, 44*, 123-130.

Assessment and
Differential Diagnosis

COLIN A. ESPIE

The aim of this chapter is to provide an overview of assessment practice in working with people with insomnia (PWI). Particular emphasis is placed upon the sleep patterns and complaints of older adults with insomnia (OAWI). Self-report, behavioral, and physiological approaches to sleep assessment are described and their advantages and disadvantages discussed. Issues of differential diagnosis in working with OAWI are introduced, and the reader is guided to apply procedures appropriate to address clinical hypotheses. Although the text is designed to be practical, the literature is referenced in some detail to help the reader pursue issues of interest.

The Assessment of Insomnia

The Sleep History

The fundamental importance of "taking a history" is widely recognized in the clinical approach to any disorder; however, there is evidence that actual practice varies widely (Platt, 1991). For example, in an inter-

TABLE 3.1 Outline Plan for a Sleep History Assessment Comprising Content Areas and Suggested Interview Questions

Content Area	Prompt Question	Supplementary Questions
Presentation of the sleep complaint		
Pattern	Can you describe the pattern of your sleep on a typical night?	Time to fall asleep? Number and duration of wakenings? Time spent asleep? Nights per week like this?
Quality	How do you feel about the quality of your sleep?	Refreshing? Enjoyable? Restless?
Daytime effects	How does your night's sleep affect your day?	Tired? Sleepy? Poor concentration? Irritable? Particular times of day?
Development of the sleep complaint	Do you remember how this spell of poor sleep started?	Events and circumstances? Dates and times? Variation since then? Exacerbating factors? Alleviating factors? Degree of impact/intrusiveness?
Lifetime history of sleep complaints	Did you used to be a good sleeper?	Sleep in childhood? Sleep in adulthood? Nature of past episodes? Dates and times? Resolution of past episodes?
General health status and medical history	Have you generally kept in good health?	Illnesses? Chronic problems? Dates and times? Recent changes in health?
Psychopathology and history of psychological functioning	Are you the kind of person who usually copes well?	Psychological problems? Anxiety or depression? Dates and times? Resourceful person? Personality type?

view-based study of a stratified, random sample of 501 general physicians, only 47% elicited any sleep history when presented with a case vignette of an OAWI (Everitt, Avorn, & Baker, 1990). Furthermore, of those who did, more than half asked less than three questions. It is interesting that there was a clear association between history taking and the likeli-

TABLE 3.1 Continued		
Content Area	*Prompt Question*	*Supplementary Questions*
Issues of differential diagnosis		
Sleep-related breathing disorder (SBD)	Are you a heavy snorer?	Interrupted breathing in sleep? Excessively sleepy in the day?
Periodic limb movements in sleep (PLMS) and restless legs syndrome (RLS)	Do your legs sometimes twitch or can't keep still?	Excessively sleepy in the day?
Circadian rhythm sleep disorders	Do you feel you want to sleep at the wrong time?	Too early? Too late?
Parasomnias	Do you sometimes act a bit strangely during your sleep?	Behavioral description? Time during night?
Narcolepsy	Do you sometimes just fall asleep without warning?	Times and places? Triggered by emotion? Poor sleep at night?
Current and previous treatments	Are you taking anything to help you sleep?	Now? In the past? Dates and times? What has worked? What have you tried yourself?

hood of lifestyle change (rather than pharmacotherapy) being regarded as the treatment of choice. Clearly, the sleep history should not be overlooked. It usually takes the form of a structured interview, often the first consultation, and enables the clinician to obtain an overview of the sleep difficulty. A number of clinical schedules have been published that are products of the experience of different centers.

A suggested format for a sleep history interview is presented in Table 3.1. This semistructured approach enables the interviewer to use general, prompt questions to focus on issues of interest, followed by more specific supplementary inquiry where required. Interviewing a spouse/partner is often helpful, especially in relation to differential diagnosis.

Measures such as the Pittsburgh Sleep Quality Index (Buysse, Reynolds, Monk, Berman, & Kupfer, 1989) and the Sleep Disorders Questionnaire (Douglass et al., 1994) are self-rated instruments that may be completed by PWI prior to attending the clinic and provide a starting point for clinical interview. The Pittsburgh Sleep Quality Index gathers descriptive data on typical sleep during the past month along with information of value in differential diagnosis. Although the derived index score of sleep quality, based on both quantitative and qualitative ratings (e.g., "depth" and "restfulness" of sleep) may be of limited validity, field development studies did comprise some samples of OAWI, and the scale is readily completed within 10 minutes. The Sleep Disorders Questionnaire also has good psychometric properties and comprises four diagnostic subscales, confirmed by discriminant function analysis, for sleep apnea, periodic limb movements in sleep (PLMS), psychiatric sleep disorders, and narcolepsy. It comprises 45 items and requires 15-20 minutes completion time. It is not in itself a diagnostic tool, but the authors suggest it may serve a confirmatory function. Specific studies on OAWI are required.

It is only during a clinical interview that the true nature, developmental course, and impact of the sleep disorder become evident. Here, factual and attributional information can be appraised. It is critically important to maintain a structure to the collection and collation of information because OAWI often have complex medical and psychiatric histories requiring careful plotting against the history of the sleep problem (see below). Current and previous interventions, including self-help strategies, should be discussed. Because the majority of assessment is conducted with a view to treatment, knowledge of what has been tried, for how long, and to what effect will be important and may affect expectations of future therapy (Morin, Gaulier, Barry, & Kowatch, 1992).

Morgan (in press) has noted the increasing use of diagnostic classification both in epidemiologic studies and in the clinical assessment of sleep disorders. The latter is particularly important in relation to later life because there are age-related changes in continuity and depth of sleep and in circadian rhythms. In terms of the former, a number of sleep disorders have significantly higher prevalence rates in late life (Ford & Kamerow, 1989; Ohayon, 1996). The differential diagnosis of insomnia will be discussed later; however, attention is drawn at this point to several clinical interview schedules that are particularly helpful in this regard.

Spielman and Anderson (1999) have developed an interview that provides an excellent structure and enables the interviewer to rate symptomatology in relation to International Classification of Sleep Disorders (*ICSD*) categories. The format of the interview leads to orderly consideration of psychological, social, and physiological determinants of sleep disturbance. Schramm et al. (1993) have reported reliability data for the Structured Interview for Sleep Disorders according to *DSM-III-R* from a sample of people aged 24 to 77 years (mean of 50.7). They suggested that the good concordance (90%) between interview diagnoses and polysomnographic data indicates that the interview might be useful as a screening instrument, especially given the average completion time of less than 30 minutes.

Lacks (1987) and Morin (1993) also have developed interview schedules. These have been widely used in psychological studies with adults and OAWI. Lacks (1987, pp. 63-69) describes a Sleep History Questionnaire that can be used as a basis for her detailed Structured Sleep History Interview, and Morin (1993, pp. 195-198) has published the format for his Insomnia Interview Schedule. The latter is particularly useful in the functional analysis of sleep behaviors but also incorporates clinical diagnostic questions. Sleep-related cognitions can be assessed on the Dysfunctional Beliefs and Attitudes About Sleep Scale, and the brief Sleep Impairment Index specifically asks the OAWI to rate the extent to which natural aging contributes to his or her sleep problem (Morin, 1993, pp. 201-204 and 199, respectively).

The Sleep Diary

The sleep diary is invaluable in the appraisal of sleep disturbance and the evaluation of treatment outcome. Whereas the sleep history provides an essential retrospective overview, the sleep diary yields night-by-night information on perceptions of sleep pattern and quality that may be obtained over many weeks. Thus, the sleep diary has become the "staple" of sleep assessment and has stood the test of time. Sleep diaries have been used since the early behavioral treatment studies (see review by Bootzin and Nicassio, 1978), and a number of commentaries on their advantages and disadvantages are available (Bootzin & Engle-Friedman, 1981; Espie, 1991; Lichstein & Riedel, 1994; Morin, 1993). The most important factors governing their use are summarized in

Table 3.2 Characteristics of the Sleep Diary

Features of Sleep Diaries	Comment
Practical usefulness	Sleep diaries are nonintrusive, inexpensive, adaptable to presenting need, and acceptable to OAWI to use. They are relatively simple to train and are completed at home.
Clinical relevance	Sleep diaries permit prolonged measurement over weeks or months. This is helpful diagnostically to establish baselines and to assess change over time and at follow-up. They are relevant to all sleep disorders.
Validity and reliability	Sleep diaries enable quantification of the presenting sleep complaint, and qualitative information and measures of daytime effects can be incorporated. When compared with PSG data, diaries provide a reasonably reliable, relative index of sleep pattern.
Treatment relevance	Sleep diaries are essentially collaborative. The OAWI is engaged actively in the assessment process, and data are shared with the therapist. This is particularly useful in cognitive-behavioral treatment. They can be used to appraise treatment benefit.

Table 3.2. OAWI do not necessarily have problems in completing diaries. Indeed, major intervention trials involving OAWI from a number of centers have used sleep diaries as a principal outcome measure (Davies, Lacks, Storandt, & Bertelson, 1986; Edinger, Hoelscher, Marsh, Lipper, & Ionescu-Pioggia, 1992; Engle-Friedman, Bootzin, Hazlewood, & Tsao, 1992; Friedman, Bliwise, Yesavage, & Salom, 1991; Morin, Kowatch, Barry, & Walton, 1993). Furthermore, diaries are widely recommended for use in general medical practice with PWI of all ages (e.g., Espie, 1993; Pearse, 1993).

Examples of two sleep diary formats are presented in Figures 3.1 and 3.2. Information on sleep parameters such as time to bed, sleep onset latency (SOL), frequency and total duration of wakenings (wake time after sleep onset; WASO), total sleep time (TST), and waking and rising time is complemented by ratings of sleep quality. The latter can be adapted to the terminology used by the OAWI. The diary in Figure 3.2 is in pictorial format. This can be useful for diagnostic assessment. The example given is of a Delayed Sleep Phase Disorder (from Spielman & Anderson, 1999). Sleep diaries should be completed for a minimum of 2 weeks for the purposes

(text continued on page 89)

ID No. _____

Name _____

Week beginning _____

Measuring the pattern of your sleep

	Day 1	Day 2	Day 3	Day 4	Day 5	Day 6	Day 7
1. At what time did you rise from bed this morning?							
2. At what time did you go to bed last night?							
3. How long did it take you to fall asleep (minutes)?							
4. How many times did you wake up *during* the night?							
5. How long were you awake during the night (in total)?							
6. About how long did you sleep altogether (hours/mins)?							
7. How much alcohol did you take last night?							
8. How many sleeping pills did you take to help you to sleep?							

Measuring the quality of your sleep

1. How well do you feel this morning? 0 1 2 3 4 not at all moderately very							
2. How enjoyable was your sleep last night? 0 1 2 3 4 not at all moderately very							

For office use only

SOL (mins)	WAKE	WASO (mins)	TST (hrs)

Figure 3.1. Example of a "Standard" Sleep Diary Incorporating Information on Sleep Pattern and Sleep Quality

NOTE: Numerical information is entered for each measure based upon the preceding night's sleep. Qualitative ratings can be personalized to suit the individual's own terminology regarding sleep.

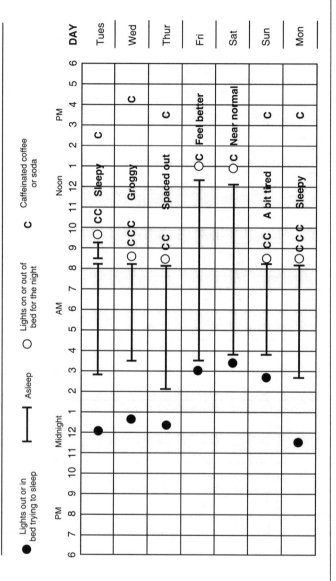

Figure 3.2. Example of a Pictorial Sleep Diary

SOURCE: From "The Clinical Interview and Treatment Planning as a Guide to Understanding the Nature of Insomnia: The CCNY Interview for Insomnia" (p. 389), Spielman and Anderson. cprcopyright 1999 by Butterworth-Heinemann. Reprinted with permission. NOTE: Information is entered on the horizontal axis for each night's sleep. The case presented is indicative of Delayed Phase Disorder, illustrating one advantage of this format of sleep diary.

88

of baseline assessment. Furthermore, training is required to familiarize the OAWI with reporting criteria and to encourage accuracy while avoiding "clock watching" (Espie, 1991; pp. 75-77). Anxiety in using sleep diaries is usually transient, and most people find them easy to use and nonintrusive.

The validity of subjective self-report has often been challenged, and a number of studies were conducted in the 1970s and 1980s comparing diary measures with EEG-defined sleep as the standard criterion (Borkovec, Grayson, O'Brien, & Weerts, 1979; Borkovec, Lane, & Van Oot, 1981; Carskadon et al., 1976; Coates et al., 1982; Frankel, Coursey, Buchbinder, & Snyder, 1976; Hauri & Olmstead, 1983; Ogilvie & Wilkinson, 1988; Schneider-Helmert, 1987). These were mainly conducted on younger adults, and it should be borne in mind that OAWI experience greater wakefulness during sleep. Nevertheless, the results of these studies can be summarized by saying that sleep diaries provide a relatively reliable index, particularly for sleep latency, total sleep time, and sleep efficiency (proportion of time in bed spent asleep). Although PWI generally overreport sleep disturbance, they tend to do so consistently (Espie, Lindsay, & Espie, 1989). There is also recent evidence that sleep time misperception forms a continuum and that generalized assumptions concerning misperceptions should be avoided, at least until diagnosis is clearly established. Edinger and Fins (1995) found that *overestimates* of sleep time were in fact quite common in PWI. Illustrating this, they pointed out that the subjective experience of repeated, brief arousals suffered, for example with PLMS, may be markedly different from prolonged wakefulness in the night as in psychophysiological insomnia. Interestingly, both of these disorders are common in OAWI. Such results strongly support the need for both quantitative and qualitative estimation in sleep diary assessment, supported by objective evaluation where appropriate. As previously mentioned, the OAWI's subjective experience may be captured on the diary by using the person's own semantics (e.g., "tossing and turning") as a construct to be rated (see also Espie, 1991, pp. 80-84 and 88-90).

Informant Report

Interviewing an observer of the OAWI's sleep can be useful for two reasons: first, to corroborate data from self-report, and second, to provide additional information that may assist diagnosis. In terms of the former, the partner may be able to confirm the frequency, severity, and intrusiveness of the sleep disorder. Partners, however, seldom will be able to provide accurate information on nighttime sleep. In a recent study of the sleep of adults with severe mental retardation, we found that carers significantly *over*estimated time slept compared with sleep EEG data (Espie et al., 1999). Other observers, such as nursing staff, have been used in hospital-based studies of poor sleepers. It has long been known, however, that observation in itself may be intrusive and precipitate sleep stage changes (Kupfer, Snyder, & Wyatt, 1970).

With respect to clinical diagnosis, partner report can be crucial; for example, in sleep-related breathing disorder (SBD) where snoring, apneic episodes, and abrupt restoration of normal breathing may have been witnessed. In OAWI, the partner should always be interviewed because of the raised incidence of (often unidentified) obstructive sleep apnea and PLMS (Ancoli-Israel et al., 1991; Enright et al., 1996; Lichstein, Riedel, Lester, & Aguillard, 1999). Partners may also provide important information on daytime functioning such as fatigue, sleepiness, and mood, and on changes in symptoms over time. Such information is complementary to their reports of sleep and again can greatly assist in diagnosis.

Polysomnography

Polysomnography provides information on the sleeping/waking brain and is the most objective means of diagnostic sleep assessment. Full polysomnographic (PSG) assessment comprises electroencephalography (EEG), electro-oculography (EOG), chin and anterior tibialis electromyography (EMG), respiratory effort, airflow, oximetry, and electrocardiography (ECG). Most assessments are laboratory based, and the first night of recording is usually discarded as comprising artifacts resulting from the novelty of the procedure and the environment. Thus, the principles of stimulus control, incorporating the interaction of brain, behavior, and environment, are recognized in practice. Because people may sleep differently in a laboratory environment and may have different attributions about their sleep, home polysomnography has been developed to provide a naturalistic alternative. The first portable PSG recordings were described by Wilkinson and Mullaney (1976). The home-based assessment of OAWI has particular advantages now that early technical problems (Ancoli-Israel, Kripke, Mason, & Messin, 1981) have largely been overcome. In insomnia research, it seems particularly important that the person sleeps in his or her own bed. Furthermore, 24-hour recording has a considerable advantage in assessing daytime sleep propensity (DeGroen, Koper, & Bergs, 1985; see McCall, Marsh, & Erwin, 1995, for review).

PSG is critical both to diagnosis in complex cases and to monitoring the effects of interventions, such as nasal continuous airways pressure (CPAP), where levels of oxygen saturation/desaturation, occurrences of apneas, and frequent arousals from sleep have to be objectively assessed before and during treatment. The complementary diagnoses of subjective and psychophysiological insomnia were first introduced to the classification system in recognition of the finding that only some PWI have reports of sleep disturbance that are objectively verifiable (Borkovec, 1979). This cannot, however, be taken to mean that people with subjective insomnia necessarily have a lesser problem. Indeed, a more extreme version of subjective insomnia has now been termed Sleep State Misperception, in which a complaint of insomnia or excessive sleepiness occurs in the absence of PSG evidence of sleep disturbance (American Sleep Disorders Association [ASDA], 1990, 1997).

American Sleep Disorders Association reviews on the use of polysomnography concur in recommending PSG assessment where there are clinical grounds to suspect SBD, PLMS, persistent circadian disorders (all conditions being likely to cause insomnia in middle to late life), precipitous arousals, or violent behavior in sleep, and in other circumstances where the diagnosis remains uncertain. Routine PSG assessment, however, is not indicated for chronic insomnia (ASDA, 1995a, 1995b; Reite, Buysse, Reynolds, & Mendelson, 1995). Clinical experience indicates that PSG will not always detect SBD and that simple assessments such as oximetry alone (monitoring of oxygen desaturation during sleep) may correctly identify a high proportion of SBD cases (Douglas, Thomas, & Jan, 1992). This latter result is interesting because oximeters may be used in conjunction with actigraphy for home-based assessment without recourse to expensive and complex technology.

Actigraphy and Other Behavioral Devices

Body movement can be used to distinguish wakefulness from sleep, and conversely, the relative absence of movement is a reasonable correlate of sleep. Actigraphy was first introduced to sleep assessment around 20 years ago (Kripke, Mullaney, Messin, & Wyborney, 1978; Mullaney, Kripke, & Messin, 1980), and contemporary devices are robust yet lightweight and provide an inexpensive, objective measure of movement over recording periods of up to 2 weeks (Hauri & Wisbey, 1992; Sadeh, Hauri, Kripke, & Lavie, 1995). The actigraph is usually attached to the nondominant wrist and worn like a wristwatch. Interface units enable the downloading of data to PC-based software for graphing and sleep analysis. Actigraphs are also used to study rest-activity patterns in older adults and in institutionalized and dementing populations where the circadian rhythm may have deteriorated (Ancoli-Israel, Clopton, Klauber, Fell, & Mason, 1997; Ancoli-Israel, Klauber, et al., 1997). Continuous monitoring across 24-hour periods permits the analysis of daytime naps. The practicability of actigraphy compared with PSG assessment is one of its greatest attractions.

An example of an actigraph trace from an OAWI is reproduced in Figure 3.3. This 68-year-old woman reported being a "light sleeper" and having intermittent arousals and unrestful, poor quality sleep. She did not experience problems in getting to sleep. Her sleep diary gave her bedtime as 11:45 p.m. and her rising time as 5:55 a.m. These parameters were used to set the "window" for sleep analysis from the actigraph data. Inspection of the trace reveals several wakenings from sleep, seven of which she identified by depressing an event marker button on the actigraph. She had relatively short sleep (4 hours, 52 mins.) and scored 73% sleep efficiency. This example illustrates the usefulness of the actigraph in confirming self-report information. Clearly, not all movement is wakefulness, and not all absence of activity is sleep. Nevertheless, comparative studies of wrist actigraphy and PSG assessment have reported greater than 90% agreement for nocturnal sleep periods (Sadeh, Sharkey, & Carskadon, 1994). The validity of actigraphic measurement has been evidenced by highly significant correlation (generally > .80) with PSG based on whole-night sleep measures, such as sleep efficiency, sleep duration, and sleep latency (Sadeh et al., 1995). Unlike PSG assessment, however, there is little evidence of first-night effects, even in OAWI (Van Hilten et al., 1993). Actigraphic evaluation is particularly useful for longitudinal study of sleep schedule disorders, but less so for SBD. Actigraphy has also been used to study age- and gender-related sleep patterns (Reyner & Horne, 1995). This study involved longitudinal wrist actigraphy in 400 adults. The most marked sleep

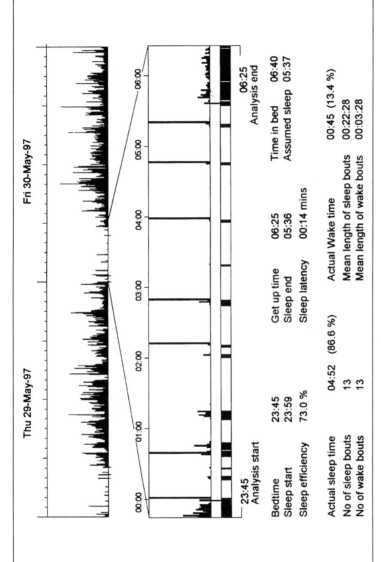

Figure 3.3. Twenty-Four-Hour Wrist-Actigraphic Trace and Sleep Summary Data From a 68-Year-Old Woman With Intermittent Wakenings

NOTE: Tall vertical lines represent perceived wakenings, entered by the subject by depressing an event marker button on the actigraph. Actiwatch® Cambridge Neurotechnology Ltd.

problems were in older women, who took longer to fall asleep than any other group. Both men and women woke earlier with increasing age. Actigraphy may also provide an index of sleep quality; it has been shown that movement during sleep is strongly related to sleep diary ratings of sleep quality (Horne, Pankhurst, Reyner, Hume, & Diamond, 1994).

Other behavioral responses can provide objective measurement of sleep patterns. Indeed, Blood, Sack, Percy, and Pen (1997) found that behavioral response monitoring (button-pressing contingent upon presentation of a low-intensity tone) was more accurate in determining sleep latency than actigraphic assessment. Both procedures, however, were sensitive to the detection of sleep. OAWI were found to require more instruction time in the use of the Sleep Assessment Device, which tape records verbal responses to preset, fixed-interval tones (Kelley & Lichstein, 1980). Nevertheless, Lichstein and Johnson (1991) found the device to be a useful and nonintrusive tool to collect objective sleep data in a sizable study of 56 women aged 60-77 years. A relatively small number of subjects withdrew from the study because of disruptive effects on sleep and spouse reactivity.

In recent years, the behavioral assessment of sleep has become increasingly established as an integral part of clinical appraisal. Actigraphy mirrors many of the advantages of sleep diary assessment (see Table 3.2), and together they represent a powerful combination of subjective and objective information for practical use. PSG assessment can then be prioritized for situations where the diagnosis remains uncertain.

Daytime Sleepiness

Evidence of daytime effects resulting from disrupted sleep has been a matter of some debate in the literature. Whereas it is now recognized that chronic insomnia will not necessarily be associated with significant daytime sequelae (Lichstein, Wilson, Noe, Aguillard, & Bellur, 1994), assessment of daytime sleepiness is medically significant because it may be a symptom of sleep apnea, narcolepsy, PLMS, circadian rhythm disorder, affective disorder, excessive drug or alcohol use, or idiopathic hypersomnolence (Moldofsky, 1992). A recent study of 4,578 adults (> 65 years of age) reported that 20% were "usually sleepy in the daytime," confirming the importance of adequately assessing daytime experiences in older adults (Whitney et al., 1998).

The experiences of tiredness and sleepiness, however, should be differentiated. The latter can involve involuntary sleep or a likelihood of sleep occurring while engaged in routine daytime activities. PWI will not always report sleepiness even after disturbed sleep. Furthermore, the older person with or without insomnia may have a greater tendency toward daytime napping irrespective of the preceding night's sleep (Metz & Bunnell, 1990). Thus, it is important to assess sleep/wakefulness longitudinally to establish an accurate picture of their interrelationship. Fatigue, by comparison, comprises tiredness, lethargy, inattention, and perhaps loss of motivation. Experimental studies investigating reaction time and word recall in younger and older PWI and normal sleepers suggest that performance is affected by sleep loss but that performance recovery is not necessarily poorer in OAWI (Berry & Webb, 1985; Bonnet & Rosa, 1987).

The Multiple Sleep Latency Test (MSLT) assesses, in a laboratory environment, the rapidity of sleep onset during daytime nap opportunities and has for long been the gold standard, objective measure of daytime sleepiness (Carskadon, Dement, Mitler, Roth, & Westbrook, 1986). The MSLT will seldom be required in the assessment of OAWI but should be used when the diagnosis of narcolepsy is suspected (Aldrich, Chervin, & Malow, 1997). Rating scale measures of sleepiness, however, can be widely used in routine practice. The best known are the Stanford Sleepiness Scale (Hoddes, Zarcone, Smythe, Phillips, & Dement, 1973), which comprises seven rank-ordered statements reflecting increasing levels of sleepiness; the Karolinska Sleepiness Scale (Akerstedt & Gillberg, 1990), a 9-point scale where 9 represents the highest level of sleepiness; and the Epworth Sleepiness Scale (ESS; Johns, 1991). The ESS is an eight-item self-report measure commonly used in research on sleep apnea and in clinical practice. It measures the likelihood of falling asleep in everyday situations such as driving and watching television. A high ESS score cannot be taken in isolation as evidence of SBD; nevertheless, where there is also a positive clinical history and a partner has witnessed apneas, the probability of SBD is significantly increased. This should then be confirmed by PSG assessment. The ESS has demonstrated reasonable validity in comparison with the MSLT (Johns, 1994). Cutoff points of > 11 for men and > 9 for women have been taken as indicative of excessive daytime sleepiness in older adults on the ESS (Whitney et al., 1998).

Differential Diagnosis
From Other Sleep Disorders

The National Institutes of Health consensus statement (1991) highlighted the importance of differential diagnosis of sleep disorders of older people. The statement called for standardization of clinical measures, assessment of the specificity and sensitivity of diagnostic procedures, and the use of "advanced skills" and "diagnostic tools" as part of the assessment process. It will be clear from the preceding section that these skills are essentially clinical; thus, the effective clinician will be working as a scientist-practitioner, using information to create and test hypotheses concerning the etiology and maintenance of the presenting sleep disorder. The "tools" available have also been described, and these range from self-report to psychophysiological. It is the integration of information from these various sources that leads to good diagnostic practice.

The International Classification of Sleep Disorders (*ICSD*) should be consulted for detailed descriptions of the full range of sleep disorders (ASDA, 1997); however, a brief summary of the major diagnostic categories is presented in Table 3.3. The majority of these have been introduced earlier in the context of specific assessment methodologies. This section, therefore, will build on that information to provide a more complete picture of differential diagnosis with particular reference to older adults.

Normal Aging

The working definition of insomnia is a persistent difficulty in initiating and/or maintaining sleep. In OAWI, however, such difficulties must be seen in the context of entirely normal, age-related changes in sleep. For example, Hoch et al. (1997) have demonstrated that quality, continuity, and depth of sleep decline over time in healthy elderly subjects aged 75-87 years. These recent results, from this important longitudinal study, confirm earlier reports of more frequent arousals (Carskadon, Brown, & Dement, 1982; Reynolds, Kupfer, & Taska, 1985), depletion of

---

Table 3.3 Simplified Classification of Sleep Disorders to Aid Differential Diagnosis of Insomnia in Older Adults

Sleep Disorder	*Summary Description of Disorder*
Insomnia	Difficulty in initiating and/or maintaining sleep occurring 4 or more nights per week and persisting for at least 3 months. Possible daytime mood and performance effects.
Normal aging	Developmentally normal changes in sleep and wakefulness.
Sleep-related breathing disorder (SBD)	Cessation of breathing (apnea), loud snoring, choking/fighting for breath during sleep. Morning headache, dry mouth, obesity, excessive daytime sleepiness/involuntary naps may present.
Periodic limb movements in sleep (PLMS) and restless legs syndrome (RLS)	Motor restlessness during sleep and relaxation, involuntary limb movements. Often excessive daytime sleepiness.
Circadian rhythm sleep disorders	Chronophysiological disorders involving misalignment between sleep pattern and local time. Delayed or advanced sleep phases produce complaints of insomnia and/or excessive sleepiness.
Narcolepsy	Irresistible sleep attacks at inappropriate times. Sometimes with cataplexy (loss of muscle tone triggered by emotion), hypnagogic hallucinations, sleep paralysis, and disturbed nighttime sleep.
Parasomnias	Abnormal behaviors in nREM sleep (e.g., sleepwalking, sleep bruxism) and REM sleep (e.g., nightmares) and in transition between wakefulness and sleep (e.g., sleep talking).
Sleep disorders associated with medical/psychiatric disorders	A wide range of disorders involve sleep symptomatology: Neurologic disorders (e.g., dementia, Parkinson's disease), other medical disorders (e.g., cardiac ischemia, pulmonary disease, gastrointestinal problems), and mental disorders (e.g., affective disorders, alcoholism).
Extrinsic sleep disorders	A wide range of exogenous causes. Includes hypnotic-, alcohol-, and stimulant-dependency sleep disorder.

SOURCE: Based on the International Classification of Sleep Disorders (American Sleep Disorders Association, 1997).

non-REM deep sleep (Bliwise, 1993), and age-related changes in the circadian rhythm (Haimov, Laudon, & Zisapel, 1994). Thus, there are developmental changes in sleep that could be misinterpreted as a clinical insomnia. Furthermore, there is evidence that only home-based PSG assessment successfully differentiates OAWI from normal sleepers (Edinger et al., 1997).

Differentiating pathological insomnia in late life from normal age-related changes in sleep, therefore, can be problematic. It is a distinction that can be made only clinically, based on evidence of the enduring impact and intrusiveness of the disorder on (a) sleep itself; (b) daytime performance, especially alertness; or (c) broader psychosocial functioning (e.g., relationships and behavior). It is wise to intervene first with a sleep educational/sleep hygiene approach, because a good response to information and simple advice probably indicates a primarily developmental problem.

Sleep-Related Breathing Disorder (SBD)

SBD refers to respiratory impairment during sleep which is commonly associated with excessive daytime sleepiness (EDS) (Table 3.3). Obstructive sleep apneas can be destructive of the continuity of sleep, of its restorative powers, and of the experience of sleep quality. Because there is known to be an increased prevalence of SBD in later life (Ancoli-Israel et al., 1991), it is important to consider this possible diagnosis where there is evidence of sleep disturbance associated with snoring and significant daytime effects measured, for example, by the Epworth Sleepiness Scale. Interviewing the partner may provide evidence of respiratory interruption. Although confirmatory diagnosis can be made only by full PSG assessment, SBD can be predicted by prudent interviewing and the calculation of body mass index (e.g., Maislin et al., 1995). Home oximetry may also be useful as a screening tool, but it is reliable only for moderate to severe cases of obstructive apnea (Yamashiro & Kryger, 1995). It is important to point out that SBD may pass undetected in samples of OAWI. Lichstein et al. (1999) have recently reported that around one third of their OAWI had undiagnosed apneas of clinical significance. This highlights the value of routine PSG assessment, particularly in older overweight males.

Restless Legs Syndrome (RLS) and Periodic Limb Movements in Sleep (PLMS)

The symptoms of these conditions are summarized in Table 3.3. RLS is primarily a condition of middle to old age, and severe symptoms do not generally present in younger adults. Nevertheless, in around one third of cases, symptoms emerge before the age of 20 years (Lavigne & Montplaisir, 1994; Walters et al., 1996). Similarly, PLMS are reported more often by older subjects and may be related to disturbance of circadian sleep-wake rhythms in the elderly (Coleman, Pollak, & Weitzman, 1980). These disorders can be associated with sleep apnea syndromes, and many people with RLS also experience PLMS (Chokroverty, 1995).

It is important, therefore, routinely to ask OAWI about movement and restlessness while asleep or relaxed. Insomnia and EDS are the most commonly reported disorders of sleep in this age group (Prinz, Vitiello, & Raskind, 1990); therefore, care should be taken to identify both the nature of the sleep disturbance and the possible etiology of any EDS. Because the sleep of partners is often interrupted by RLS/PLMS, the partner should be interviewed. Full PSG assessment normally provides accurate diagnosis and establishes possible co-presentation with SBD.

Circadian Disorders

Haimov and Lavie (1997) have recently reported age-related trends toward lower circadian amplitude and advanced phase disorder. In this study, sleep propensity in young adults was still high at 7 a.m., whereas in the 17 elderly males in the study it began to decline at 5 a.m. Older adults also demonstrated increases in sleepiness during the period from 7 to 9 p.m. With advancing age, fragmented sleep can lead to daytime napping, and this further contributes to disorganization of circadian rhythms. O'Connor, Mahowald, and Ettinger (1995) recommend monitoring sleep-wake patterns on a sleep diary for 2 weeks to assist in differential diagnosis of sleep-phase disorders. As previously mentioned, the diary format in Figure 3.2 is useful for this assessment task. O'Connor et al. (1995) also present actigraphic examples of normal and chaotic sleep-wake patterns over consecutive 24-hour periods that demonstrate the usefulness of the actigraph as a diagnostic tool for circadian disorder. Disorders of the sleep-wake schedule are also common in dementing and institutionalized older adults (see the section below on sleep problems associated with medical/psychiatric disorders).

Narcolepsy

OAWI typically complain of inadequate sleep; therefore, one might not expect to have problems in differential diagnosis from hypersomnia. People with narcolepsy, however, often sleep poorly at night. MSLT assessment can be helpful here and may provide information suggestive of narcolepsy such as sleep onset REM periods (Dement, Rechtschaffen, & Gulevich, 1966). Hudson et al. (1992), however, completed a meta-analysis of PSG measurement in insomnia, depression, and narcolepsy which suggested that PSG alone may not be sufficient to differentiate these conditions, particularly in older adults. They noted that depressives show a greater change with age than nondepressed people on most component measures of sleep disturbance (e.g., Gillin et al., 1981). Although Hudson et al.'s "unitary" view of sleep disturbance is less popular than a pluralistic hypothesis, care should be taken in differential diagnosis. The case of narcolepsy highlights the importance of a good clinical history. This will generally reveal a peak age of onset of irresistible sleep episodes and EDS at around 15 and 25 years, with the nighttime sleep disturbance of narcolepsy becoming progressively more problematic with advancing age (Billiard, Besset, & Cadhilac, 1993).

Parasomnias

Parasomnias are behavioral phenomena occurring during sleep and may be disorders of arousal, partial arousal, or sleep-stage transition. The most common parasomnias in older adults are REM sleep behavior disorder, sleepwalking, and night terrors. REM sleep behavior disorder is characterized by the intermittent restoration of muscle tone during REM sleep and the appearance of elaborate motor activity (e.g., punching, kicking, leaping from bed) associated with apparent dream enactment. Although parasomnias normally first present in childhood or adolescence, sudden onset (particularly of REM sleep behavior disorder) in late life may indicate an acute neurological problem (Culebras & Magana, 1987). Parasomnias, however, will seldom be confused with insomnia.

Sleep Problems Associated With Medical/Psychiatric Disorders

The International Classification of Sleep Disorders recognizes a large number of primary medical and psychiatric diagnoses that are associated with sleep disturbance. The importance of a medical and drug history in older adults has been particularly stressed by Chokroverty (1995), who recommends using the interview guidelines developed by Kales and coworkers (Kales & Kales, 1984; Kales, Soldatos, & Kales, 1980). Some examples of common illness etiologies are presented in Table 3.3.

Sleep disturbance also features in a wide range of psychiatric disorders, most notably in depression (Buysse et al., 1997; Gillin et al., 1981; Gillin, Sitaram, & Wehr, 1984), although there also is an association with other disorders such as panic (Stein, Enns, & Kryger, 1993) and generalized anxiety (Fuller, Waters, Binks, & Anderson, 1997). The differentiation of primary depression from primary sleep disturbance may be best addressed by structured psychiatric interview (Buysse et al., 1997) or through the use of one of the many available range of symptom rating scales for depression. Where insomnia is secondary to major depression, other evidence of biobehavioral disturbance is usually found (e.g., appetite and moti vational drive), and negativity in mood is more global and severe, rather than attributed specifically to poor sleep. Although sleep disturbance can be an early sign of the onset of depression, a careful history of any previous episodes may indicate amelioration in sleep problems as the depression is treated. Where insomnia is being treated as the primary disorder and associated depressive symptoms persist or worsen, the focus of treatment should be altered to address these, either pharmacologically or with cognitive-behavior therapy. PSG assessment may also help to differentiate major depression (Thase et al., 1996), and a composite measure of sleep disturbance based on REM latency, REM density, and sleep efficiency has been suggested. Around 50% of depressed outpatients, however, have normal sleep studies.

It should also be noted that both mental state and age can affect presenting sleep pattern (Ancoli-Israel, Klauber et al., 1997; Jacobs, Ancoli-Israel, Parker, & Kripke, 1989). This has been confirmed by longitudinal study of sleep-activity patterns in nursing home populations, where disturbed sleep with night wandering, sleep fragmentation, and circadian disorder are relatively common. Thus, people with dementia and institutionalized elderly people require special consideration in diagnosis, because both neurological and environmental factors can influence sleep.

Extrinsic Sleep Disorders

Difficulty in initiating and maintaining sleep in OAWI may arise from drugs taken for illnesses common in this age group (e.g., central nervous system stimulants, beta blockers, and antihypertensives). Benzodiazepine hypnotics have long been contraindicated for OAWI because of their direct effects on sleep structure and their association with drug withdrawal insomnia (Consensus Conference, 1984). Alcohol is the most frequent form of self-medication and is known to worsen sleep disturbance and can exacerbate any existing SBD. Clearly, differential diagnosis requires an accurate history and monitoring of drug use in parallel with sleep diary reports.

Clinical Formulation of
the Sleep Problem

It is important to place assessment and differential diagnosis in context. It is clear that a good sleep assessment will carefully consider possible explanatory hypotheses concerning the etiology and maintenance of the sleep disorder. In older adults, these possibilities are wide ranging. It is also clear that valid and reliable assessment may involve subjective and objective methods, as well as the gathering of information from a partner where appropriate. The central purpose of the assessment process, however, is clinical formulation. The interpretation and integration of evidence from these various sources should lead to a working model that guides intervention. An understanding of the impact and intrusiveness of the sleep problem, along with appraisal of treatment-related change in these and other target variables, should represent a collaborative agenda for the older adult and the clinician to follow. Although this chapter necessarily has focused on the assessment of sleep per se, it should be noted that other chapters will consider aspects of the assessment process that are especially relevant to psychological management, such as attributional style, readiness to implement change, and expectations of treatment effectiveness.

References

Akerstedt, T., & Gillberg, M. (1990). Subjective and objective sleepiness in the active individual. *International Journal of Neuroscience, 52*, 29-37.

Aldrich, M. S., Chervin, R. D., & Malow, E. A. (1997). Value of the Multiple Sleep Latency Test (MSLT) for the diagnosis of narcolepsy. *Sleep, 20*, 620-629.

American Sleep Disorders Association. (1990). *The International Classification of Sleep Disorders: Diagnostic and coding manual*. Rochester, MN: Author.

American Sleep Disorders Association. (1995a). Practice parameters for the use of actigraphy in the clinical assessment of sleep disorders. *Sleep, 18*, 285-287.

American Sleep Disorders Association. (1995b). Practice parameters for the use of polysomnography in the evaluation of insomnia. *Sleep, 18*, 55-57.

American Sleep Disorders Association. (1997). *International Classification of Sleep Disorders: Diagnostic and coding manual*. Rochester, MN: Author.

Ancoli-Israel, S., Clopton, P., Klauber, M. R., Fell, R., & Mason, W. (1997). Use of wrist activity for monitoring sleep/wake in demented nursing-home patients. *Sleep, 20*, 24-27.

Ancoli-Israel, S., Klauber, M. R., Williams Jones, D., Kripke, D. F., Martin, J., Mason, W., Pat-Horenczyk, R., & Fell, R. (1997). Variations in circadian rhythms of activity, sleep, and light exposure related to dementia in nursing-home residents. *Sleep, 20*, 18-23.

Ancoli-Israel, S., Kripke, D. F., Klauber, M. R., Mason, W. J., Fell, R., & Kaplan, O. (1991). Sleep disorder breathing in community-dwelling elderly. *Sleep, 14*, 486-495.

Ancoli-Israel, S., Kripke, D. F., Mason, W., & Messin, S. (1981). Comparisons of home sleep recordings and polysomnograms in older adults with sleep disorder. *Sleep, 4*, 283-291.

Berry, D.T.R., & Webb, W. B. (1985). Sleep and cognitive functions in normal older adults. *Journal of Gerontology, 40*, 331-335.

Billiard, M., Besset, A., & Cadhilac, J. (1983). The clinical and polygraphic development of narcolepsy. In C. Guilleminault and E. Lugaresi (Eds.), *Sleep/wake disorders: Natural history, epidemiology and long-term evaluation* (pp. 187-199). New York: Raven.

Bliwise, D. (1993). Sleep in normal ageing and dementia. *Sleep, 16*, 40-81.

Blood, M. L., Sack, R. L., Percy, D. S., & Pen, J. C. (1997). A comparison of sleep detection by wrist actigraphy, behavioral response, and polysomnography. *Sleep, 20*, 388-395.

Bonnet, M. H., & Rosa, R. R. (1987). Sleep and performance in young adults and older normals and insomniacs during acute sleep loss and recovery. *Biological Psychiatry, 25*, 153-172.

Bootzin, R. R., & Engle-Friedman, M. (1981). The assessment of insomnia. *Behavioral Assessment, 3*, 107-126.

Bootzin, R. R., & Nicassio, P. M. (1978). Behavioural treatments for insomnia. In M. Hersen, R. M. Eisler, & P. M. Miller (Eds.), *Progress in behaviour modification* (Vol. 6, pp. 1-45). New York: Academic Press.

Borkovec, T. D. (1979). Pseudo-(experiential) insomnia and idiopathic (objective) insomnia: Theoretical and therapeutic issues. *Advances in Behaviour Research and Therapy, 2,* 27-55.

Borkovec, T. D., Grayson, J. B., O'Brien, G. T., & Weerts, T. C. (1979). Relaxation treatment of pseudoinsomnia and idiopathic insomniac: An electroencephalographic evaluation. *Journal of Applied Behavioural Analysis, 12,* 37-54.

Borkovec, T. D., Lane, T. W., & Van Oot, P. A. (1981). Phenomenology of sleep among insomniacs and good sleepers: Wakefulness experience when cortically asleep. *Journal of Abnormal Psychology, 90,* 607-609.

Buysse, D. J., Reynolds, C. F., Kupfer, D. J., Thorpy, M. J., Bixler, E., Kales, A., Manfredi, R., Vgontzas, A., Stepanski, E., Roth, T., Hauri, P., & Stapf, D. (1997). Effects of diagnosis on treatment recommendations in chronic insomnia—A report from the APA/NIMH DSM-IV field trial. *Sleep, 20,* 542-552.

Buysse, D. J., Reynolds, C. F., Monk, T. H., Berman, S. R., & Kupfer, D. J. (1989). The Pittsburgh Sleep Quality Index: A new instrument for psychiatric practice and research. *Psychiatry Research, 28,* 193-213.

Carskadon, M. A., Brown, E. D., & Dement, W. C. (1982). Sleep fragmentation in the elderly: Relationship to daytime sleep tendency. *Neurobiology of Aging, 3,* 321-327.

Carskadon, M. A., Dement, W. C., Mitler, M. M., Guilleminault, C., Zarcone, V. P., & Spiegel, R. (1976). Self-report versus sleep laboratory findings in 122 drug-free subjects with complaints of chronic insomnia. *American Journal of Psychiatry, 133,* 1382-1388.

Carskadon, M. A., Dement, W. C., Mitler, M. M., Roth, T., & Westbrook, P. R. (1986). Guidelines for the multiple sleep latency test (MSLT): A standard measure of sleepiness. *Sleep, 9,* 519-524.

Chokroverty, S. (1995). Sleep disorders in elderly persons. In S. Chokroverty (Ed.), *Sleep disorders medicine: Basic science, technical considerations and clinical aspects* (pp. 401-415). Newton, MA: Butterworth-Heinemann.

Coates, T. J., Killen, J. D., Marchini, E., Silverman, S. S., Hamilton, S., & Thoresen, C. E. (1982). Discriminating good sleepers from insomniacs using all-night polysomnograms conducted at home. *Journal of Nervous and Mental Disease, 170,* 224-230.

Coleman, R. M., Pollak, C. P., & Weitzman, E. D. (1980). Periodic movements in sleep (nocturnal myoclonus): Relation to sleep-wake disorders. *Annals of Neurology, 8,* 416-421.

Consensus Conference. (1984) Drugs and insomnia: The use of medication to promote sleep. *Journal of the American Medical Association, 251,* 2410-2414.

Culebras, A., & Magana, R. (1987). Neurologic disorders and sleep disturbances. *Seminars in Neurology, 7,* 277-285.

Davies, R., Lacks, P., Storandt, M., & Bertelson, A. D. (1986). Countercontrol treatment of sleep-maintenance insomnia in relation to age. *Psychology and Aging, 1,* 233-238.

DeGroen, J.H.M., Koper, H., & Bergs, E.P.E. (1985). Ambulatory sleep-wake polygraphy in narcolepsy. *Electroencephalography and Clinical Neurophysiology, 60,* 420-422.

Dement, W., Rechtschaffen, A., & Gulevich, G. (1966). The nature of the narcoleptic sleep attack. *Neurology, 16,* 18-33.

Douglas, N. J., Thomas, S., & Jan, M. A. (1992). Clinical value of polysomnography. *Lancet, 339,* 347-350.

Douglass, A. B., Bornstein, R., Nino-Murcia, G., Keenan, S., Miles, L., Zarcone, V. P., Guilleminault, C., & Dement, W. C. (1994). The Sleep Disorders Questionnaire I: Creation and multivariate structure of SDQ. *Sleep, 17,* 160-167.

Edinger, J. D., & Fins, A. I. (1995). The distribution and clinical significance of sleep time misperceptions among insomniacs. *Sleep, 18,* 232-239.

Edinger, J. D., Fins, A. I., Sullivan, R. J., Marsh, G. R., Dailey, D. S., Hope, T. V., Young, M., Shaw, E., Carlson, D., & Vasilas, D. (1997). Sleep in the laboratory and sleep at home: Comparisons of older insomniacs and normal sleepers. *Sleep, 20,* 1119-1126.

Edinger, J. D., Hoelscher, T. J., Marsh, G. R., Lipper, S., & Ionescu-Pioggia, M. (1992). A cognitive-behavioral therapy for sleep-maintenance insomnia in older adults. *Psychology and Aging, 7,* 282-289.

Engle-Friedman, M., Bootzin, R. R., Hazlewood, L., & Tsao, C. (1992). An evaluation of behavioral treatments for insomnia in the older adult. *Journal of Clinical Psychology, 48,* 77-90.

Enright, P. L., Newman, A. B., Wahl, P. W., Manolio, T. A., Haponik, E. F., & Boyle, P.J.R. (1996). Prevalence and correlates of snoring and observed apneas in 5201 older adults. *Sleep, 19,* 531-538.

Espie, C. A. (1991). *The psychological treatment of insomnia.* Chichester, UK: J. Wiley and Sons.

Espie, C. A. (1993). The practical management of insomnia: Cognitive and behavioural techniques. *British Medical Journal, 306,* 509-511.

Espie, C. A., Lindsay, W. R., & Espie, L. C. (1989). Use of the Sleep Assessment Device (Kelley and Lichstein, 1980) to validate insomniacs' self-report of sleep pattern. *Journal of Psychopathology and Behavioral Assessment, 11,* 71-79.

Espie, C. A., Paul, A., McFie, J., Amos, P., Hamilton, D., McColl, J. H., Tarassenko, L., & Pardey, J. (1998). Sleep studies of adults with severe or profound mental retardation and epilepsy. *American Journal on Mental Retardation, 103,* 47-59.

Everitt, D. E., Avorn, J., & Baker, M. W. (1990). Clinical decision-making in the evaluation and treatment of insomnia. *The American Journal of Medicine, 89,* 357-363.

Ford, D. E., & Kamerow, D. B. (1989). Epidemiological study of sleep disturbances in psychiatric disorders. *Journal of the American Medical Association, 262,* 1479-1484.

Frankel, B. L., Coursey, R. D., Buchbinder, R., & Snyder, F. (1976). Recorded and reported sleep in primary chronic insomnia. *Archives of General Psychiatry, 33,* 615-623.

Friedman, L., Bliwise, D. L., Yesavage, J. A., & Salom, S. R. (1991). A preliminary study comparing sleep restriction and relaxation treatments for insomnia in older adults. *Journal of Gerontology, 46,* 1-8.

Fuller, K. H., Waters, W. F., Binks, P. G., & Anderson, T. (1997). Generalized anxiety and sleep architecture: A polysomnographic investigation. *Sleep, 20,* 370-376.

Gillin, J. C., Duncan, W. C., Murphy, D. L., Post, R. M., Wehr, T. A., Goodwin, F. K., Wyatt, R. J., & Bunney, W. E. (1981). Age-related changes in sleep in depressed and normal subjects. *Psychiatry Research, 4,* 73-78.

Gillin, J. C., Sitaram, N., & Wehr, T. (1984). Sleep and affective illness. In R. M. Post & J. C. Ballinger (Eds.), *Neurobiology of mood disorders* (pp. 157-189). Baltimore: Williams and Wilkins.

Haimov, I., Laudon, M., & Zisapel, N. (1994). Sleep disorders and melatonin rhythms in elderly people. *British Medical Journal, 309,* 167.

Haimov, I., & Lavie, P. (1997). Circadian characteristics of sleep propensity function in healthy elderly: A comparison with young adults. *Sleep, 20,* 294-300.

Hauri, P. J., & Olmstead, E. (1983). What is the moment of sleep-onset for insomniacs? *Sleep, 6,* 10-15.

Hauri, P. J., & Wisbey, J. (1992). Wrist actigraphy in insomnia. *Sleep, 15,* 293-301.

Hoch, C. C., Dew, M. A., Reynolds, C. F., Buysse, D. J., Noel, P. D., Monk, T. H., Mazumdar, S., Borland, M. D., Miewald, J., & Kupfer, D. J. (1997). Longitudinal changes in diary- and laboratory-based sleep measures in healthy "old old" and "young old" subjects: A three year follow up. *Sleep, 20,* 192-202.

Hoddes, E., Zarcone, V., Smythe, H., Phillips, R., & Dement, W. C. (1973). Quantification of sleepiness: A new approach. *Psychophysiology, 10,* 431-436.

Horne, J. A., Pankhurst, F. P., Reyner, L. A., Hume, K., & Diamond, I. (1994). A field study of sleep disturbance: Effects of aircraft noise and other factors on 5,742 nights of actimetrically monitored sleep in a large subject sample. *Sleep, 17,* 146-159.

Hudson, J. I., Pope, H. G., Sullivan, L. E., Waternaux, C. M., Keck, P. E., & Broughton, R. J. (1992). Good sleep, bad sleep: A meta-analysis of polysomnographic measures in insomnia, depression and narcolepsy. *Biological Psychiatry, 32,* 958-975.

Jacobs, D., Ancoli-Israel, S., Parker, L., & Kripke, D. F. (1989). Twenty-four-hour sleep-wake patterns in a nursing home population. *Psychology and Aging, 4,* 352-356.

Johns, M. W. (1991). A new method for measuring daytime sleepiness: The Epworth Sleepiness Scale. *Sleep, 14,* 540-545.

Johns, M. W. (1994). Sleepiness in different situations measured by the Epworth Sleepiness Scale. *Sleep, 17,* 703-710.

Kales, A., & Kales, J. D. (1984). *Evaluation and treatment of insomnia.* New York: Oxford University Press.

Kales, A., Soldatos, C. R., & Kales, J. D. (1980). Taking a sleep history. *American Family Physician, 22,* 101-108.

Kelley, J. E., & Lichstein, K. L. (1980). A sleep assessment device. *Behavioral Assessment, 2,* 135-146.

Kripke, D. F., Mullaney, D. J., Messin, S., & Wyborney, V. G. (1978). Wrist actigraphic measures of sleep and rhythms. *Electroencephalography and Clinical Neurophysiology, 44,* 674-676.

Kupfer, D. J., Snyder, F., & Wyatt, R. J. (1970). Comparison between electroencephalographic and nursing observations of sleep in psychiatric patients. *Journal of Nervous and Mental Disease, 151,* 361-368.

Lacks, P. (1987). *Behavioral treatment for persistent insomnia.* New York: Pergamon.

Lavigne, G. J., & Montplaisir, J. Y. (1994). Restless legs syndrome and sleep bruxism: Prevalence and association among Canadians. *Sleep, 17,* 739-743.

Lichstein, K. L., & Johnson, R. S. (1991). Older adults' objective self-recording of sleep in the home. *Behavior Therapy, 22,* 531-549.

Lichstein, K. L., & Riedel, B. W. (1994). Behavioral assessment and treatment of insomnia: A review with an emphasis on clinical application. *Behavior Therapy, 25,* 659-688.

Lichstein, K. L., Riedel, B. W., Lester, K. W., & Aguillard, R. N. (1999). Occult sleep apnea in a recruited sample of older adults with insomnia. *Journal of Consulting and Clinical Psychology, 67,* 405-410.

Lichstein, K. L., Wilson, N. M., Noe, S. L., Aguillard, R. N., & Bellur, S. N. (1994). Daytime sleepiness in insomnia: Behavioral, biological and subjective indices. *Sleep, 17,* 693-702.

Maislin, G., Pack, A. I., Kribbs, M. B., Smith, P. L., Schwartz, K. R., Kline, L. R., Schwab, R. J., & Dinges, D. F. (1995). A survey screen for prediction of apnea. *Sleep, 18,* 158-166.

McCall, W. V., Marsh, G. R., & Erwin, C. W. (1995). Ambulatory cassette polysomnography. In S. Chokroverty (Ed.), *Sleep disorders medicine: Basic science, technical considerations and clinical aspects* (pp. 141-149). Newton, MA: Butterworth-Heinemann.

Metz, M. E., & Bunnell, D. E. (1990). Napping and sleep disturbances in the elderly. *Family Practice Research Journal, 10,* 47-56.

Moldofsky, H. (1992). Evaluation of daytime sleepiness: A review. *Clinics in Chest Medicine, 13,* 417-425.

Morgan, K. (in press). Sleep and insomnia in later life. In J. C. Brocklehurst, R. C. Tallis, & H. M. Fillit (Eds.), *Textbook of geriatric medicine and gerontology* (5th ed.). London: Churchill Livingstone.

Morin, C. M. (1993). *Psychological management of insomnia.* New York: Guilford.

Morin, C. M., Gaulier, B., Barry, T., & Kowatch, R. (1992). Patients' acceptance of psychological and pharmacological therapies for insomnia. *Sleep, 15,* 302-305.

Morin, C. M., Kowatch, R. A., Barry, T., & Walton, E. (1993). Cognitive-behavior therapy for late-life insomnia. *Journal of Consulting and Clinical Psychology, 61,* 137-146.

Mullaney, D. J., Kripke, D. F., & Messin, S. (1980). Wrist-actigraphic estimation of sleep time. *Sleep, 3,* 83-92.

National Institutes of Health. (1991). Consensus development conference statement: The treatment of sleep disorders of older people, March 26-28, 1990. *Sleep, 14,* 169-177.

O'Connor, K. A., Mahowald, M. W., & Ettinger, M. G. (1995). Circadian rhythm disorders. In S. Chokroverty (Ed.), *Sleep disorders medicine: Basic science, technical considerations and clinical aspects* (pp. 369-379). Newton, MA: Butterworth-Heinemann.

Ogilvie, R. D., & Wilkinson, R. T. (1988). Behavioral versus EEG-based monitoring of all-night sleep/wake patterns. *Sleep, 11,* 139-155.

Ohayon, M. M. (1996). Epidemiological study on insomnia in a general population. *Sleep, 19,* S7-S15.

Pearse, P.A.E. (1993). Use of the sleep diary in the management of patients with insomnia. *Australian Family Physician, 22,* 744-748.

Platt, F. W. (1991). Research in medical interviewing. *Annals of Internal Medicine, 94,* 405-407.

Prinz, P. N., Vitiello, M. V., & Raskind, M. A. (1990). Geriatrics: Sleep disorders and aging. *New England Journal of Medicine, 323,* 520-526.

Reite, M., Buysse, D., Reynolds, C., & Mendelson, W. (1995). The use of polysomnography in the evaluation of insomnia. *Sleep, 18,* 58-70.

Reyner, A., & Horne, J. A. (1995). Gender- and age-related differences in sleep determined by home-recorded sleep logs and actimetry from 400 adults. *Sleep, 18,* 127-134.

Reynolds, C. F., Kupfer, D. J., & Taska, L. S. (1985). Sleep of healthy seniors: A revisit. *Sleep, 8,* 20-29.

Sadeh, A., Hauri, P. J., Kripke, D. F., & Lavie, P. (1995). The role of actigraphy in the evaluation of sleep disorders. *Sleep, 18,* 288-302.

Sadeh, A., Sharkey, M., & Carskadon, M. A. (1994). Activity-based sleep-wake identification: Clinical tests of methodological issues. *Sleep, 17,* 201-207.

Schneider-Helmert, D. (1987). Twenty-four-hour sleep-wake function and personality patterns in chronic insomniacs and healthy controls. *Sleep, 10,* 452-462.

Schramm, E., Hohagen, F., Grasshoff, U., Reimann, D., Hajak, G., Weeß, H-G., & Berger, M. (1993). Test-retest reliability and validity of the structured interview for sleep disorders according to DSM-III-R. *American Journal of Psychiatry, 150,* 867-872.

Spielman, A. J., & Anderson, M. W. (1999). The clinical interview and treatment planning as a guide to understanding the nature of insomnia: The CCNY Interview for Insomnia. In S. Chokroverty (Ed.), *Sleep disorders medicine: Basic science, technical considerations and clinical aspects* (2nd ed., pp. 385-426). Boston: Butterworth-Heinemann.

Stein, M. B., Enns, M. W., & Kryger, M. H. (1993). Sleep in nondepressed patients with panic disorder: II. Polysomnographic assessment of sleep architecture and sleep continuity. *Journal of Affective Disorders, 28,* 1-6.

Thase, M. E., Kupfer, D. J., Fasiczka, A. J., Buysse, D. J., Simons, A. D., & Frank, E. (1996). Identifying an abnormal electroencephalographic sleep profile to characterise major depressive disorder. *Biological Psychiatry, 41,* 964-973.

Van Hilten, Braat E.A.M., Van Der Velde, E. A., Middelkoop, H.A.M., Kerkhoff, G. A., & Kamphuisen, H.A.C. (1993). Ambulatory activity monitoring during sleep: An evaluation of internight and intra-subject variability in healthy persons aged 50-98. *Sleep, 16,* 146-150.

Walters, A. S., Hickey, K., Maltzman, J., Verrico, T., Joseph, D., Hening, W., Wilson, V., & Chokroverty, S. (1996). A questionnaire study of 138 patients with restless legs syndrome: The "Night-Walkers" survey. *Neurology, 46,* 92-95.

Whitney, C. W., Enright, P. L., Newman, A. B., Bonekat, W., Foley, D., & Quan, S. F. (1998). Correlates of daytime sleepiness in 4,578 elderly persons: The cardiovascular health study. *Sleep, 21,* 27-36.

Wilkinson, R. T., & Mullaney, D. (1976). Electroencephalogram recording of sleep in the home. *Postgraduate Medicine, 52,* 92-96.

Yamashiro, Y., & Kryger, M. H. (1995). Nocturnal oximetry: Is it a screening tool for sleep disorders? *Sleep, 18,* 167-171.

PART II

Intervention Strategies

4

Treatment Overview

KENNETH L. LICHSTEIN
CHARLES M. MORIN

The separate chapters of this book describe particular methods of assessment and treatment of older adults with insomnia (OAWI). The present chapter is intended to provide a cohesive, integrative analysis. It will explore clinical and methodological concerns that cut across multiple interventions, it will fill gaps, and it will provide a summary view.

Normal Developmental Changes

Advancing age may bring on unwelcome sleep changes that easily can be misconstrued as insomnia. These are discussed in great detail in Chap-

AUTHORS' NOTE: The first author received support in the preparation of this chapter from grant AG12136 from the National Institute on Aging, from the H. W. Durham Foundation, from Methodist Healthcare, and from the Department of Psychology's Center for Applied Psychological Research, part of the state of Tennessee's Center of Excellence Grant program. The second author received support in the preparation of this chapter from the National Institute of Mental Health (MH 55469).

ter 1. Briefly, older adults can expect to have lighter sleep and to have more awakenings during the night than they did in their middle years. Total sleep time may also be decreased. Further, a circadian shift often occurs, advancing the natural sleep period to earlier in the evening and ending earlier in the morning (Hoch, Buysse, Monk, & Reynolds, 1992).

These changes should be considered by the client and the clinician in two ways. First, in estimating the severity of the insomnia, the normal standard should not be the sleep of the client in earlier years. Most often, individuals come to conclude they have insomnia by noticing sleep deterioration over time. In the case of older adults, however, some portion of this deterioration is normal and may be misinterpreted as insomnia. Age-appropriate norms should serve as the expected sleep profile against which the individual's sleep is compared. Second, treatment outcome expectations similarly must be age adjusted. Successful treatment will improve sleep but will not recover individuals' sleep experience of their middle years. Typically, treatment for OAWI will consolidate sleep, reduce excess awake time in bed, and enhance the restorative value of sleep but will do little to improve the depth of sleep and may not increase total sleep time.

Common Interventions

Five established psychological interventions have been employed with OAWI, and these are the focus of the remaining chapters of this section of the book. By way of introduction, we will begin with a brief description of each and follow this with some general recommendations as to their coordinated application.

Sleep hygiene (Chapter 5) refers to a collection of lifestyle practices that are known to influence nighttime sleep. As examples, engaging in behaviors such as late afternoon napping or omitting behaviors such as regular exercise may adversely affect sleep, and individuals are encouraged to adopt a lifestyle that is consistent with good sleep hygiene to promote optimal sleep.

Sleep restriction (Chapter 6) is a collection of methods that focuses directly on excess awake time in bed during the night. OAWI may extend time in bed with the incorrect expectation that this will reap more sleep time. Instead, excess time in bed distributes sleep over a longer period, fragments sleep, and fosters frustration. Sleep restriction aims to shrink the boundaries between bedtime and morning awake time so that the sleep period conforms to one's biological sleep capacity.

Stimulus control (Chapter 7) seeks to establish the bedroom as a discriminative stimulus for sleep. For some, the bedroom becomes infused with a variety of activities (such as doing paperwork) and thoughts (such as worrying) that are incompatible with sleep. At bedtime, these associations instigate cognitive or physiological arousal that is sleep obstructing. Stimulus control procedures rid the bedroom of nonsleep-related activities, including awake time in bed, to strengthen the expectation that sleep will come swiftly at bedtime.

Relaxation (Chapter 8) refers to a collection of procedures that share common procedural (focus on pleasant thoughts in a quiet environment) and outcome (physiological and experiential calm) characteristics. When practicing relaxation at bedtime, cognitive and somatic arousal barriers to sleep are diminished.

Cognitive therapy (Chapter 9) addresses cognitive arousal born of distorted, exaggerated thoughts and attitudes about sleep and its consequences. Drawing on conventional cognitive therapy, as that of Beck, it seeks to correct faulty cognitions to relieve daytime worrying and bedtime arousal.

Additional interventions (e.g., drug therapy) for sleep disturbance in late life are also covered in this book, but the main focus of our discussion here is the selection of a nonpharmacological treatment for primary insomnia. Specific issues surrounding the indications and contraindications, as well as the risks and benefits, of pharmacotherapy for late-life insomnia are discussed in Chapter 10.

Some Issues in Clinical Procedure

Selecting Treatments

Armed with five insomnia treatments, how does the therapist select treatments for different kinds of insomnia? The research literature provides some general guidance but no definitive answers. For example, the

Table 4.1 Matching Common Treatments With Common Insomnia
Characteristics Based on Likelihood of Success

	Insomnia Type		Insomnia Cause		Insomnia Effect
Common Treatments	Onset Insomnia	Maintenance Insomnia	Cognitive Arousal	Somatic Arousal	Impaired Daytime Functioning
Sleep hygiene	X	X	X	X	X
Sleep restriction	X	X			
Stimulus control	X	X	X	X	X
Relaxation	X		X	X	X
Cognitive therapy	X	X	X		X

few insomnia studies that matched different methods of treatment with different client characteristics were unsuccessful in identifying reliable matches (Espie, Brooks, & Lindsay, 1989; Sanavio, 1988). We can, however, glean from the large body of insomnia research that some treatments are expected to work better with some types of clients, and these data can help guide treatment decisions. The following recommendations derive from such data, from our clinical experience, and from educated guesses. Treatment selection decisions cannot be delayed until an adequate empirical foundation surfaces.

Table 4.1 will serve as a heuristic for this discussion. Insomnia clients will vary with respect to age, gender, personality, cause, symptoms, severity, duration, and other factors. The number of therapeutically relevant characteristics present in a given client are great in number, and most of these are probably undiscovered. Table 4.1 therefore cannot be viewed as a comprehensive accounting of relevant factors, but rather is a simplified guide based on typical molar characteristics. The explanation of Table 4.1 that follows is a starting point for the kind of reasoning engaged in by therapists in reaching clinical decisions. It is important to restate that this decision-making process is concerned mainly with primary insomnia. For secondary insomnia, it is generally recognized that the first line of treatment should focus on removing the underlying pre-cipitating conditions (e.g., medical, drug, psychological). If this approach fails to resolve the sleep disturbance, the addition of a sleep-focused treatment would then be indicated. As pointed out in Chapter 12, however, a growing body of evidence shows that even secondary insomnia is treatment responsive.

The columns of Table 4.1 refer to broad categories of variables that are generally considered in making treatment decisions. The two insomnia types refer to individuals whose problem is mainly getting to sleep (onset) or staying asleep (maintenance). Although problems maintaining sleep (i.e., nocturnal awakenings and early morning awakening) are more frequent in older adults, not uncommonly, individuals have mixed insomnia: difficulty getting to sleep and staying asleep. The causes of insomnia are highly idiosyncratic, and at times their number seems to equal the number of people who have insomnia. The use of two categories is intended to provide only the most general guidance. Under cognitive arousal are included individuals whose thoughts are agitated at bedtime only, individuals who are agitated all day including bedtime, and individuals battling anxiety and depression that stirs their thoughts. Cognitive arousal includes reviewing the day's experiences, nonworrisome planning about future events, worrying about the future, and worrying about being able to go to sleep. Under somatic arousal are included physical discomfort, fidgetiness, sweating, and tossing and turning. More serious elevations in heart rate and blood pressure are possible but uncommon. In general, somatic arousal is probably less common than cognitive arousal (Lichstein & Rosenthal, 1980). The effects of insomnia are highly varied, but there is little basis for matching insomnia treatments with specific types of effects. The general category of daytime impairment distinguishes individuals with poor sleep who are sleepy, inattentive, or grumpy during the day from those who function fine despite poor sleep. Objective findings of daytime impairment (e.g., short sleep latencies on the multiple sleep latency test, impaired memory, inattentiveness) in people with insomnia (PWI) including OAWI are uncommon, but subjective complaints of diminished quality of life attributed to the insomnia are routine (Riedel & Lichstein, in press).

Looking now at the treatments, Xs within the body of the table indicate the kind of OAWI we expect would profit from this treatment. The same pattern would probably occur with PWI of any age. There is no rea-

son to withhold sleep hygiene instructions from any PWI. These are simply good suggestions, and it is difficult to anticipate when they will have
beneficial effects. For example, not all PWI will enjoy improved sleep
from starting up an exercise program, but some surely will. Sleep restriction is recommended for either type of PWI but is not marked for either
of the causes because it has no specific effect on either. There is no reason,
however, to withhold it from individuals experiencing either cognitive
or somatic arousal. On the other hand, sleep restriction may prove problematic for individuals experiencing nontrivial daytime impairment.
The sleep restriction procedure may itself induce some sleep deprivation, sometimes intentionally to promote sleepiness at bedtime, producing further daytime impairment (Glovinsky & Spielman, 1991). This
would be a rare instance in which a nonpharmacological sleep treatment
could potentially cause harm by impairing alertness, judgment, or motor
skills. Stimulus control has proven to be an effective intervention for virtually every kind of PWI. The same can be said for relaxation and cognitive therapy. Relaxation is not checked for maintenance insomnia because some data suggest that it is not as effective for these individuals
(Morin, Culbert, & Schwartz, 1994). Cognitive therapy is not checked for
somatic arousal because it has no specific effect for such disturbance. If
somatic arousal is the primary cause, cognitive therapy is probably not
the best treatment choice.

Multicomponent Treatments

Table 4.1 yields the immediate conclusion that most insomnia treatments are fit for most PWI. What is not obvious from the table, but
equally true, is that these treatments are all brief and compatible. Unlike
the treatment of some other disorders, there is little pressure to select one
of these treatments to the exclusion of others in the clinical setting. Consequently, insomnia treatments are often bundled to offer a set of treatments to clients. In contrast, this situation may be compared with the
treatment of depression, as an example. Therapists may consider
psychodynamic or cognitive therapy. The two are incompatible, and
each requires a fairly long-term commitment to present the therapy. For
depression, the decision to choose a treatment is consequential and
exclusionary. For insomnia, there is inadequate data to guide the deci-

sion to select unitary interventions, and there is little advantage to making the effort.

Multicomponent treatments should receive serious consideration in insomnia treatment. The composition of multicomponent treatments will vary, but they commonly include some of or even all the above treatments. This approach has several advantages.

1. Because most insomnia treatments are compatible with one another and each is relatively brief to present, multicomponent treatments usually can be efficiently presented in 10 sessions or fewer.
2. Clients may emphasize those treatments that best suit them.
3. When the insomnia assessment is imperfect, the multicomponent treatment increases the likelihood that unrecognized aspects of the insomnia will not be therapeutically neglected.
4. Multicomponent treatments are, on the average, 20% more effective than unitary treatments (Morin, Culbert, et al., 1994).

Multicomponent treatments can be presented in clusters or in series. For example, stimulus control and relaxation do not take long to introduce and can be initiated in the same session. Even when treatments are introduced in bundles, however, some sequencing decisions must be made. Although there is no research to guide our decision making on sequencing, several strategies should be considered. Clinical experience suggests that cognitive therapy is a good starting strategy when a patient displays a high level of sleep-related anxiety (e.g., fear of the detrimental consequences of insomnia on health, fear of never being able to sleep again). Cognitive therapy is likely to provide reassurance about the circumscribed consequences of insomnia and to alleviate the underlying performance anxiety. Relaxation therapy could also be indicated with an anxious patient, although clinical benefits with this treatment may take longer to become noticeable. For an older person with unrealistic sleep expectations, simple education about age-appropriate norms would seem the most effective initial strategy. In general, sleep restriction will yield quick results, which may make an older person more receptive to other clinical procedures during the course of treatment. Finally, when combining sleep restriction and stimulus control therapy, it makes more sense logistically to implement sleep restriction first, and only when increasing the sleep window (i.e., time in bed) would the stimulus control procedures become relevant (i.e., going to bed only when sleepy and getting out of bed when unable to sleep).

Number of Treatment Sessions

Once a treatment or combination of treatments is chosen, how many sessions constitute an adequate treatment course? This may vary with the number of treatments presented, the severity and etiology of the insomnia, and the degree of motivation and adherence of the client, but generally, 6 to 10 sessions are needed. Although some individuals will attain maximum therapeutic benefits in fewer than 6 sessions, our clinical experience and research suggest that this is insufficient for others (Carlson & Hoyle, 1993; Morin, Stone, et al., 1994). Given that insomnia is often a recurrent condition, maintenance therapy in the form of periodic booster sessions may be necessary for some OAWI.

Treatment Implementation

Typically, research methodologies have been more attentive to the quality of the dependent variables than that of the independent variables, but asserting the adequacy of the treatment (independent variable) is central to obtaining strong outcomes and fairly judging the treatment. The term *treatment implementation* may be used to refer to the set of dimensions constituting adequate exposure of the independent variable. Conducting fair clinical trials and maximizing treatment effectiveness in the clinical domain both require that the intervention be fully implemented. The assumption that full implementation has occurred is often not merited, and when there is partial treatment implementation, the clinical outcome will likely suffer.

We (KLL) have proposed a treatment implementation model as one way of determining if the goal of full implementation has been achieved (Lichstein, Riedel, & Grieve, 1994). Independent treatment components—termed delivery, receipt, and enactment—must be adequately represented to conclude that proper treatment occurred. The delivery component refers to the accuracy of treatment presentation (also called treatment integrity), receipt refers to the accuracy of the client's comprehension of treatment, and enactment refers to the extent of out-of-session application initiated by the client (this component is equivalent to the usual meaning of adherence).

Inadequate implementation of any component may derive from numerous sources and will cause the client to deviate from the intended treatment. As examples, delivery faults may arise from poorly trained therapists, receipt faults from inattentive clients, and enactment faults from poorly motivated clients. From this perspective, incomplete implementation may arise from faults in the therapist, the client, or both. To illustrate the implications of this model, errors in delivery or receipt will lead to adherence to the wrong treatment, which is functionally equivalent to nonadherence, and problems arising from this particular process would occur even with highly motivated, "compliant" clients. Each treatment implementation component requires independent attention to achieve overall adequate implementation, and we have provided methods for inducing (methods of increasing the likelihood that satisfactory implementation occurred) and assessing each component (Lichstein et al., 1994).

A recent review of psychological treatments for OAWI found a total of 15 studies (Lichstein, Riedel, & Means, 1999). Of these, only 2 (Morin & Azrin, 1988; Riedel, Lichstein, & Dwyer, 1995) induced and assessed all treatment implementation components, a most disappointing finding. Assessment is more critical than induction in demonstrating that a fair clinical trial was conducted because it is the assessment process that verifies that the independent variable is intact. Induction is needed only to increase the likelihood that the assessment will yield satisfactory findings. Turning the focus to assessment, besides the two studies mentioned above, no study assessed all three treatment components. Receipt assessment was neglected the most, leaving indeterminate the question of how much of the treatment clients mastered. Further, nearly two-thirds of the studies did not assess delivery, in which case the exact content of treatment cannot be confirmed.

The following assessment and induction strategies were used most often. For assessment, supervision or review of audiotapes was employed for delivery, discussion with the participant or written quizzes for receipt, and discussion or home diaries for enactment. For induction, therapist training sessions and treatment manuals were employed for delivery, written descriptions of treatment procedures for receipt, and written reminders and practice aids (like relaxation tapes) for enactment.

With specific reference to treating OAWI, our experience suggests that the following induction strategies may prove helpful. Researchers can improve treatment receipt and enactment by considering communication obstacles common to older adults. Many older adults experience impaired visual and auditory acuity that, for example, may affect their understanding of the intervention. Strategies to facilitate communication with older adults require little effort and involve such steps as conducting sessions in a well-lighted, quiet environment and providing written materials in large, bold print (Campbell & Lancaster, 1988). Consent forms should be brief and easily understandable. Other suggestions for therapists include speaking clearly and concisely, proceeding at the client's pace, and confirming that the conveyed message was understood.

Matters of treatment implementation are no less critical in clinical settings than they are to fair evaluations of clinical research. Treatments that are poorly delivered, poorly understood, or minimally enacted will yield smaller therapeutic benefits. When clinicians employ the same induction strategies as researchers, they are more likely to achieve clearer and more efficient treatments that are comprehended well by their clients and practiced well at home.

Outcome Issues

There is currently no consensus as to how treatment effectiveness should be measured and what should be the optimal outcome when treating late-life insomnia. Clinical studies, with both younger and older adults, have documented treatment outcomes almost exclusively in terms of symptom reductions (e.g., time required to fall asleep, duration of awakenings, and total sleep time). Although these sleep variables are important markers of progress and should be part of outcome evaluation, they provide a very narrow focus of treatment effectiveness. Insomnia is more than just a complaint about poor sleep; the perceived consequences (e.g., fatigue, impaired functioning) and associated emotional distress, rather than sleep loss per se, often prompt individuals to seek treatment. Thus, measurement of successful outcome should incorporate other indices of improvements such as measures of functional impairments, mood disturbances and psychological well-being, and even usage of hypnotic medications. These measures would provide more clinically meaningful indices of treatment impact.

A related issue concerns what should be the optimal outcome when treating OAWI. Several factors must be considered to answer this important question. As noted earlier, normal developmental changes occur in sleep as a person ages. For this reason, when working with seniors, treatment goals should be defined according to age-appropriate norms. Even within the segment of the older population, treatment goals may need to be adjusted as a function of comorbid medical or psychiatric conditions. What might be an optimal outcome for a healthy 70-year-old person (e.g., sleeping 6.5 hours per night with one or two awakenings of 15-20 min each) may be totally unrealistic for a more frail elderly person of the same age who suffers from severe cognitive impairments (i.e., dementia). In the latter case, minimizing nighttime wandering and reducing usage of sedating drugs might be more appropriate goals (see Chapter 13). Another illustration of the need to remain flexible in setting treatment goals concerns the use of sleep medications. Although a hypnotic medication may be indicated temporarily for an older person in grief, for another person who has been dependent on sleeping pills for many years, the goal may simply be to discontinue this medication. As noted by Bliwise and Breus in Chapter 13, what may be a desired outcome for a given patient may be much less meaningful for another individual of the same age. Thus, the optimal treatment outcome needs to be adjusted for the particular circumstances of every patient.

Are there moderators of treatment outcome? Several patient (demographic and clinical) and treatment-related variables (format, delivery mode) have been examined as potential moderators of treatment response. Few, if any, have been reliably associated with outcome. Although one early study (Alperson & Biglan, 1979) reported that older adults were less responsive to self-help treatments for insomnia than younger persons, the evidence from two meta-analyses indicate that older and younger adults with insomnia exhibit a comparable treatment response (Morin et al., 1994; Murtagh & Greenwood, 1995). This is particularly true when older adults are well screened for medical and sleep disorders such as sleep apnea and periodic limb movements. One exception may be for relaxation and imagery training, which appear less effective with older than with younger adults with insomnia (Friedman, Bliwise, Yesavage, & Salom, 1991; Lichstein & Johnson, 1993; Morin & Azrin, 1988). Among older adults with primary insomnia, there is little evidence that initial insomnia severity influences treatment response; however, because insomnia severity is also mediated by the presence of comorbid medical and psychiatric disorders, patients with secondary insomnia may not respond as well to treatment. One clinical replication series (Morin, Stone, McDonald, & Jones, 1994) showed that sleep improvements were similar in patients with primary and secondary insomnia, although the latter group often continued to display significant sleep disturbances even after treatment. Some studies have shown that individuals using hypnotic medications do not respond to behavioral treatment as well as unmedicated insomniacs (Morawetz, 1989; Morin & Azrin, 1988; Riedel et al., 1998). It could be, however, that lack of change in sleep (lack of deterioration) is a positive outcome for medicated individuals.

OAWI seen in clinical practice typically are treated on an individual basis, but there are as many outcome studies in which treatment was implemented in a group format as there are of individual treatment. Although there is a slight advantage in symptom reduction favoring individual therapy (Morin, Culbert, et al., 1994), there are certainly other advantages (e.g., cost-effectiveness) to implementing treatment in a group format. With the increasing popularity of self-help treatment manuals, recent studies have examined the benefits of such a treatment format for insomnia. Some studies have shown that self-help treatment is equally effective, with or without therapist guidance, for unmedicated insomniacs (Mimeault & Morin, 1999; Morawetz, 1989), although medicated participants benefited less from the self-help treatment alone. Another study conducted with older adults (Riedel et al., 1995) showed that therapist-assisted treatment yielded a more favorable outcome than self-administered treatment without therapist guidance.

Conclusions

Treating sleep problems in older adults can be a very challenging task for clinicians, but it can also be a very rewarding and successful experience. Increasing evidence shows that insomnia is treatable, even in late life. Several treatment options are available to choose from and, given the multifaceted nature of late-life sleep disturbances, clinicians do not have to and should not restrict their interventions to a single treatment modality. Multicomponent approaches should be considered to optimize therapeutic benefits. Outcome expectations may need to be adjusted to the particular circumstances (e.g., age, health status) of each older person. In addition, treatment effectiveness will vary as a function of several factors, including the nature of the intervention and the quality of its implementation. Despite significant progress made in the last decade, we must remain humble because treatment outcome for late-life insomnia is still far from ideal. Most treatment studies have focused on healthy, medication-free, and community-residing, ambulatory older adults. Much more research is needed to document the generalizability of the findings to medically ill, hypnotic-dependent, and more frail, institutionalized elderly persons.

References

Alperson, J., & Biglan, A. (1979). Self-administered treatment of sleep onset insomnia and the importance of age. *Behavior Therapy, 10,* 347-356.

Campbell, J. M., & Lancaster, J. (1988). Communicating effectively with older adults. *Family and Community Health, 11*(3), 74-85.

Carlson, C. R., & Hoyle, R. H. (1993). Efficacy of abbreviated progressive muscle relaxation training: A quantitative review of behavioral medicine research. *Journal of Consulting and Clinical Psychology, 61,* 1059-1067.

Espie, C. A., Brooks, D. N., & Lindsay, W. R. (1989). An evaluation of tailored psychological treatment of insomnia. *Journal of Behavior Therapy and Experimental Psychiatry, 20,* 143-153.

Friedman, L., Bliwise, D. L., Yesavage, J. A., & Salom, S. R. (1991). A preliminary study comparing sleep restriction and relaxation treatments for insomnia in older adults. *Journal of Gerontology, 46,* 1-8.

Glovinsky, P. B., & Spielman, A. J. (1991). Sleep restriction therapy. In P. J. Hauri (Ed.), *Case studies in insomnia* (pp. 49-63). New York: Plenum.

Hoch, C. C., Buysse, D. J., Monk, T. H., & Reynolds, C. F., III. (1992). Sleep disorders and aging. In J. E. Birren, R. B. Sloane, & G. D. Cohen (Eds.), *Handbook of mental health and aging* (2nd ed., pp. 557-581). San Diego, CA: Academic Press.

Lichstein, K. L., & Johnson, R. S. (1993). Relaxation for insomnia and hypnotic medication use in older women. *Psychology and Aging, 8,* 103-111.

Lichstein, K. L., Riedel, B. W., & Grieve, R. (1994). Fair tests of clinical trials: A treatment implementation model. *Advances in Behaviour Research and Therapy, 16,* 1-29.

Lichstein, K. L., Riedel, B. W., & Means, M. K. (1999). Psychological treatment of late-life insomnia. In R. Schulz, G. Maddox, & M. P. Lawton (Eds.), *Annual review of gerontology and geriatrics: Vol. 18. Focus on interventions research with older adults* (pp. 74-110). New York: Springer.

Lichstein, K. L., & Rosenthal, T. L. (1980). Insomniacs' perceptions of cognitive versus somatic determinants of sleep disturbance. *Journal of Abnormal Psychology, 89,* 105-107.

Mimeault, V., & Morin, C. M. (1999). Self-help treatment for insomnia: Bibliotherapy with and without professional guidance. *Journal of Consulting and Clinical Psychology, 67,* 511-517.

Morawetz, D. (1989). Behavioral self-help treatment for insomnia: A controlled evaluation. *Behavior Therapy, 20,* 365-379.

Morin, C. M., & Azrin, N. H. (1988). Behavioral and cognitive treatments of geriatric insomnia. *Journal of Consulting and Clinical Psychology, 56,* 748-753.

Morin, C. M., Culbert, J. P., & Schwartz, S. M. (1994). Nonpharmacological interventions for insomnia: A meta-analysis of treatment efficacy. *American Journal of Psychiatry, 151,* 1172-1180.

Morin, C. M., Stone, J., McDonald, K., & Jones, S. (1994). Psychological treatment of insomnia: A clinical replication series with 100 patients. *Behavior Therapy, 25,* 159-177.

Murtagh, D.R.R., & Greenwood, K. M. (1995). Identifying effective psychological treatments for insomnia: A meta-analysis. *Journal of Consulting and Clinical Psychology, 63,* 79-89.

Riedel, B. W., & Lichstein, K. L. (in press). Insomnia and daytime functioning. *Sleep Medicine Reviews.*

Riedel, B. W., Lichstein, K. L., & Dwyer, W. O. (1995). Sleep compression and sleep education for older insomniacs: Self-help vs. therapist guidance. *Psychology and Aging, 10,* 54-63.

Riedel, B. W., Lichstein, K. L., Peterson, B. A., Epperson, M. T., Means, M. K., & Aguillard, R. N. (1998). A comparison of the efficacy of stimulus control for medicated and nonmedicated insomniacs. *Behavior Modification, 22,* 3-28.

Sanavio, E. (1988). Pre-sleep cognitive intrusions and treatment of onset-insomnia. *Behaviour Research and Therapy, 26,* 451-459.

5

Sleep Hygiene

BRANT W. RIEDEL

ood sleep hygiene involves practicing behaviors that are conducive to sleep and avoiding behaviors that impede sleep. Sleep hygiene instructions for people with insomnia typically emphasize five behaviors affecting sleep: (a) caffeine consumption, (b) smoking, (c) alcohol use, (d) exercise, and (e) napping. Recommendations include eliminating caffeine consumption, smoking, and alcohol use or at least avoiding use of these sleep-disruptive substances close to bedtime. Exercise that is not too close to bedtime is encouraged, and napping is generally discouraged. In addition to these five major areas of concern, other topics that can be included under the general rubric of sleep hygiene include the following: irregular wake-up times and bedtimes, excessive amount of time in bed, and discomfort of the bed or bedroom (e.g., too hot or cold).

The International Classification of Sleep Disorders (*ICSD*; American Sleep Disorders Association, 1990) includes a diagnostic category termed Inadequate Sleep Hygiene. Inadequate Sleep Hygiene is defined as "a sleep disorder due to the performance of daily living activities that are inconsistent with the maintenance of good quality sleep and full daytime alertness" (American Sleep Disorders Association, 1990, p. 73). The diagnosis requires the presence of insomnia or excessive sleepiness and at least 1 of 11 listed behaviors that are considered poor sleep hygiene.

In clinical and research settings, sleep hygiene instruction usually is not presented alone as a treatment for insomnia but often is combined with other cognitive-behavioral strategies such as relaxation, stimulus control, and sleep restriction. The sleep hygiene treatment component generally focuses on some of or all the five major areas listed above. Other sleep-related behaviors listed in the *ICSD*'s description of Inadequate Sleep Hygiene disorder are often addressed through cognitive-behavioral treatments presented in conjunction with sleep hygiene instructions. For example, sleep restriction and stimulus control discourage excessive time in bed, and sleep restriction promotes a consistent sleep schedule. Stimulus control prevents use of the bed for activities unrelated to sleep, and relaxation therapy combats sleep-impeding mental activities (e.g., planning).

This chapter will include a separate literature review for each of the five major sleep hygiene behaviors, emphasizing studies with older adults. In addition, the few treatment studies that have included multiple sleep hygiene strategies will be reviewed. Based on the literature and clinical experience, clinical recommendations for delivering sleep hygiene instructions to older adults will be outlined. Finally, recommendations for future research will be presented.

Empirical Evidence for Sleep Hygiene Instructions

Caffeine

Caffeine is a stimulant that disrupts sleep. In their self-help book, Hauri and Linde (1991) provide useful tables detailing the amount of caffeine found in various foods, beverages, and medication. Brewed coffee, iced tea, and soft drinks average approximately 115 mg, 70 mg, and 30-60 mg of caffeine per serving respectively (Hauri & Linde, 1991). Certain pain relief medications, diuretics, and cold and allergy formulas also contain significant amounts of caffeine. Smaller amounts of caffeine are found in chocolate products such as milk chocolate (6 mg per ounce).

Caffeine consumption in the range of 100-400 mg has been shown to produce significant changes in sleep measured through polysomnography (PSG), including increased sleep latency, decreased total sleep time, increased number of awakenings and arousals, increased Stage 1 sleep, and decreased Stages 2 and 4 sleep (Bonnet & Arand, 1992; Roehrs & Roth, 1997). Bonnet and Arand (1992) found that some of these effects dissipated after a week of daily caffeine administration, but Stage 4 sleep remained reduced and number of arousals was still increased over baseline after a week of caffeine use. Multiple studies suggest that withdrawal from or reduction of caffeine use will produce immediate sleep benefits (Bonnet & Arand, 1992; Edelstein, Keaton-Brasted, & Burg, 1984; Lader, Cardwell, Shine, & Scott, 1996). One study found that on the first night after caffeine withdrawal, amount of Stage 4 sleep and number of arousals improved significantly over the previous evening (Bonnet & Arand, 1992); however, unpleasant effects such as headaches, tiredness, increased depressive symptoms, and confusion have been reported during the initial period of caffeine withdrawal (Bonnet & Arand, 1992; Lader et al., 1996).

There appears to be substantial variability in caffeine sensitivity across individuals (Nehlig, Daval, & Debry, 1992; Swift & Tiplady, 1988). In particularly sensitive adults, caffeine may continue to exert its effect up to 10 hours after consumption (Roehrs & Roth, 1997), and therefore caffeine consumed relatively early in the day could still negatively affect nighttime sleep. There is also evidence that older adults are more sensitive to the effects of caffeine (Nehlig et al., 1992; Swift & Tiplady, 1988). A decreased rate of caffeine clearance in older adults could contribute to this increased sensitivity (Schnegg & Lauterburg, 1986). In addition, psychotropic agents may produce greater effects in older adults because of increased central nervous system (CNS) receptor-site sensitivity (Salzman & Nevis-Olesen, 1992).

Furthermore, a study comparing good sleepers and poor sleepers found that after the same dosage of caffeine, poor sleepers exhibited a higher maximum saliva caffeine concentration (Tiffin, Ashton, Marsh, & Kamali, 1995). Poor sleepers also showed greater variability on measures of caffeine clearance and half-life, with a trend toward slower caffeine elimination than the good sleepers (Tiffin et al., 1995). Therefore, older adults who are poor sleepers may be especially vulnerable to the effects of caffeine.

Studies comparing the level of caffeine use between older adults with and without sleep difficulties have produced mixed results. One study of a large group of older adults found that participants who used medication containing caffeine were significantly more likely than nonusers to report difficulty falling asleep (Brown et al., 1995). Another investigation found that older adults with poor sleep reported higher levels of tea consumption than age-matched normal sleepers (Morgan, Healey, & Healey, 1989). Morgan et al. hypothesized that tea consumption could contribute to insomnia through its stimulant or diuretic properties. In contrast, other studies of older good and poor sleepers have found no difference in reported caffeine consumption between the groups (Bliwise, 1992; Libman, Creti, Amsel, Brender, & Fichten, 1997). The finding by some studies that caffeine use does not predict sleep quality may reflect the substantial variability in caffeine sensitivity across individuals.

Smoking

Epidemiological studies have provided evidence that sleep disturbance is associated with smoking. From a survey of more than 3,500 adults ages 20 to 69, Wetter and Young (1994) found that smoking was associated with difficulty initiating sleep. For males, smoking was also associated with nightmares. Another investigation of more than 400 individuals found that smokers were significantly more likely than nonsmokers to report difficulty initiating and maintaining sleep (Phillips & Danner, 1995). The authors report that the relationship between smoking and sleep difficulty was consistent across age groups, including those greater than 50 years old (Phillips & Danner, 1995). In a study focusing on older adults, Foley et al. (1995) found that being a current smoker was associated with self-reported sleep difficulties in two of the three communities surveyed. Soldatos, Kales, Scharf, Bixler, and Kales (1980) offer further evidence that smoking is associated with sleep difficulties. Comparing smokers with a matched group of nonsmokers, the investigators found that smokers spent more time awake at night and had greater difficulty initiating sleep.

Several studies have investigated the effect of smoking cessation on sleep. Studies employing self-report measures of sleep have found that nocturnal awakenings increase during the acute period after smoking cessation (Hatsukami, Hughes, Pickens, & Svikis, 1984; Hughes & Hatsukami, 1986). One study explored the effect of a 2-day smoking abstinence on several variables in younger (ages 25 to 35) and older (ages 55 to 65) females. Self-reported sleep quality decreased from the smoking phase to the abstinence phase of the study, but no age by abstinence interaction was observed (Kos, Hasenfratz, & Battig, 1997). Smoking cessation studies using objective sleep measures have produced conflicting results. Soldatos et al. (1980) found that PSG-measured sleep latency and total awake time decreased during the first few days after smoking cessation. In contrast, another investigation using PSG observed an increase in nocturnal sleep fragmentation and daytime sleepiness during an acute period of abstinence from smoking (Prosise, Bonnet, Berry, & Dickel, 1994).

Two studies have explored the sleep effects of smoking cessation with and without transdermal nicotine replacement (TNR). Wetter, Fiore, Baker, and Young (1995) randomly assigned smokers ranging in age from 20 to 65 to one of three conditions: continued smoking, quit smoking and active TNR, or quit smoking and placebo TNR. Sleep was assessed with PSG and sleep diaries at baseline and during the week immediately following cessation. Those who continued smoking showed no sleep changes across time. Individuals receiving active TNR experienced decreased sleep fragmentation and more deep sleep during the cessation period according to PSG. The active TNR group, however, self-reported increased awakenings and time awake and decreased sleep quality during the cessation period. PSG and self-report measures showed significant sleep deterioration among placebo TNR participants during smoking abstinence. The PSG sleep improvement in the active TNR group was somewhat surprising because nicotine is thought to be the mechanism by which smoking disturbs sleep. Wetter et al. hypothesized that the low, consistent dose of nicotine provided by TNR may be less disruptive of sleep than the typical smoking pattern of a large dose of nicotine prior to bedtime followed by a steep drop in blood nicotine level during the night.

Wolter et al. (1996) randomly assigned smokers attempting cessation to one of three doses of active TNR or a placebo TNR group. Each group participated in a 1-week inpatient smoking cessation treatment program. Immediately following the inpatient program, placebo TNR was switched to active TNR, and all groups participated in 7 more weeks of outpatient TNR treatment before TNR was withdrawn. Wrist actigraphy was used to assess sleep during baseline, inpatient treatment, the last week of TNR, the first week off TNR, and 6-month follow-up. No significant change in sleep efficiency from baseline was observed at any assessment point. These results contrast with two findings of Wetter et al. (1995): (a) smoking cessation without TNR produces sleep deterioration, and (b) smoking cessation with TNR results in sleep improvement.

Most studies have addressed only the acute effects of smoking cessation. The exception is Wolter et al.'s study, which included a 6-month follow-up. These results suggest that smoking cessation has no long-term effect on sleep. Epidemiological data suggest that smoking cessation may have positive long-term sleep effects. Wetter and Young (1994) found that self-reported sleep of former smokers did not differ from those who had never smoked, but former smokers reported significantly better sleep than current smokers. There is a lack of studies of smoking and sleep that focus on older adults; however, the studies that have included older and younger adults have generally found no age-related differences (Kos et al., 1997; Phillips & Danner, 1995).

Alcohol

Survey data suggest that many older adults use alcohol to cope with sleep difficulties (Johnson, 1997). Empirical studies, however, indicate that alcohol is harmful rather than helpful to sleep. In nonalcoholic sleepers, bedtime alcohol use decreases sleep latency but increases wakefulness during the latter part of the sleep period (Roehrs & Roth, 1997). Increased wakefulness and increased REM sleep during the second half of the sleep period are probably a rebound effect resulting after ethanol has been eliminated from the body (Roehrs & Roth, 1997). In individuals with alcoholism, sleep disruption tends to increase over time, and sleep disruption may continue for several weeks or months during periods of abstinence (Le Bon et al., 1997; Roehrs & Roth, 1997; Williams & Rundell, 1981).

Alcohol use also may fragment sleep by producing sleep-disordered breathing. Studies have shown that alcohol consumption increases the frequency of apneas and hypopneas during the sleep of older and younger adults (Guilleminault, Silvestri, Mondini, & Coburn, 1984; Mitler, Dawson, Henriksen, Sobers, & Bloom, 1988; Scrima, Broudy, Nay, & Cohn, 1982). In addition to the acute effects of alcohol, chronic alcohol abuse may contribute to sleep-disordered breathing. During abstinence, older males with alcoholism show greater oxygen desaturation during sleep than nonalcoholic males in the same age group (Vitiello et al., 1987). Another study found a relationship between alcohol consumption and periodic limb movements during sleep (PLMS). In a sample of sleep clinic patients, clinically significant PLMS was more likely to be observed in individuals who consumed at least two alcoholic beverages a day than in participants who drank less than two alcoholic beverages a day (Aldrich & Shipley, 1993); however, the causal direction of the relationship between alcohol and PLMS cannot be determined from this study.

Exercise

An early narrative review of the sleep and exercise literature suggested that exercise is associated with increased deep sleep (Torsvall, 1981), but a more recent narrative review concluded that the majority of studies have not found a relationship between deep sleep and exercise (Trinder, Montgomery, & Paxton, 1988). A recent meta-analysis found statistically significant but modest increases in deep sleep and total sleep time following acute exercise (Youngstedt, O'Connor, & Dishman, 1997). In comparison to control groups, the median increase in deep sleep and total sleep time was 1.4 min and 10 min respectively after exercise (Youngstedt et al., 1997). The timing of exercise appears to be critical. Torsvall's review suggested that exercise close to bedtime produced increased wakefulness. Similarly, Youngstedt et al. found that exercise 4-8 hours prior to bedtime was associated with decreased sleep latency and wake time after sleep onset, whereas exercise within 4 hours of bedtime was linked to increased sleep latency and less improvement for wake time after sleep onset.

Few studies of exercise and sleep have focused on older adults, and therefore results from literature reviews may or may not generalize to older adults. One study of older normal sleepers used PSG to examine sleep in physically fit and sedentary males following acute exercise and no exercise. A main effect was found for fitness, with physically fit participants exhibiting shorter sleep latencies, less wake time after sleep onset, less Stage 1 sleep, and more slow waves suggestive of deep sleep (Edinger et al., 1993). No significant results were found for the exercise versus no exercise comparison or the interaction of exercise condition and fitness status. Because of the cross-sectional design of the study, a causal relationship between fitness and sleep quality cannot be assumed.

Two longitudinal studies have examined the sleep effects of a structured exercise program on older normal sleepers. Vitiello, Prinz, and Schwartz (1994) randomly assigned older adults to an aerobic training condition or a control group that received stretching/flexibility training. After the 6-month training period, only participants in the aerobic training condition showed a significant increase in Stages 3 and 4 sleep. Neither group improved on other sleep variables such as total sleep time, sleep latency, or sleep efficiency. Another research group randomly assigned healthy older adults to a 9-month low- or moderate-intensity exercise program. At the end of the exercise program, both exercise groups self-reported significant sleep improvement over baseline, but no control group was included for comparison purposes (Stevenson & Topp, 1990).

Other studies have focused on the impact of exercise on older adults with sleep complaints. Singh, Clements, and Fiatarone (1997) randomly assigned older adults with depression or dysthymia to a 10-week program of progressive resistance training or a control group. Most participants reported poor sleep at baseline, and participants in the exercise group showed significantly more subjective sleep improvement than the control group at the end of the study. Improvement in an individual's Geriatric Depression Scale score was a significant predictor of improved sleep, suggesting the possibility that exercise may have indirectly improved sleep by reducing depressive symptoms. Another exercise study focused on older adults with moderate sleep complaints and no psychiatric disorder accounting for the sleep complaints (King, Oman, Brassington, Bliwise, & Haskell, 1997). In comparison to control group participants, individuals assigned to a 16-week exercise program self-reported greater improvement in sleep quality, sleep latency, and sleep duration, which increased by nearly an hour over baseline. Significant exercise versus control group sleep differences that were observed after 16 weeks were not evident after 8 weeks, suggesting that a substantial period of regular exercise may be necessary for sleep improvement (King et al., 1997).

In summary, research focusing on older adults suggests significant sleep benefits resulting from exercise. A consistent finding of the current literature is that an acute period of exercise cannot be expected to have a substantial sleep benefit (Edinger et al., 1993; King et al., 1997; Youngstedt et al., 1997). Fitness appears to be a better predictor of good sleep, and therefore establishing an ongoing exercise routine that increases fitness may produce significant sleep improvement (King et al., 1997; Stevenson & Topp, 1990; Vitiello et al., 1994).

Napping

Napping is prevalent in older adults. In one survey of older adults, the majority of participants indicated that they habitually napped during the day (Hohagen et al., 1994), and an epidemiological study of older adults found that approximately 25% reported getting so sleepy during the day or evening that they had to take a nap (Foley et al., 1995). A study directly comparing napping behavior in older and younger adults found that older adults took more daytime naps (Buysse et al., 1992). Studies to date have produced mixed results regarding whether older adults are sleepier during the day than younger adults, and therefore age-related increases in napping could be due to factors other than excessive sleepiness, such as social changes (e.g., retirement) (Bliwise, 1993).

Multiple studies have compared napping behavior in older good and poor sleepers. Several of these studies have found no relationship between nocturnal sleep variables and tendency to nap during the day (Bliwise, 1992; Hohagen et al., 1994; Morgan et al., 1989). In contrast, other studies of older adults have found that frequent nappers are more likely to have nighttime sleep complaints (Hays, Blazer, & Foley, 1996) and that napping duration is negatively correlated with nocturnal sleep duration (Beh, 1994). The cross-sectional nature of these studies, however, prevents one from making causal conclusions regarding a relationship between napping and nocturnal sleep.

A few studies have experimentally manipulated napping behavior to examine its impact on nighttime sleep. One study included 16 older adults without sleep complaints and compared PSG-measured nocturnal sleep after no daytime nap and following a 1-hour afternoon (3:15 to 4:15 p.m.) nap opportunity. No significant difference in nocturnal sleep variables was found between the no nap and the afternoon nap conditions (Aber & Webb, 1986). Three studies with younger adults have compared a no nap condition to a late afternoon or early evening 2-hour nap

opportunity, and each of these studies found that the nap opportunity resulted in a significant reduction in Stage 4 sleep at night (Feinberg et al.,
1985; Karacan, Williams, Finley, & Hursch, 1970; Werth, Dijk,
Achermann, & Borbely, 1996). Karacan et al. also found that nocturnal
Stage 4 sleep was reduced after a condition that provided both a 1-hour
morning nap opportunity and a 1-hour afternoon nap opportunity. The
remaining two studies observed that in comparison to the no nap condition, sleep after the 2-hour nap opportunity was characterized by a longer sleep onset latency and shorter total sleep time (Feinberg et al., 1985;
Werth et al., 1996).

The reason for the discrepancy between the findings of Aber and
Webb (1986) and the remaining studies is not clear. One possibility is that
daytime naps have less of an effect on the nocturnal sleep of older adults
as compared to younger adults. This attenuated impact of napping on
nocturnal sleep could represent a floor effect. Older adults already experience reduced Stage 4 sleep at night, so there is limited room for further
reduction of deep sleep after a nap. Another explanation is that the
shorter nap opportunity in Aber and Webb's study prevented the disruptive sleep effects observed in the other studies. Unfortunately, all
these studies focused on individuals without sleep complaints, raising
the question of whether these results can be generalized to people with
insomnia.

Multicomponent Sleep Hygiene Interventions

A limited number of studies have evaluated a sleep hygiene treatment
package consisting of several sleep hygiene recommendations (e.g., reduce caffeine, nicotine, and alcohol). A treatment study involving a
mixed-age sample (range = 28-75 years) compared sleep hygiene instruction alone to stimulus control treatment plus sleep hygiene and meditation treatment plus sleep hygiene (Schoicket, Bertelson, & Lacks, 1988).
The sleep hygiene treatment included instructions regarding alcohol,
caffeine, exercise, napping, nonspecific relaxing behavior at bedtime,
not going to bed hungry, and bedroom comfort. Significant improvement was observed in all three treatment groups, but no significant difference was observed between groups for wake time after sleep onset or
number of awakenings. However, despite comparable quantitative
sleep maintenance improvement, the participants using sleep hygiene

alone were more likely than the other two groups to still consider themselves to have insomnia after treatment.

There are 15 published studies evaluating cognitive-behavioral insomnia treatment that have focused on older adults (see Lichstein, Riedel, & Means, 1999, for a review). Four of these studies reported using sleep hygiene instructions in their treatment packages (Engle-Friedman, Bootzin, Hazlewood, & Tsao, 1992; Friedman, Bliwise, Yesavage, & Salom, 1991; Morin, Colecchi, Ling, & Sood, 1995; Morin, Kowatch, Barry, & Walton, 1993), but only one study isolated sleep hygiene from other cognitive-behavioral treatments (Engle-Friedman et al., 1992). Engle-Friedman et al. (1992) randomly assigned participants to one of four groups: (a) support and sleep hygiene; (b) support, sleep hygiene, and progressive relaxation; (c) support, sleep hygiene, and stimulus control; or (d) a measurement control group. The sleep hygiene and support group produced positive initial treatment gains relative to the measurement control group. Feeling refreshed upon awakening improved across time for the sleep hygiene plus support group and the relaxation group but not the measurement control group. Also, the sleep hygiene plus support group and the relaxation group reported significantly more restful sleep than the control group at 3-week follow-up. There was evidence, however, that the addition of relaxation or stimulus control to sleep hygiene instruction produced better long-term results on certain sleep variables. At 2-year follow-up, the relaxation group reported feeling more refreshed in the morning than the remaining groups, and the stimulus control group reported the highest sleep quality and the shortest sleep latency among the groups (Engle-Friedman et al., 1992).

Clinical Recommendations

Assessment

The assessment process should begin with a thorough clinical interview. During this interview, detailed information can be obtained regarding sleep hygiene issues. For example, if the patient uses alcohol, questions would address how much alcohol is being used, how often it is being consumed, and what time of day it is being used. Because global self-report provided during a clinical interview could contain errors, the patient should be asked to monitor sleep and sleep hygiene behavior on a daily basis for 1 to 2 weeks. Hauri and Linde (1991) suggest completing a sleep diary and a day log simultaneously. The sleep diary contains standard questions such as going to bed and arising time, time to fall asleep, and time awake during the night. The day log contains a row for each day of the week and a column for each sleep-related behavior a patient would like to explore. For example, a patient could monitor caffeine use and exercise. On a daily basis, the patient would make detailed notes in the day log regarding timing and amount of caffeine use and exercise. The day log would then be compared with sleep diary data to ascertain any relationships between daytime behaviors and nighttime sleep.

The day log/sleep diary method is probably ideal for documenting a relationship between lifestyle factors and sleep quality; however, a lack of adherence to the day log requirements may occur in some patients because the day log requires detailed documentation on a daily basis. For these patients, adherence to the assessment procedure may be enhanced by substituting a simple checklist of sleep hygiene behaviors for the day log. An example of a sleep hygiene checklist is provided in Figure 5.1. The patient simply checks the sleep hygiene–related behaviors that were followed each day for a 2-week period. The checklist can then be compared with 2 weeks of sleep diaries to determine if particular behaviors are affecting sleep quality. Assessment of sleep and sleep hygiene practices should continue throughout the treatment period to determine adherence to treatment recommendations and the effectiveness of particular recommendations.

Treatment

A good method for starting sleep hygiene treatment is to provide the patient with a handout that lists basic sleep hygiene rules and the rationale behind each rule. If a handout is used, it is important that the handout be presented in a manner that tailors treatment to the individual patient. Components of sleep hygiene instruction that are helpful for one individual will not be valuable for others (Hauri, 1991). Using baseline assessment results as a guide, the clinician can discuss the handout with the patient, emphasizing behaviors that seem to be particularly problematic for the patient. Any questions that arise can be addressed at this

SLEEP HYGIENE CHECKLIST

Name _____

Please record each day's date along the top row. For each day, please check the instructions that you followed. For instructions that you did not follow, leave the appropriate space blank.

Date	(1)	(2)	(3)	(4)	(5)	(6)	(7)
1. Avoid caffeine after noon							
2. Avoid naps past noon							
3. Avoid exercise within 2 hr of bedtime							
4. Avoid smoking within 2 hr of bedtime							
5. Avoid alcohol within 2 hr of bedtime							
6. Avoid heavy meals within 2 hr of bedtime							

Date	(8)	(9)	(10)	(11)	(12)	(13)	(14)
1. Avoid caffeine after noon							
2. Avoid naps past noon							
3. Avoid exercise within 2 hr of bedtime							
4. Avoid smoking within 2 hr of bedtime							
5. Avoid alcohol within 2 hr of bedtime							
6. Avoid heavy meals within 2 hr of bedtime							

Figure 5.1. Sleep Hygiene Checklist for Recording Daily Adherence to Sleep Hygiene Instructions

point, and patients will have a written document that they can take home and refer to in the future when necessary.

In some cases, a patient will generally practice good sleep hygiene and only one or two behaviors will need to be addressed. In other cases, multiple lifestyle factors may need to be modified. If the patient is not willing to modify a number of behaviors simultaneously, the clinician will be forced to make decisions regarding the sequencing of these modifications. Also, it may be desirable to introduce behavioral changes one at a time rather than simultaneously to allow the clinician and patient to determine which behavioral changes are having a positive sleep impact. Based on the literature and clinical experience, the following sequencing of sleep hygiene components is recommended.

Alcohol and caffeine reduction. Alcohol and caffeine reduction is recommended as an ideal first step because this could produce an immediate, positive impact on sleep. In contrast, beginning an exercise program may not show immediate effects (King et al., 1997), and smoking cessation may have a detrimental impact on sleep initially (Prosise et al., 1994). If immediate gains are not acquired or short-term sleep deterioration occurs, the patient could lose faith in behavioral approaches, and adherence to future recommendations could be reduced. Although beginning an exercise program is not expected to produce immediate gains, moving exercise that is too close to bedtime should be considered early in treatment along with alcohol and caffeine reduction.

If chronic alcohol abuse is suspected, this problem should receive immediate attention; however, the patient and clinician should not expect immediate sleep improvement even if the alcohol abuser becomes abstinent (Williams & Rundell, 1981). For patients who are not abusing alcohol but are habitually using alcohol close to bedtime, the sleep outlook is more positive. To ensure adherence by the patient, the clinician must provide a good rationale for eliminating a bedtime alcoholic beverage. Most patients have probably observed that alcohol tends to decrease their sleep onset latency; therefore, the clinician must emphasize the detrimental impact of alcohol on sleep maintenance. One way of emphasizing this relationship is to use the patient's sleep diaries and sleep hygiene questionnaire to demonstrate a correlation between alcohol use and sleep maintenance and sleep quality problems. Because sleep maintenance difficulty rather than sleep initiation problems is the most frequent complaint among older sleepers, this rationale may be especially relevant to their concerns. Also, patients should be made aware that they may develop a tolerance to the sleep initiation effects of alcohol, leaving only its detrimental effects. The relationship between alcohol and sleep-disordered breathing should also be discussed.

In contrast to eliminating or reducing alcohol, eliminating caffeine close to bedtime may not be sufficient. Because of the variability in sensitivity to caffeine and the decreased clearance rate in older adults, caffeine use much earlier in the day may still affect sleep. If a patient is willing to eliminate caffeine altogether, this is ideal. Noncaffeinated versions of coffee, tea, and soft drinks can be substituted for caffeinated beverages. The clinician should be sure that the patient is aware that some medications contain caffeine. If the patient is using prescribed medications containing caffeine, the clinician and patient can work with the prescribing physician to find acceptable substitute medications that are caffeine free.

Other patients may demand a less dramatic or more gradual withdrawal schedule. For these patients, caffeine use in the late afternoon or early evening should be eliminated first. Later, any caffeine use after noon can be eliminated. When providing a rationale for caffeine reduction, it should be emphasized that a vicious cycle can develop involving caffeine and sleep disruption. Some caffeine users will consume caffeine in an attempt to maintain alertness after a poor night of sleep. This caffeine consumption may lead to another poor night of sleep, which tempts one to use caffeine the next day. Breaking this cycle may lead to better nighttime sleep and improved daytime functioning.

Elimination of napping. Focusing on napping is the next recommended step. Elimination of napping could also produce an immediate sleep benefit, but the empirical support for this benefit is less convincing than the literature on alcohol and caffeine and sleep. Studies of younger adults indicate that napping disrupts nocturnal sleep. In older adults, a consistent relationship between napping and nocturnal sleep disruption has not been found. There may be a great deal of variability across patients, with napping negatively affecting the sleep of some individuals but not others. Hauri (1993) reports that a minority of patients will actually sleep better on a night following a short nap. Patients should be encouraged to experiment with reducing naps while simultaneously observing the effect on nighttime sleep.

Timing and duration of naps appears to be important. If a patient is unwilling to eliminate napping altogether, he or she should be encouraged to avoid long naps and naps in the late afternoon or early evening. A nap opportunity should not last more than 30 minutes. Many individuals experience an increased level of sleepiness in the mid- to late afternoon (Haimov & Lavie, 1997), and it can be tempting to nap during this period. Unlike younger adults, who are often prevented from afternoon napping by their occupations, older adults who are retired may have difficulty fighting the urge to nap. To combat this urge to nap, the clinician and patient can discuss planned activities that the older adult can engage in during this "high risk" period to prevent napping.

Begin an exercise program. Exercise should be introduced to the patient as a long-term rather than short-term strategy for improving sleep. Improved fitness based on a habitual exercise program is the ultimate goal. To improve adherence to this recommendation, the clinician will want to emphasize that a strenuous program of exercise is not required. Instead, commitment to a moderate- or low-intensity exercise program for several months may produce substantial sleep gains. Prior to embarking on an exercise program, the patient should be required to submit to a thorough physical examination to determine if particular exercise protocols are contraindicated. In designing an exercise program for sleep improvement, a crucial component to consider is the timing of exercise. The exercise literature suggests that 4-8 hours prior to bedtime is the optimal exercise time (Youngstedt et al., 1997). The interventions that have been shown to be helpful for older adults have generally involved 30-60 minute exercise sessions three or four times per week for at least 10 weeks (King et al., 1997; Singh et al., 1997; Stevenson & Topp, 1990; Vitiello et al., 1994). A variety of exercises have shown beneficial sleep results, including progressive resistance training, low-impact aerobics combined with brisk walking or stationary cycling, and stationary cycling combined with slow walking. An exercise program therefore can be individually tailored to match the patient's preferences. Because the exercise program will require long-term adherence, strategies that improve exercise adherence such as enlisting social support (e.g., spouse participates also) (Wallace, Raglin, & Jastremski, 1995) should be incorporated into the overall plan.

Smoking cessation. In contrast to other sleep hygiene strategies that may immediately help sleep or have no immediate impact on sleep, smoking cessation may initially disrupt sleep (Kos et al., 1997; Prosise et al., 1994; Wetter et al., 1995). The patient therefore should be warned of a possible acute period of sleep disruption before sleep improves. There is evidence that use of transdermal nicotine replacement can combat the initial sleep-disruptive effects of cessation, so this strategy should be considered (Wetter et al., 1995); however, although objective sleep measures improved, participants using TNR still subjectively experienced sleep deterioration during smoking cessation (Wetter et al., 1995). Referral to a supportive smoking cessation group may be helpful. For patients who are unwilling to give up smoking, some sleep benefit may be derived from eliminating smoking close to bedtime. Patients can experiment with not smoking within 2 hours of bedtime and document the effects of this strategy on sleep.

Other strategies. Hauri (1991) suggests other sleep hygiene–related strategies such as hiding the bedroom clock and eating a light bedtime snack. The bedroom clock may become a source of anxiety when individuals with insomnia check the clock and think about how long they have been awake and how little time is left before their scheduled arising time. In a sleep clinic sample of people with insomnia, 40% reported that hiding their bedroom clock was a helpful strategy after 1 month of treatment (Hauri, 1993). A light bedtime snack (e.g., cheese and crackers) will help some patients by eliminating hunger and possibly inducing sleepiness; however, a large meal or spicy food close to bedtime could disrupt sleep and should be avoided. Passive body heating via a warm bath late in the afternoon or early in the evening appears to have a beneficial effect on sleep (Horne & Reid, 1985). For those patients who have a highly variable sleep schedule at baseline, establishing consistent bedtimes and waking times may be helpful (Hauri, 1993).

Future Research Recommendations

First, more research focusing on older adults is needed. Most sleep hygiene studies to date have included younger samples or mixed-age samples. Clinical experience suggests that sleep complaints differ between older and younger adults (i.e., more maintenance versus initiation complaints in older adults). Also, age-related physiological changes could influence the relationship between sleep hygiene behaviors and sleep. Specifically, older adults show a reduced rate of metabolism and clearance for many psychotropic drugs, and increased CNS receptor-site sensitivity can alter the effects of psychotropic agents. The sleep effects of caffeine, nicotine, and alcohol found in younger samples therefore may not generalize to older adults.

Second, further study is needed on people with insomnia. Much sleep hygiene–related research has examined normal sleepers. For example, the experimental studies that have examined the relationship between napping and nocturnal sleep have excluded people with insomnia. Similarly, the majority of empirical data regarding exercise's impact on sleep is based on normal sleepers. It may be inappropriate to generalize results from normal sleepers to people with insomnia.

Third, future studies should document the long-term outcome of sleep hygiene strategies. Although several researchers have studied the acute effects of smoking cessation, little information exists regarding the long-term effects of abstinence from smoking. Also, what are the long-term effects of recommendations to exercise? Do older adults continue to adhere to exercise recommendations 2 or 3 years later, and does exercise continue to positively affect sleep quality at this point? In addition, the role of sleep hygiene instructions in the overall insomnia treatment picture should be explored. Can sleep hygiene instructions alone produce significant sleep benefits in older adults with insomnia? Does the addition of sleep hygiene instructions to other cognitive-behavioral treatments improve outcome? Are there certain sleep hygiene instructions that are more beneficial to older adults with insomnia and consequently should be emphasized during treatment?

In conclusion, the current sleep hygiene literature provides the clinician with basic treatment guidelines. Future sleep hygiene studies that focus on older adults with insomnia and include a long-term follow-up would broaden the knowledge base that clinicians can use to design effective treatment approaches.

References

Aber, R., & Webb, W. B. (1986). Effects of a limited nap on night sleep in older subjects. *Psychology and Aging, 1*, 300-302.

Aldrich, M. S., & Shipley, J. E. (1993). Alcohol use and periodic limb movements of sleep. *Alcoholism: Clinical and Experimental Research, 17*, 192-196.

American Sleep Disorders Association. (1990). *The International Classification of Sleep Disorders: Diagnostic and coding manual*. Rochester, MN: Author.

Beh, H. C. (1994). A survey of daytime napping in an elderly Australian population. *Australian Journal of Psychology, 46*, 100-106.

Bliwise, D. L. (1993). Sleep in normal aging and dementia. *Sleep, 16*, 40-81.

Bliwise, N. G. (1992). Factors related to sleep quality in healthy elderly women. *Psychology and Aging, 7*, 83-88.

Bonnet, M. H., & Arand, D. L. (1992). Caffeine use as a model of acute and chronic insomnia. *Sleep, 15*, 526-536.

Brown, S. L., Salive, M. E., Pahor, M., Foley, D. J., Corti, M. C., Langlois, J. A., Wallace, R. B., & Harris, T. B. (1995). Occult caffeine as a source of sleep problems in an older population. *Journal of the American Geriatrics Society, 43*, 860-864.

Buysse, D. J., Browman, K. E., Monk, T. H., Reynolds, C. F., III, Fasiczka, A. L., & Kupfer, D. J. (1992). Napping and 24-hour sleep/wake patterns in healthy elderly and young adults. *Journal of the American Geriatrics Society, 40*, 779-786.

Edelstein, B. A., Keaton-Brasted, C., & Burg, M. M. (1984). Effects of caffeine withdrawal on nocturnal enuresis, insomnia, and behavior restraints. *Journal of Consulting and Clinical Psychology, 52*, 857-862.

Edinger, J. D., Morey, M. C., Sullivan, R. J., Higginbotham, M. B., Marsh, G. R., Dailey, D. S., & McCall, W. V. (1993). Aerobic fitness, acute exercise and sleep in older men. *Sleep, 16*, 351-359.

Engle-Friedman, M., Bootzin, R. R., Hazlewood, L., & Tsao, C. (1992). An evaluation of behavioral treatments for insomnia in the older adult. *Journal of Clinical Psychology, 48*, 77-90.

Feinberg, I., March, J. D., Floyd, T. C., Jimison, R., Bossom-Demitrack, L., & Katz, P. H. (1985). Homeostatic changes during post-nap sleep maintain baseline levels of delta EEG. *Electroencephalography and Clinical Neurophysiology, 61*, 134-137.

Foley, D. J., Monjan, A. A., Brown, S. L., Simonsick, E. M., Wallace, R. B., & Blazer, D. G. (1995). Sleep complaints among elderly persons: An epidemiologic study of three communities. *Sleep, 18*, 425-432.

Friedman, L., Bliwise, D. L., Yesavage, J. A., & Salom, S. R. (1991). A preliminary study comparing sleep restriction and relaxation treatments for insomnia in older adults. *Journal of Gerontology, 46*, P1-P8.

Guilleminault, C., Silvestri, R., Mondini, S., & Coburn, S. (1984). Aging and sleep apnea: Action of benzodiazepine, acetazolamide, alcohol, and sleep deprivation in a healthy elderly group. *Journal of Gerontology, 39*, 655-661.

Haimov, I., & Lavie, P. (1997). Circadian characteristics of sleep propensity function in healthy elderly: A comparison with young adults. *Sleep, 20*, 294-300.

Hatsukami, D. K., Hughes, J. R., Pickens, R. W., & Svikis, D. (1984). Tobacco withdrawal symptoms: An experimental analysis. *Psychopharmacology, 84*, 231-236.

Hauri, P. J. (1991). Sleep hygiene, relaxation therapy, and cognitive interventions. In P. J. Hauri (Ed.), *Case studies in insomnia* (pp. 65-84). New York: Plenum.

Hauri, P. J. (1993). Consulting about insomnia: A method and some preliminary data. *Sleep, 16*, 344-350.

Hauri, P. J., & Linde, S. (1991). *No more sleepless nights.* New York: Wiley.

Hays, J. C., Blazer, D. G., & Foley, D. J. (1996). Risk of napping: Excessive daytime sleepiness and mortality in an older community population. *Journal of the American Geriatrics Society, 44*, 693-698.

Hohagen, F., Kappler, C., Schramm, E., Rink, K., Weyerer, S., Riemann, D., & Berger, M. (1994). Prevalence of insomnia in elderly general practice attenders and the current treatment modalities. *Acta Psychiatrica Scandinavica, 90*, 102-108.

Horne, J. A., & Reid, A. J. (1985). Night-time sleep EEG changes following body heating in a warm bath. *Electroencephalography and Clinical Neurophysiology, 60*, 154-157.

Hughes, J. R., & Hatsukami, D. (1986). Signs and symptoms of tobacco withdrawal. *Archives of General Psychiatry, 43*, 289-294.

Johnson, J. E. (1997). Insomnia, alcohol, and over-the-counter drug use in old-old urban women. *Journal of Community Health Nursing, 14*, 181-188.

Karacan, I., Williams, R. L., Finley, W. W., & Hursch, C. J. (1970). The effects of naps on nocturnal sleep: Influence on the need for stage-1 REM and stage 4 sleep. *Biological Psychiatry, 2*, 391-399.

King, A. C., Oman, R. F., Brassington, G. S., Bliwise, D. L., & Haskell, W. L. (1997). Moderate-intensity exercise and self-rated quality of sleep in older adults: A randomized controlled trial. *Journal of the American Medical Association, 277*, 32-37.

Kos, J., Hasenfratz, M., & Battig, K. (1997). Effects of 2-day abstinence from smoking on dietary, cognitive, subjective, and physiologic parameters among younger and older female smokers. *Physiology and Behavior, 61*, 671-678.

Lader, M., Cardwell, C., Shine, P., & Scott, N. (1996). Caffeine withdrawal symptoms and rate of metabolism. *Journal of Psychopharmacology, 10*, 110-118.

Le Bon, O., Verbanck, P., Hoffmann, G., Murphy, J. R., Staner, L., De Groote, D., Mampunza, S., Den Dulk, A., Vacher, C., Kornreich, C., & Pelc, I. (1997). Sleep in detoxified alcoholics: Impairment of most standard sleep parameters and increased risk for sleep apnea, but not for myoclonias—A controlled study. *Journal of Studies on Alcohol, 58*, 30-36.

Libman, E., Creti, L., Amsel, R., Brender, W., & Fichten, C. S. (1997). What do older good and poor sleepers do during periods of nocturnal wakefulness? The sleep behaviors scale: 60+. *Psychology and Aging, 12*, 170-182.

Lichstein, K. L., Riedel, B. W., & Means, M. K. (1999). Psychological treatment of late-life insomnia. In R. Schulz, G. Maddox, & M. P. Lawton (Eds.), *Annual review of gerontology and geriatrics: Vol. 18. Focus on interventions research with older adults* (pp. 74-110). New York: Springer.

Mitler, M. M., Dawson, A., Henriksen, S. J., Sobers, M., & Bloom, F. E. (1988). Bedtime ethanol increases resistance of upper airways and produces sleep apneas in asymptomatic snorers. *Alcoholism: Clinical and Experimental Research, 12*, 801-805.

Morgan, K., Healey, D. W., & Healey, P. J. (1989). Factors influencing persistent subjective insomnia in old age: A follow-up study of good and poor sleepers aged 65 to 74. *Age and Ageing, 18*, 117-122.

Morin, C. M., Colecchi, C. A., Ling, W. D., & Sood, R. K. (1995). Cognitive behavior therapy to facilitate benzodiazepine discontinuation among hypnotic-dependent patients with insomnia. *Behavior Therapy, 26*, 733-745.

Morin, C. M., Kowatch, R. A., Barry, T., & Walton, E. (1993). Cognitive-behavior therapy for late-life insomnia. *Journal of Consulting and Clinical Psychology, 61*, 137-146.

Nehlig, A., Daval, J., & Debry, G. (1992). Caffeine and the central nervous system: Mechanisms of action, biochemical, metabolic and psychostimulant effects. *Brain Research Reviews, 17,* 139-170.

Phillips, B. A., & Danner, F. J. (1995). Cigarette smoking and sleep disturbance. *Archives of Internal Medicine, 155,* 734-737.

Prosise, G. L., Bonnet, M. H., Berry, R. B., & Dickel, M. J. (1994). Effects of abstinence from smoking on sleep and daytime sleepiness. *Chest, 105,* 1136-1141.

Roehrs, T., & Roth, T. (1997). Hypnotics, alcohol, and caffeine: Relation to insomnia. In M. R. Pressman & W. C. Orr (Eds.), *Understanding sleep: The evaluation and treatment of sleep disorders* (pp. 339-355). Washington, DC: American Psychological Association.

Salzman, C., & Nevis-Olesen, J. (1992). Psychopharmacologic treatment. In J. E. Birren, R. B. Sloane, & G. D. Cohen (Eds.), *Handbook of mental health and aging* (2nd ed., pp. 721-762). San Diego, CA: Academic Press.

Schnegg, M., & Lauterburg, B. H. (1986). Quantitative liver function in the elderly assessed by galactose elimination capacity, aminopyrine demethylation and caffeine clearance. *Journal of Hepatology, 3,* 164-171.

Schoicket, S. L., Bertelson, A. D., & Lacks, P. (1988). Is sleep hygiene a sufficient treatment for sleep-maintenance insomnia? *Behavior Therapy, 19,* 183-190.

Scrima, L., Broudy, M., Nay, K. N., & Cohn, M. A. (1982). Increased severity of obstructive sleep apnea after bedtime alcohol ingestion: Diagnostic potential and proposed mechanism of action. *Sleep, 5,* 318-328.

Singh, N. A., Clements, K. M., & Fiatarone, M. A. (1997). A randomized controlled trial of the effect of exercise on sleep. *Sleep, 20,* 95-101.

Soldatos, C. R., Kales, J. D., Scharf, M. B., Bixler, E. O., & Kales, A. (1980). Cigarette smoking associated with sleep difficulty. *Science, 207,* 551-552.

Stevenson, J. S., & Topp, R. (1990). Effects of moderate and low intensity long-term exercise by older adults. *Research in Nursing and Health, 13,* 209-218.

Swift, C. G., & Tiplady, B. (1988). The effects of age on the response to caffeine. *Psychopharmacology, 94,* 29-31.

Tiffin, P., Ashton, H., Marsh, R., & Kamali, F. (1995). Pharmacokinetic and pharmacodynamic responses to caffeine in poor and normal sleepers. *Psychopharmacology, 121,* 494-502.

Torsvall, L. (1981). Sleep after exercise: A literature review. *Journal of Sports Medicine and Physical Fitness, 21,* 218-225.

Trinder, J., Montgomery, I., & Paxton, S. J. (1988). The effect of exercise on sleep: The negative view. *Acta Physiologica Scandinavica, 133*(Suppl. 574), 14-20.

Vitiello, M. V., Prinz, P. N., Personius, J. P., Nuccio, M. A., Ries, R. K., & Koerker, R. M. (1987). History of chronic alcohol abuse is associated with increased nighttime hypoxemia in older men. *Alcoholism: Clinical and Experimental Research, 11,* 368-371.

Vitiello, M. V., Prinz, P. N., & Schwartz, R. S. (1994, June). *Slow wave sleep but not overall sleep quality of healthy older men and women is improved by increased aerobic fitness.* Paper presented at the meeting of the Association of Professional Sleep Societies, Boston.

Wallace, J. P., Raglin, J. S., & Jastremski, C. A. (1995). Twelve month adherence of adults who joined a fitness program with a spouse vs. without a spouse. *The Journal of Sports Medicine and Physical Fitness, 35,* 206-213.

Werth, E., Dijk, D., Achermann, P., & Borbely, A. A. (1996). Dynamics of the sleep EEG after an early evening nap: Experimental data and simulations. *American Journal of Physiology, 271,* R501-R510.

Wetter, D. W., Fiore, M. C., Baker, T. B., & Young, T. B. (1995). Tobacco withdrawal and nicotine replacement influence objective measures of sleep. *Journal of Consulting and Clinical Psychology, 63*, 658-667.

Wetter, D. W., & Young, T. B. (1994). The relation between cigarette smoking and sleep disturbance. *Preventive Medicine, 23*, 328-334.

Williams, H. L., & Rundell, O. H., Jr. (1981). Altered sleep physiology in chronic alcoholics: Reversal with abstinence. *Alcoholism: Clinical and Experimental Research, 5*, 318-325.

Wolter, T. D., Hauri, P. J., Schroeder, D. R., Wisbey, J. A., Croghan, I. T., Offord, K. P., Dale, L. C., & Hurt, R. D. (1996). Effects of 24-hr nicotine replacement on sleep and daytime activity during smoking cessation. *Preventive Medicine, 25*, 601-610.

Youngstedt, S. D., O'Connor, P. J., & Dishman, R. K. (1997). The effects of acute exercise on sleep: A quantitative synthesis. *Sleep, 20*, 203-214.

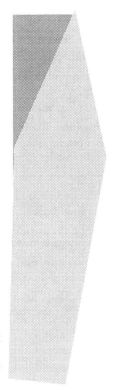

6

Sleep
Restriction
Therapy

WILLIAM K. WOHLGEMUTH
JACK D. EDINGER

S leep restriction therapy (SRT) is a behavioral insomnia therapy wherein sleep improvements are
achieved primarily by limiting/restricting the time allotted for sleep
each night. As noted herein, this simple, straightforward technique is
surprisingly powerful and effective. This chapter is designed to provide
both a theoretical and a practical understanding of the SRT approach. In
the ensuing two sections, we discuss the presumed mechanism by which
SRT reduces sleep difficulty and consider its applicability to the insomnia problems of older adults. Subsequently, we review the literature supporting the efficacy of this technique among insomnia sufferers in general and specifically among older adults with insomnia (OAWI).
Following this review, we provide detailed instructions for implementing SRT and *troubleshooting* treatment compliance problems. We also
present some case examples that highlight the range of responses OAWI
may display when treated with SRT. In the concluding section of the
chapter, we consider some potential pitfalls inherent in SRT therapy and
provide suggestions for future research with this technique.

Theoretical Rationale for
Sleep Restriction Therapy

To understand the mechanism whereby SRT addresses insomnia, it is useful to consider those factors presumed to govern sleep's duration and quality. In this regard, Borbely (1982) has hypothesized that sleep propensity is governed both by a circadian system and by a homeostatic process. The circadian system is controlled by an internal pacemaker in the brain's hypothalamus and allows sleepiness and alertness to wax and wane in approximately a 24-hour rhythm. Maximal alertness typically occurs in the daytime, and maximal sleepiness occurs at night. In contrast, the homeostatic process gives rise to a sleep drive that provides progressively increasing motivation throughout extended periods of wakefulness for individuals to seek sleep. Although the circadian and homeostatic regulators presumably are independently controlled by distinct underlying mechanisms (Dijk, Beersma, Daan, & Lewy, 1989), they interact to determine the manifest level of sleepiness or alertness at any given time. Nevertheless, interventions that increase either homeostatic sleep drive or circadian sleep/wake rhythmicity should lead to overall sleep improvements among those with chronic sleep difficulties.

In the case of SRT, sleep improvements result presumably as a result of this treatment's effects on the homeostatic sleep mechanism. As first suggested by Spielman and colleagues (Spielman, Saskin, & Thorpy, 1987), SRT may result in mild sleep deprivation. Because the time-in-bed (TIB) prescription used in SRT is based on subjective estimates from sleep logs and because insomniacs typically underestimate their sleep time (Edinger & Fins, 1995), it is likely that many OAWI will initially spend less time in bed than they truly require. This mild sleep deprivation, however, should enhance the subsequent sleep drive and help the OAWI overcome nocturnal sleeplessness. If daytime sleepiness persists following consolidation of nocturnal sleep, increases in TIB can be made until daytime sleepiness diminishes. In general, the more time spent awake out of bed, the higher the sleep drive will be. Ideally, the amount of time allotted for sleep at night (i.e., time spent in bed) should approximate an individual's biologically determined personal sleep requirement. Furthermore, the remainder of the 24-hour day would best be spent alert and out of bed to ensure that the optimal homeostatic drive may develop to facilitate sleep during the ensuing night. When a consistent sleep-wake pattern is not maintained, disruption of nocturnal sleep and subsequent daytime alertness might be expected as a result. When insomnia inter-feres with the normal sleep process, OAWI may adapt to their sleep diffi-culty by spending more time in bed than they biologically require so as to recover lost sleep. Spending too much time in bed to recover lost sleep can lead to fragmented, nonrestorative sleep and perpetuate insomnia. For the OAWI, this process can become an established habit leading to chronic insomnia.

Why SRT May Be Particularly Useful Among Older Insomnia Sufferers

Unfortunately, in the older adult, the mechanism that generates sleep drive may not perform as efficiently as it does in the younger sleeper. In-deed, sleep typically becomes increasingly fragmented and shallow as a function of aging (Bliwise, 1993; Carskadon, Brown, & Dement, 1982). Although research has been equivocal regarding the impact of the circa-dian system on sleep in the elderly (Campbell & Murphy, 1998; Carrier, Monk, Buysse, & Kupfer, 1996; Monk, Buysse, Reynolds, Kupfer, & Houck, 1995), the homeostatic sleep drive does decline with increasing age (Buysse et al., 1993). This compromise in the homeostatic system, in turn, ostensibly contributes to an enhanced vulnerability for insomnia among older adults. As a consequence, SRT, which is specifically de-signed to maximize the biological sleep drive, may be particularly appli-cable to many older adults who present insomnia complaints.

In addition, SRT may prevent or reverse common sleep-disruptive practices that often develop among those older adults who face increas-ing sleep difficulty. After experiencing several nights of fragmented, un-satisfying sleep, the OAWI may take the apparently sensible step and stay in bed longer to make up for the perceived loss of sleep. Although this response most typically perpetuates both nocturnal sleep fragmen-tation (Levine, Lumley, Roehrs, Zorick, & Roth, 1988; Monk, Buysse, Billy, Kennedy, & Kupfer, 1997) and reduced daytime function (Roehrs, Merlotti, Petrucelli, Stepanski, & Roth, 1994; Bonnet, 1989), the intuitive appeal of this self-corrective action often overrides its actual lack of effi-cacy and allows this practice to persist. When this occurs, the broken sleep may become worse. Moreover, by spending time awake in bed while struggling to go to sleep, the poor sleeper may begin to experience negative emotions as well as elevated physiological and cognitive arousal. Such a scenario is an ideal paradigm for the development of conditioned arousal that further confounds sleep attempts. Hence, in addition to enhancing sleep drive per se, SRT may prevent or reverse sleep-disruptive practices and conditioned arousal that often help perpetuate the sleep difficulties of untreated OAWI.

Because spending too much time in bed can interfere with sleep consolidation, an important step in treating OAWI is that of assessing their true sleep needs. Although normative data describing the population distribution of sleep needs are not presently available, it is well recognized that individuals vary in the amount of sleep required to function optimally while awake. The commonly given and accepted recommendation of 8 hours may not be appropriate for everyone. As discussed later in this chapter, it is usually helpful to observe an individual's sleep over a period of time to derive a reasonable estimate of this sleeper's actual sleep requirement. Judgments about the time to be allotted for sleep can then be made more easily and effectively when implementing SRT.

In summary, among older adults, both biological and behavioral factors may contribute to a form of insomnia that is particularly responsive to the SRT technique. Because SRT leads to enhanced sleep drive, this treatment compensates for the older adult's weakened homeostatic sleep system. In addition, SRT reverses the sleep-disruptive practice of staying in bed longer to recover lost sleep so commonly seen among OAWI as they wrestle with their continued sleep fragmentation. In turn, this technique eliminates the frustration, anxiety, anger, and other negative emotions that often develop when extended periods of time in bed fail to rectify the sleep problem. The simple strategy of reducing time spent in bed to match the older individual's true sleep need ostensibly is effective because it addresses all these perpetuating mechanisms simultaneously.

Efficacy of Sleep Restriction Therapy: Empirical Findings

Although SRT seems a logical and sensible approach for treating OAWI, its intuitive appeal is not sufficient justification for its routine clinical use. Fortunately, however, the empirical literature has generally supported the efficacy of this approach. The first empirical support for this technique came from a report by Spielman et al. (1987), in which they provided a detailed description of the SRT approach as well as treatment results for a mixed group ($n = 35$) of predominantly middle-aged ($M_{Age} =$ 46 years; $SD = 13$ years) insomnia sufferers. The specific SRT approach used in this study consisted of first having individuals maintain baseline sleep logs for 2 weeks to derive subjective estimates of their respective average total sleep times (ATSTs). Treatment was then initiated by reducing each individual's time in bed (TIB) to the ATST shown on the baseline sleep log. During treatment, these individually tailored TIB prescriptions were increased by 15 minutes whenever the individual's sleep log showed a mean sleep efficiency percentage, or MSE% (i.e., total sleep time/TIB × 100%) ≥ 90% over the 5 previous days. In contrast, TIB was reduced whenever the individual's MSE% fell below 85% over a period of 5 consecutive days. Finally, no TIB changes were initiated when the individual's MSE% remained between 85% and 90%.

Results of this investigation showed that study participants, on average, increased their total sleep time (TST) by 33 minutes per night, reduced their total wake time (TWT) by 108 minutes per night, and increased their sleep efficiency (SE%) by 20% per night over the course of an 8-week treatment program. Moreover, the subgroups of individuals suffering from psychophysiological insomnia ($n = 12$), insomnia associated with a comorbid psychiatric condition ($n = 21$), and insomnia due to other causes ($n = 2$) showed reasonably similar pre- to posttreatment improvements on these measures. In addition, the 23 treated individuals who also completed a subsequent follow-up occurring, on average, 36 weeks ($SD = 20.5$ weeks) after the end of treatment showed only mild deterioration in TWT and SE% measures and virtually no decline in TST. Unfortunately, these authors failed to include a control group against which their SRT effects could be compared. Nevertheless, these initial results suggested that SRT might be particularly effective for reducing the excessive middle-of-the-night nocturnal wake time that often characterizes late-life insomnia (Bliwise, 1993; Dement, Miles, & Carskadon, 1982).

Subsequent to this initial study, there have been several published reports describing the use of SRT as the sole or primary treatment of OAWI. These investigations have generally supported the particular efficacy of this treatment for this patient group. Lichstein (1988), for example, used a *sleep compression* technique, a modified version of SRT, to successfully reduce nocturnal wake time in a 59-year-old retired man whose sleep expectations far exceeded his apparent nocturnal sleep needs. The sleep compression technique was used again by Riedel, Lichstein, and Dwyer (1995) both with and without therapist guidance. Those without therapist guidance received a self-help video. Results demonstrated that the outcome for those with therapist guidance was better than for the self-help group, and both treatment groups had better outcome than a wait list control. Subsequently, Rubinstein et al. (1990) used a modified SRT protocol to treat seven older (M_{Age} = 57.9 years) adults who collectively reported an average wake time after sleep onset (WASO) of 136.2 minutes per night. Using a strategy in which TIB was initially set at each patient's baseline ATST and then increased weekly based on a mathematical algorithm rather than made contingent on improvements, these authors found that such treatment resulted in 64% reductions in WASO, 12.3% increases in TST, and 16.4% enhancement of SE% over 6 weeks of treatment. More recently, however, Anderson, Zendell, Rubinstein, and Spielman (1994) found that this modified SRT protocol produced significant sleep improvements in older adults (M_{Age} = 65.2 years; SD = 9 years) with objectively confirmed insomnia complaints but led to decrements in both nighttime sleep and objectively measured daytime alertness among older (M_{Age} = 57 years; SD = 7 years) individuals whose insomnia complaints could not be verified by objective nocturnal sleep recordings.

In addition to these findings, there appears to be emerging evidence that SRT is among the more effective behavioral insomnia treatments in general. Data reported in the two most recent meta-analytic reviews (Morin, Culbert, & Schwartz, 1994; Murtagh & Greenwood, 1995) have suggested that SRT is generally more effective than relaxation therapies and perhaps as effective as stimulus control therapy (SCT) (see Chapter 7 for full discussion), the intervention long considered to be the "gold standard" behavioral insomnia treatment. In addition, studies including direct experimental comparisons of SRT and other behavioral treatments generally have supported these meta-analytic impressions. Specifically, such studies have shown that SRT is superior to progressive muscle relaxation therapy, or RT (Bliwise, Friedman, Nekich, & Yesavage, 1995; Friedman, Bliwise, Yesavage, & Salom, 1991), and is comparable to SCT (Anderson et al., 1988) for ameliorating nocturnal sleep disruption among OAWI. One recent study (Lichstein & Riedel, 1998), however, failed to show that SRT was more efficacious than either RT or a placebo intervention among older individuals with chronic insomnia complaints. Although the results of this most recent study are discouraging, such findings stand in stark contrast to the remaining clinical trials that employed the SRT technique.

Furthermore, indirect support for SRT's efficacy has come from various studies in which SRT strategies were incorporated into omnibus treatment packages to address the sleep complaints of OAWI. Among the first in a series of such investigations was the multiple-baseline, case-series study reported by Hoelscher and Edinger (1988). In this early study, these investigators treated four older (ages ≥ 55 years) adults suffering from severe sleep-maintenance insomnia (mean baseline WASO > 103 minutes per night by sleep diary) using a 4-week treatment program consisting of (a) sleep education designed to correct common misconceptions that perpetuate sleep disturbance; (b) common SCT strategies; and (c) an SRT approach in which initial TIB prescriptions were based on baseline sleep log/diary estimates of ATST plus an amount of time consistent with age-appropriate norms for wake time in bed (derived from normative data reported by Williams, Karacan, & Hursch, 1974). Results of this investigation showed that three of the study's participants manifested clinically significant subjective (sleep diary) and objective (measures derived from a sleep assessment device, or SAD) reductions in their sleep-maintenance difficulties, whereas the remaining subject had only a modest treatment response. This latter subject's unimpressive response appeared attributable to an occult severe periodic limb movement disorder found during a posttreatment nocturnal sleep recording.

Over the past decade, several additional studies have supported the efficacy of this combined treatment approach. In a follow-up study, Edinger, Hoelscher, Marsh, Lipper, and Ionescu-Pioggia (1992) found that a group of seven OAWI (M_{Age} = 61.9 years) treated first with RT and then with a cognitive-behavioral therapy (CBT) consisting of sleep education, SCT, and SRT showed significantly greater gains with the latter treatment than they did with the former. Similarly, in their randomized clinical trial, Morin, Kowatch, Barry, and Walton (1993) showed that a similar CBT that included SRT was superior to a waiting list condition among individuals with late-life insomnia. More recently, Edinger, Radtke, Wohlgemuth, Marsh, and Quillian (1997) found the above-described CBT approach far superior to both placebo and RT for addressing the complaints of older adults with severe sleep-maintenance insomnia. Admittedly, these studies of *treatment packages* provide no information about SRT's relative contribution to the observed treatment outcome. Indeed, additional studies designed to isolate specific effects of the various treatment components will be needed to determine SRT's relative value within these multicomponent approaches. Nevertheless, these promising findings provide impetus for further clinical tests among older insomnia sufferers of treatment packages that include SRT.

In addition, investigators have begun to successfully implement SRT among more diverse populations, not just those with primary insomnia. For example, McCurry, Logsdon, Vitiello, and Teri (1998) used sleep hygiene, stimulus control, and sleep compression to treat the sleep difficulties of elderly caregivers of dementia patients. Significant improvements in sleep were found at posttreatment and 3-month follow-up. In addition, behavioral treatment of insomnia, including SRT, has been used successfully to facilitate the discontinuation of sleeping pills (Morin, Colecchi, Ling, & Sood, 1995). The behavioral treatment was used in addition to a supervised medication taper. During the course of the taper, sleep tended to deteriorate; however, sleep efficiency returned to baseline at 3-month follow-up.

The SRT Approach:
Step by Step Instructions

SRT consists of a fairly straightforward approach in which the therapist recommends eliminating daytime napping and restricting TIB at night. This treatment is appropriate whenever there is evidence of frequent daytime napping or that excessive TIB is a perpetuating factor in a particular individual's insomnia complaint. This is often the case for patients meeting *DSM-IV* criteria for primary insomnia. For such individuals, SRT may be considered as either the sole or an essential treatment strategy. Patients with insomnia caused by a medical or psychiatric condition are not immune to poor sleep hygiene practices such as sleep-disruptive languishing in bed. In these cases, SRT might be considered an important *ingredient* in the overall insomnia management approach used.

When historical data suggest that SRT may be a useful treatment strategy, it is necessary to obtain some reliable (stable) estimate of the patient's underlying sleep requirement. Admittedly, there are no universally accepted practice parameters for obtaining this estimate; however, we (Wohlgemuth, Edinger, Fins, & Sullivan, 1999) have found that 2 to 3 weeks of some form of sleep monitoring may be required to obtain stable sleep measures. Of course, this time requirement makes such procedures as nocturnal electronic sleep monitoring too costly and cumbersome to consider. In contrast, the more subjective, albeit less accurate, approach of having the patient complete a sleep log or diary for a 2- to 3-week period appears the most practical method to assess an individual's underlying sleep requirement. Moreover, this is the approach that has been used in all the above-cited empirical studies of SRT. Usually such sleep logs/diaries require the patient to record bed and rising time and to provide estimates of sleep onset latency and both the number and duration of nocturnal awakenings. Typically, the patient is instructed to complete the sleep log upon arising each morning. A sample of the sleep log we use for this purpose is shown in Figure 6.1. An alternative to sleep logs for deriving sleep estimates may be to use actigraphy (Brooks, Friedman, Bliwise, & Yesavage, 1993). An actigraph can provide inexpensive objective sleep estimates over multiple nights and may be a useful alternative to the subjective estimates most commonly used.

After the patient has maintained a subjective sleep record for 2 to 3 weeks, the TST obtained each night is calculated from the information recorded. Subsequently, the ATST across the entire monitoring period is computed. One of two methods may then be employed for deriving a TIB prescription for the patient in question. Specifically, the initial TIB prescription may be set either at the ATST or at a value equal to the ATST plus an amount of time that is deemed to represent normal nocturnal wakefulness (NNW). Both of these approaches have been used in clinical studies, but the latter approach may be more consistent with normative sleep findings (Williams et al., 1974) inasmuch as such data indicate that some limited amount of nocturnal wakefulness is normal. For simplicity's sake, we typically begin with a TIB prescription equal to the patient's baseline ATST plus 30 minutes. Unless there is persuasive evidence to suggest that the patient has an unusually low sleep requirement, however, we do not make initial TIB prescriptions below 5 hours per night.

Once the initial TIB prescription is determined, it is important to help the patient choose a standard wake-up time and earliest bedtime so that the prescription can be followed. In doing so, it is important to have the patient consider both ends of the night. A patient may initially decide that 7:00 a.m. is a desirable wake-up time; however, if the initial TIB prescription were 6 hours, this wake-up time would result in an earliest bedtime of 1:00 a.m. Upon discovering this fact, the patient may wish to select an earlier wake-up time so that bedtime can be earlier during the night. Whatever wake-up and bed times are chosen, it is important to involve the patient in this decision-making process. Compliance with the TIB prescription will usually be best when the patient takes an active role in selecting bed and wake-up times.

When assigning this initial TIB prescription, it is important to note that the ATST shown during pretreatment sleep log monitoring may not represent the patient's optimal *dose* of nocturnal sleep. Because this estimate typically is obtained during a period when the subject's sleep is markedly disturbed, it is likely that the ATST shown prior to treatment misrepresents the patient's actual sleep needs. Furthermore, it is well recognized that individuals with insomnia tend to underestimate their TST when providing sleep log estimates (Edinger & Fins, 1995; Frankel, Coursey, Buchbinder, & Snyder, 1976). Given these considerations, it is likely that the patient's actual sleep need may be somewhat higher than the estimated ATST initially obtained.

Fortunately, SRT includes provisions for making subsequent adjustments in the initial TIB prescription used with each patient. Most published reports suggest that such adjustment should be made contingent on the patient's response to the initial prescription provided. It is noteworthy that one group (i.e., Rubinstein et al., 1990) reported successful treatment outcome using an SRT approach in which TIB prescriptions changed noncontingently during treatment. Nevertheless, most typically the TIB prescription is raised in 15- to 30-minute increments each week the patient shows an average sleep efficiency percentage, or SE% (TST/TIB × 100%), ≥ 90% and reports residual daytime fatigue/sleepiness. Conversely, the TIB prescription is lowered in 15- to 30-minute increments each week the patient shows a mean SE < 85%. Although this represents the most common approach used in SRT treatment, it should be recognized that there are no universally accepted standards that indicate what minimum value of SE% represents a successful treatment outcome. Thus, currently it is probably best to consider the patient's overall satisfaction with nocturnal sleep and waking functioning in determining the optimal TIB prescription.

At the conclusion of treatment, the patient may ask whether it will be necessary to continue restricting TIB to avoid future bouts of insomnia. Perhaps the best answer to this question is a qualified "yes." It is likely, however, that patients have varying tolerances to the loosening of the

SAMPLE

DAY OF THE WEEK	Monday							For Clinic Use Only
CALENDAR DATE	3/25/96							
1. Yesterday I napped from ____ to ____. (Note time of all naps.)	1:30-2:45 p.m.							
2. Last night I took ____ mg of ____ or ____ of alcohol as a sleep aid.	Ambien 5 mg							
3. Last night I turned off the lights and attempted to fall asleep at ____. (a.m. or p.m.?)	11:30 p.m.							
4. After turning off the lights it took me about ____ minutes to fall asleep.	40 min							
5. I woke from sleep ____ times. (Do not count your final awakening here.)	2 times							
6. My awakenings lasted ____ minutes. (List each awakening separately.)	25 min 40 min							
7. Today I woke up at ___. (a.m. or p.m.?) NOTE: This is your final awakening	6:30 a.m.							
8. Today I got out of bed for the day at ___. (a.m. or p.m.?)	7:15 a.m.							
9. I would rate the quality of last night's sleep as: 1 = very poor 4 = good 2 = poor 5 = excellent 3 = fair	3							
10. When I awoke today I felt: 1 = not at all rested 4 = rested 2 = slightly rested 5 = well rested 3 = somewhat rested	2							

Figure 6.1. Sample Sleep Log

strict SRT protocol. Some patients may show little deterioration of their sleep with modest relaxation of the SRT protocol, whereas others may require strict adherence to maintain treatment gains. Nevertheless, by the conclusion of treatment, patients generally should have a sufficient understanding of the SRT approach so that they can independently assess the effects of their variation from the SRT protocol and decide their optimal long-term maintenance strategies. Indeed, consistent with other sleep experts (Hauri, 1997), we invite each patient to serve as a "co-scientist" in treatment and determine what eventual TIB prescription works best.

Special Considerations and Troubleshooting Compliance Difficulties Among OAWI

OAWI represent a unique clinical population with specific demographic considerations that require attention in the treatment process. Multiple life changes including retirement from long-term employment, chronic medical illness, loss of a loved one, and reduced social contacts, individually or in combination, may dramatically alter the rest-activity cycle of the older insomnia sufferer. Indeed, it is not uncommon for such individuals to increasingly use sleep as a means of combating boredom and/or occupying time. Many such individuals may set aside too much time for sleep each night, both going to bed far too early each evening and arising far too late each morning. For such patients, SRT treatment requires much more than merely reducing TIB and establishing an optimal TIB prescription. When treating these patients, it is usually necessary to identify additional waking activities in which they can engage to occupy their time and/or reduce their chronic boredom. Without such attention to the waking period, such patients are likely to resist efforts to reduce the time they typically spend in bed. Common suggestions include becoming more involved with hobbies (e.g., playing golf, playing cards, knitting), volunteering, spending more time with family and friends, and completing projects around the house. There is no magic suggestion, and clinical skill is required to overcome resistance.

In addition to these factors, it is not uncommon to encounter attitudes or beliefs that may perpetuate sleep disturbances among OAWI (Morin, Stone, Trinkle, Mercer, & Remsberg, 1993). Common to many older retired insomnia patients is a sense of *sleep entitlement*. Specifically, many such individuals will state that because they are retired, they now should be able to sleep as long as they wish. Alternatively, some patients may mistakenly believe that all adults require 8 hours of sleep per night. In either case, efforts to reduce TIB may encounter resistance from the patient. Because of this possibility, it is usually helpful to educate OAWI about the range of human sleep requirements and the negative effects of too much time in bed before introducing the SRT protocol. Indeed, our anecdotal observations suggest that this education enhances patients' acceptance of and compliance with SRT.

Frequently, patients who have experienced chronic insomnia have made several attempts to help themselves sleep better. Recommendations for better sleep are often promulgated through the media, doctors' offices, the Internet, and other sources. Those OAWI who present clinically typically have not been successful in their self-treatment efforts. Because of their failed attempts to help themselves, these individuals often lose confidence in their ability to be able to sleep; that is, they do not have a strong sense of *sleep self-efficacy*. Part of the process of successful treatment is to restore this self-efficacy or confidence in the individual's inherent ability to sleep. This initial lack of self-efficacy, however, may be a hurdle to the initiation of treatment. Continuous tracking of sleep changes through daily logs is important to document positive changes made in sleep patterns and to provide positive feedback to enhance self-efficacy.

Once treatment is initiated, it may become necessary for the practitioner to engage in troubleshooting activities to determine the cause of a less-than-expected treatment response. Often, a lack of treatment response is traceable to the patient's misunderstanding of or noncompliance with treatment recommendations. By far the most common compliance problems are patients' failures to adhere to a standard wake-up time and propensities to engage in unintentional sleeping during the daytime. A careful review of sleep logs should be employed to identify noncompliance with prescribed wake-up times. Also, specific questioning of the patient to ascertain the occurrence of daytime dozing episodes and extended periods of wakefulness spent in bed may be useful. When such problems are identified, the behavioral regimen should be reviewed with the patient and methods to help the patient avoid these practices in the future should be discussed.

In some cases, introduction of SRT leads to enhanced anxiety and resultant treatment compliance difficulties. This may occur because some patients may interpret the increased daytime sleepiness that often occurs at the beginning of SRT as a sign that the treatment is making their sleep problems worse. In contrast, prescribed reductions in TIB may enhance the sleep-related performance anxiety of some patients. In rare cases, a power struggle over the TIB prescription may emerge between the patient and the practitioner. When any of these problems arises, some modification of the SRT protocol might be necessary to enhance patient compliance and increase the chances for a successful treatment outcome. Generally speaking, relaxation of the SRT protocol and allowing the patient to have a greater sense of involvement in and control over the TIB prescription usually is effective in overcoming such problems.

Case Examples

Case 1

A 78-year-old woman presented to the clinic complaining that she often awakened 3 to 4 hours earlier than she desired several mornings each week. She claimed that this had been a problem for several years but had become worse after the death of her husband 1 year earlier. She reported no symptoms of depression; in fact, she was quite active socially. She was taking dancing lessons and spending several months during the summer taking care of her granddaughter. She reported no trouble relaxing her body or mind at bedtime, and she could not pinpoint any reason for her sleeping difficulty.

This patient had a sleep pattern commonly found in older adults with sleep-maintenance insomnia. During a baseline evaluation, she fell asleep each night in 10 minutes or less; however, on four of the baseline nights she awoke earlier than she desired and could not go back to sleep. On one night, she woke up at 3:00 a.m., did not return to sleep, and finally got out of bed at 7:00 a.m. Her TIB ranged from 6.5 to 9 hours. By using her baseline sleep log, we determined that she spent, on average, 6.5 hours asleep per night. Using this estimate and adding an additional 30 minutes, we allocated 7 hours for her TIB prescription. She decided that she would go to bed at 11:00 p.m. each night and get out of bed at 6:00 a.m. each morning. This congenial woman offered no resistance and readily agreed to the treatment recommendation. Within 3 weeks, she had consolidated sleep on 6 nights out of 7. She woke up an hour early on

3 of 7 nights, but she did not stay in bed. After 6 weeks of adhering to her new sleep schedule, she continued to have consolidated sleep on 6 of 7 nights and was sleeping until her allocated wake-up time. She was quite satisfied with her treatment and felt much better during the day.

Case 2

A 64-year-old man presented to our sleep center with a complaint of sleep-maintenance insomnia. Evaluation of this patient suggested that he typically allotted too much time for sleep each night and, as a result, often experienced extended periods of wakefulness in bed. He was, thus, provided a course of behavioral treatment that included SRT. After 1 week of this treatment, he reported back to our center noting little improvement. From a review of his sleep logs and a discussion with him, it was discovered that he failed to adhere to a standard wake-up time as instructed. In fact, on three of the nights during the first week of treatment, he stayed in bed more than 2 hours beyond his prescribed wake-up time, reportedly to compensate for periods of wakefulness during the night. Although he adamantly denied daytime napping, he did admit to some unintentional dozing around 7:00 each evening while he was reclining on a couch watching TV.

To correct the patient's sleep problem, the therapist first explained the deleterious effect the noted noncompliance would continue to have on his sleep. Subsequently, the patient and therapist jointly decided that the patient would place his alarm clock in a location so that he could not reach it while in bed. This measure was used to force the patient to get out of bed at the selected wake-up time. In addition, the patient was encouraged to refrain from reclining while watching TV in the evening and to have his wife help him remain awake during the early evening hours. At a follow-up session 1 week later, the patient showed markedly improved compliance and a reduction in his sleep maintenance difficulty.

Case 3

Ms. C. was a 66-year-old retired female who presented with severe sleep-maintenance insomnia that developed after her retirement. Following an assessment that suggested a diagnosis of primary insomnia, she was begun on a course of SRT. After 2 weeks of following this regimen, she returned to the clinic anxiously explaining that her sleep had gotten worse. Furthermore, she reported that the strict behavioral regimen made her very anxious and that she felt under too much pressure to sleep. To address this problem, a more lenient TIB prescription was established, and the patient was allowed to take a brief (30 min) daytime nap each day if she felt the need to do so. With these changes, the patient was able to relax and gradually showed nocturnal sleep improvements over the ensuing month of treatment.

Case 4

The final case was a 66-year-old woman who participated in a recent clinical trial of cognitive-behavioral therapy for insomnia. She had no current or past history of psychiatric or medical conditions that would cause insomnia. As part of the research protocol, she was evaluated with an overnight sleep study, which indicated that she did not have periodic limb movement disorder or sleep apnea. She recalls having had difficulty sleeping throughout her entire adult life and claimed that she never felt that she experienced a good night's rest. On her baseline sleep log evaluation, she averaged 90 minutes of time awake at night. She fell asleep easily each night but woke up, on average, more than three times each night. She was spending, on average, 7.5 hours in bed each night; however, this ranged from 5.5 hours to 10 hours. We determined from her baseline that she averaged 6 hours of sleep time each night and allocated 6.5 hours of TIB. Hesitantly, she decided that she would go to bed at midnight and get out of bed at 6:30 a.m.

Following the first week of treatment, this patient complained of excessive sleepiness and wanted more sleep time. She was allocated 15 more minutes per the study protocol. In the subsequent weeks, 30 more minutes were added to her TIB prescription. She did not, however, believe that her sleep was getting any better and thus decided to drop out of the protocol after 4 weeks. She also asserted that getting up at 6:30 was far too early, and she wanted to sleep later than that. During her active participation, she improved at the beginning of treatment, but then her sleep began to deteriorate as wake time began to encroach into her allocated TIB. This research participant was persuaded to keep records of her sleep after she dropped out of the study. Interestingly, her sleep began to improve once again. This case illustrates an important problem in using SRT, namely a power struggle between the therapist and patient. This struggle may be focused on the bedtime and wake time or the length of time allocated for bed. In this case, once the woman decided to drop out of the study protocol and there was no longer a power struggle with the therapist, her sleep improved. It is important for the therapist to be flexible with the SRT protocol in OAWI who appear resistant to treatment. Sometimes "bending the rules" slightly or increasing the patient's perceived control over treatment may be required to ensure an acceptable outcome.

Summary and Future Directions

In conclusion, SRT offers a powerful and effective solution to a common sleep complaint among OAWI. Although the technique is straightforward, its success depends on adherence to the treatment recommendations. Treatment compliance may be confounded by the beliefs and attitudes held by the OAWI, by performance anxiety, and/or by power struggles between the patient and therapist. Successful treatment may require both that OAWI suspend judgment of the therapy until they have tried it for several weeks and that the therapist exercise a flexible, negotiating approach in providing treatment prescriptions.

In considering the available research, it appears that SRT may be regarded as an efficacious treatment for OAWI; nevertheless, many questions remain to be answered in future studies of this technique. As a starting point, more research is needed to identify and empirically validate the hypothesized mechanisms in SRT. In most cases, SRT is used in combination with stimulus control therapy. By combining these two treatments, both circadian factors and homeostatic sleep drive factors are addressed simultaneously, and the mechanisms are confounded. A study isolating the effects of treating only circadian factors (e.g., controlling sleep-wake times but not length of time in bed) versus treating only homeostatic sleep drive (e.g., controlling length of time in bed but not sleep-wake times) may provide insight into the mechanisms of SRT.

Also, it would be useful to determine the characteristics of those OAWI most suited for SRT and to identify those subtypes who may benefit little from this approach. Furthermore, we have yet to study dosing factors (e.g., number of treatment sessions, amount of time in treatment) and modes of delivery (individual vs. group treatment) so that we can determine the most cost-effective method of administering this treatment. Because chronic insomnia is such a widespread problem, affecting 10% of the population, determining the most effective, efficient method of delivery is an important goal. In addition, because recent studies (Chang, Ford, Mead, Cooper-Patrick, & Klag, 1997; Dement & Pelayo, 1997; Simon & VonKorff, 1997; Weissman, Greenwald, Nino-Murcia, & Dement, 1997) have suggested that insomnia may significantly increase health care utilization and risk for other medical and mental disorders, it would be useful to determine if successful SRT treatment is associated with improvements in functional measures other than those merely reflecting nocturnal sleep quality. Finally, because recent research has indicated that having the symptom of insomnia puts one at risk of developing depression and other psychiatric disorders (Chang et al., 1997), it will be important to learn if reducing the prevalence of insomnia will reduce the risk of developing a subsequent psychiatric disorder. The treatment of insomnia may become an important preventive health measure. Given current market pressures (e.g., managed care) and the emerging epidemiological findings documenting the costs and risks associated with insomnia, it is important that future studies of SRT begin addressing many of these questions.

References

Anderson, M. W., Zendell, S. M., Rosa, D. P., Rubinstein, M. L., Herrera, C. O., Simons, O., Caruso, L., & Spielman, A. J. (1988). Comparison of sleep restriction therapy and stimulus control in older insomniacs: An update. *Sleep Research, 17,* 141.

Anderson, M. W., Zendell, S. M., Rubinstein, M. L., & Spielman, A. J. (1994). Daytime alertness in chronic insomnia: Diagnostic differences and response to behavioral treatment. *Sleep Research, 23,* 217.

Bliwise, D. L. (1993). Sleep in normal aging and dementia. *Sleep, 16,* 40-81.

Bliwise, D. L., Friedman, L., Nekich, J. C., & Yesavage, J. A. (1995). Prediction of outcome in behaviorally based insomnia treatments. *Journal of Behavior Therapy and Experimental Psychiatry, 26,* 17-23.

Bonnet, M. H. (1989). Infrequent periodic sleep disruption: Effects on sleep, performance, and mood. *Physiology & Behavior, 45,* 1049-1055.

Brooks, J. O., III, Friedman, L., Bliwise, D. L., & Yesavage, J. A. (1993). Use of the wrist actigraph to study insomnia in older adults. *Sleep, 16*, 151-155.

Buysse, D. J., Monk, T. H., Reynolds, C. F., III, Mesiano, D., Houck, P. R., & Kupfer, D. J. (1993). Patterns of sleep episodes in young and elderly adults during a 36-hour constant routine. *Sleep, 16*, 632-637.

Campbell, S. S., & Murphy, P. J. (1998). Relationships between sleep and body temperature in middle-aged and older subjects. *Journal of the American Geriatrics Society, 46*, 458-462.

Carrier, J., Monk, T. H., Buysse, D. J., & Kupfer, D. J. (1996). Amplitude reduction of the circadian temperature and sleep rhythms in the elderly. *Chronobiology International, 13*, 374-386.

Carskadon, M. A., Brown, E. D., & Dement, W. C. (1982). Sleep fragmentation in the elderly: Relationship to daytime sleep tendency. *Neurobiology of Aging, 3*, 321-327.

Chang, P. P., Ford, D. E., Mead, L. A., Cooper-Patrick, L., & Klag, M. J. (1997). Insomnia in young men and subsequent depression: The Johns Hopkins Precursors Study. *American Journal of Epidemiology, 146*, 105-114.

Dement, W. C., Miles, L. E., & Carskadon, M. A. (1982). "White paper" on sleep and aging. *Journal of the American Geriatrics Society, 30*, 25-50.

Dement, W. C., & Pelayo, R. (1997). Public health impact and treatment of insomnia. *European Psychiatry, 12*, 31S-39S.

Dijk, D. J., Beersma, D. G., Daan, S., & Lewy, A. J. (1989). Bright morning light advances the human circadian system without affecting NREM sleep homeostasis. *American Journal of Physiology, 256*, R106-R111.

Edinger, J. D., & Fins, A. I. (1995). The distribution and clinical significance of sleep time misperceptions among insomniacs. *Sleep, 18*, 232-239.

Edinger, J. D., Hoelscher, T. J., Marsh, G. R., Lipper, S., & Ionescu-Pioggia, M. (1992). A cognitive-behavioral therapy for sleep-maintenance insomnia in older adults. *Psychology and Aging, 7*, 282-289.

Edinger, J. D., Radtke, R. A., Wohlgemuth, W. K., Marsh, G. R., & Quillian, R. E. (1997). The efficacy of cognitive-behavioral therapy for sleep-maintenance insomnia. *Sleep Research, 26*, 357.

Frankel, B. L., Coursey, R. D., Buchbinder, R., & Snyder, F. (1976). Recorded and reported sleep in chronic primary insomnia. *Archives of General Psychiatry, 33*, 615-623.

Friedman, L., Bliwise, D. L., Yesavage, J. A., & Salom, S. R. (1991). A preliminary study comparing sleep restriction and relaxation treatments for insomnia in older adults. *Journal of Gerontology, 46*, P1-P8.

Hauri, P. J. (1997). Can we mix behavioral therapy with hypnotics when treating insomniacs? *Sleep, 20*, 1111-1118.

Hoelscher, T. J., & Edinger, J. D. (1988). Treatment of sleep-maintenance insomnia in older adults: Sleep period reduction, sleep education and modified stimulus control. *Psychology and Aging, 3*, 258-263.

Levine, B., Lumley, M., Roehrs, T., Zorick, F., & Roth, T. (1988). The effects of acute sleep restriction and extension on sleep efficiency. *International Journal of Neuroscience, 43*, 139-143.

Lichstein, K. L. (1988). Sleep compression treatment of an insomnoid. *Behavior Therapy, 19*, 625-632.

Lichstein, K. L., & Riedel, B. W. (1998). Placebo-controlled treatment of insomnia in older adults. *Sleep, 21*, 99.

McCurry, S. M., Logsdon, R. G., Vitiello, M. V., & Teri, L. (1998). Successful behavioral treatment for reported sleep problems in elderly caregivers of dementia patients: A controlled study. *Journal of Gerontology: Psychological Sciences, 53B*, P122-P129.

Monk, T. H., Buysse, D. J., Billy, B. D., Kennedy, K. S., and Kupfer, D. J. (1997). The effects on human sleep and circadian rhythms of 17 days of continuous bedrest in the absence of daylight. *Sleep, 17*, 438-443.

Monk, T. H., Buysse, D. J., Reynolds, C. F. III, Kupfer, D. J., & Houck, P. R. (1995). Circadian temperature rhythms of older people. *Experimental Gerontology, 30*, 455-474.

Morin, C. M., Colecchi, C. A., Ling, W. D., & Sood, R. K. (1995). Cognitive behavior therapy to facilitate benzodiazepine discontinuation among hypnotic-dependent patients with insomnia. *Behavior Therapy, 26*, 733-745.

Morin, C. M., Culbert, J. P., & Schwartz, S. M. (1994). Nonpharmacological interventions for insomnia: A meta-analysis of treatment efficacy. *American Journal of Psychiatry, 151*, 1172-1180.

Morin, C. M., Kowatch, R. A., Barry, T., & Walton, E. (1993). Cognitive-behavior therapy for late-life insomnia. *Journal of Consulting and Clinical Psychology, 61*, 137-147.

Morin, C. M., Stone, J., Trinkle, D., Mercer, J., & Remsberg, S. (1993). Dysfunctional beliefs and attitudes about sleep among older adults with and without insomnia complaints. *Psychology and Aging, 8*, 463-467.

Murtagh, D. R., & Greenwood, K. M. (1995). Identifying effective psychological treatments for insomnia: A meta-analysis. *Journal of Consulting and Clinical Psychology, 63*, 79-89.

Riedel, B. W., Lichstein, K. L., & Dwyer, W. O. (1995). Sleep compression and sleep education for older insomniacs: Self-help versus therapist guidance. *Psychology and Aging, 10*, 54-63.

Roehrs, T., Merlotti, L., Petrucelli, N., Stepanski, E., & Roth, T. (1994). Experimental sleep fragmentation. *Sleep, 17*, 438-443.

Rubinstein, M. L., Rothenberg, S. A., Maheswaran, S., Tsai, J. S., Zozula, R., & Spielman, A. J. (1990). Modified sleep restriction therapy in middle-aged and elderly chronic insomniacs. *Sleep Research, 19*, 276.

Simon, G. E., & VonKorff, M. (1997). Prevalence, burden, and treatment of insomnia in primary care. *American Journal of Psychiatry, 154*, 1417-1423.

Spielman, A. J., Saskin, P., & Thorpy, M. J. (1987). Treatment of chronic insomnia by restriction of time in bed. *Sleep, 10*, 45-55.

Weissman, M. M., Greenwald, S., Nino-Murcia, G., & Dement, W. C. (1997). The morbidity of insomnia uncomplicated by psychiatric disorders. *General Hospital Psychiatry, 19*, 245-250.

Williams, R. L., Karacan, I., & Hursch, C. J. (1974). *Electroencephalography (EEG) of human sleep: Clinical applications*. New York: John Wiley & Sons.

Wohlgemuth, W. K., Edinger, J. D., Fins, A. I., & Sullivan, R. J., Jr. (1999). How many nights are enough? The short-term stability of sleep parameters in elderly insomniacs and normal sleepers. *Psychophysiology, 36*, 233-244.

7

Stimulus Control

RICHARD R. BOOTZIN
DANA R. EPSTEIN

Stimulus control instructions (SC) for insomnia were proposed by Bootzin (1972) in a case study of the treatment of a person with insomnia (PWI). The instructions were expanded during the next couple of years (Bootzin, 1973, 1975) and have remained unchanged in the intervening 25 years. Reviews and meta-analyses of studies from many different investigators indicate that SC is one of the most effective, if not the most effective, single-component therapies for insomnia (Lacks & Morin, 1992; Morin, Culbert, & Schwartz, 1994; Murtagh & Greenwood, 1995).

SC for insomnia is based primarily on an operant learning analysis of sleep:

In this analysis, falling asleep is conceptualized as an instrumental act emitted to produce reinforcement (i.e., sleep). Thus, stimuli associated with sleep become discriminative stimuli for the occurrence of reinforcement. Difficulty in falling asleep, then, may be due to inadequate stimulus control. Strong discriminative stimuli for sleep may not have been established and/or discriminative stimuli for activities incompatible with sleep may be present. (Bootzin & Nicassio, 1978, p. 29)

In the late 1960s and early 1970s, stimulus control treatments were used as a means of helping individuals change various problem behaviors. Among the most thorough and promising analyses at the time were stimulus control interventions for overeating. To reduce the number of discriminative stimuli for eating, Ferster, Nurnberger, and Levitt (1962) proposed that eating should be made a pure experience so that discriminative stimuli for eating were not discriminative stimuli for other activities. An individual wanting to eat could do so if she or he did not engage in some other activity at the same time that might inadvertently reinforce eating. Eating could not be paired with reading, watching television, listening to music, and talking with others. Furthermore, eating should occur in a place away from routine activities to further separate cues from other activities. Programs for weight reduction that focused on SC were found to be highly effective (e.g., Stuart, 1967).

Bootzin (1972) proposed a similar stimulus control analysis for insomnia. In overeating, there are many cues associated with the problem behavior, and the goal is to reduce the cues for eating as a means of decreasing the frequency of overeating. In insomnia, the goal is to increase the frequency of quickly falling asleep by strengthening the cues for sleep as well as decreasing the cues for behaviors that are incompatible with sleep.

> Bed and bedtime may become cues for behaviors that are incompatible with falling asleep. . . . This can include a variety of activities such as watching television, reading, eating, and worrying. Such activities may be well-established habits begun long before the onset of the sleeping difficulties, or they may be activities engaged in to distract the insomniac from his or her primary concern, being unable to sleep. Many insomniacs seem to organize their entire existence around their bedroom, with television, telephone, books, and food within easy reach. For others, bedtime is the first quiet time during the day available to rehash the day's events and to worry and plan for the next day. Under these conditions, bed and bedtime become cues for arousal rather than cues for sleep. (Bootzin & Nicassio, 1978, p. 29)

The role of discriminative stimuli in facilitating or interfering with sleep is not the only learning principle that can affect sleep. Pavlovian conditioning is also important in that the bed and bedroom can become cues for the anxiety and frustration associated with *trying* to fall asleep (Bootzin & Nicassio, 1978). Internal cues, such as mind-racing, anticipatory anxiety, and physiological arousal can become interoceptive cues for further arousal and sleep disruption. SC reduces cues associated with arousal as well as cues that are discriminative stimuli for activities that are incompatible with sleep.

Recent research has found that many PWI are hyperaroused as indicated by 24-hour metabolism (Bonnet & Arand, 1995), autonomic measures (Freedman & Sattler, 1982; Monroe, 1967), and auditory event–related EEG activity during sleep (Loewy & Bootzin, 1998). Although this might suggest that methods of directly reducing arousal, such as relaxation training, should be highly effective treatments for insomnia, they typically are not. Relaxation-based interventions are of moderate effectiveness and generally have been found to be less effective than SC (for reviews, see Morin, Mimeault, & Gagne, 1999; Murtagh & Greenwood, 1995). SC produces reductions in sleep-related arousal such as sleep anticipatory anxiety as well as producing improvement in sleep (Bootzin, Lack, & Wright, 1999).

SC is intended to help the PWI relearn how to fall asleep quickly in bed. It consists of a set of instructions designed to (a) establish a consistent sleep-wake rhythm, (b) strengthen the bed and bedroom as cues for sleep, and (c) weaken them as cues for activities that might interfere with or are incompatible with sleep. The same instructions are followed if the PWI either has difficulty falling asleep initially or wakes up in the middle of the night and has difficulty falling back to sleep. Figure 7.1 lists the stimulus control instructions (Bootzin, 1972; Bootzin, Epstein, & Wood, 1991) as modified for older adults.

Most outcome studies evaluating behavioral treatments for insomnia have been done with young and middle-aged adults. Until recently, the developmental sleep findings of more frequent awakenings and decreased slow-wave sleep in the elderly led to an assumption that psychosocial interventions for insomnia in the elderly would be ineffective. Outcome studies on the treatment of insomnia in the elderly have begun to accumulate. Contrary to expectations held earlier, age has not been found to be related to treatment effectiveness in studies of behavioral treatments (Morin, Mimeault, et al., 1999). The elderly show the same degree of improvement in response to behavioral treatments of insomnia as do younger adults.

SC, singly and in multicomponent interventions, has been found to be effective for older adults. It is effective for the type of insomnia most of-

1. Lie down intending to go to sleep only when you are sleepy.
2. Do not use your bed for anything except sleep; that is, do not read, watch television, eat, or worry in bed. Sexual activity is the only exception to this rule. On such occasions, the instructions are to be followed afterward when you intend to go to sleep.
3. If you find yourself unable to fall asleep, get up and go into another room. This instruction should be followed whenever during the night you have difficulty falling asleep. It should be followed if you have difficulty falling to sleep initially, and it should also be followed if you wake up in the middle of the night and have difficulty falling back to sleep. Stay up as long as you wish and then return to the bedroom to sleep. Although we do not want you to watch the clock, we want you to get out of bed if you do not fall asleep immediately. Remember that the goal is to associate your bed with falling asleep quickly! If you are in bed more than about 15 to 20 minutes without falling asleep and have not gotten up, you are not following this instruction.
4. If you still cannot fall asleep, repeat Step 3. Do this as often as is necessary throughout the night.
5. Set your alarm and get up at the same time every morning irrespective of how much sleep you got during the night. This will help your body acquire a consistent sleep rhythm.
6. Do not nap during the day.

Figure 7.1. Stimulus Control Instructions for Older Adults

ten found in the elderly, sleep maintenance insomnia (Edinger, Hoelscher, Marsh, Lipper, & Ionescu-Pioggia, 1992; Engle-Friedman, Bootzin, Hazlewood, & Tsao, 1992; Epstein, 1994; Hoelscher & Edinger, 1988; Morin & Azrin, 1987, 1988; Morin, Kowatch, Berry, & Walton, 1993) as well as for sleep onset insomnia (Engle-Friedman et al., 1992; Puder, Lacks, Bertelson, & Storandt, 1983).

Multicomponent Treatments Involving Stimulus Control Instructions

SC is compatible with other behavioral approaches to insomnia and can be implemented within a treatment package. A multicomponent treatment consisting of SC, sleep restriction, cognitive restructuring, and sleep education has been found to be effective for adult (Chambers &

Alexander, 1992; Morin, Stone, McDonald, & Jones, 1994) and elderly insomniacs (Edinger et al., 1992; Morin et al., 1993). Epstein (1994) used SC, sleep restriction therapy, and sleep education with 22 older PWI in a 6-week treatment program following a small-group format. Treatment was implemented in six weekly sessions: four small group meetings followed by two telephone interventions. After treatment, there was significant improvement in wake after sleep onset, sleep efficiency, and total sleep time. Posttreatment improvement was maintained at 3-month and 2-year follow-ups. Multicomponent treatments that included SC also have been used effectively for the sleep problems of elderly caregivers of dementia patients (McCurry, Logsdon, Vitiello, & Teri, 1998) and for the treatment of insomnia in the general population through the use of a televised treatment program in the mass media (Oosterhuis & Klip, 1997).

Stimulus Control Instructions and Psychopharmacology

The prescription of sedative/hypnotics is the most frequently used treatment for insomnia. Many insomniacs who seek treatment when pharmacotherapy has become ineffective are reluctant to withdraw from hypnotics for fear that their sleep will become substantially worse. This fear is not entirely unfounded; benzodiazepine withdrawal symptoms have been well documented and may last as long as 4 or 5 weeks following abrupt discontinuation (Espie, Lindsay, & Brooks, 1988; Rickels, Schweizer, Case, & Greenblatt, 1990).

Behavioral treatment, including SC, has been shown to be effective when patients either withdraw from hypnotics or maintain a consistent dose of the hypnotic throughout the behavioral treatment (Espie, Lindsay, Brooks, Hood, & Turvey 1989). An accumulating literature indicates that behavioral treatments can be used to both help patients withdraw from hypnotics and improve their sleep. In a study of SC, the investigators found that SC plus withdrawal of medication was more effective than medication withdrawal alone at producing significant improvement in total sleep, sleep efficiency, and sleep quality at a 2-month follow-up (Riedel et al., 1998).

Few controlled studies have directly compared a hypnotic with a nonpharmacological treatment. In a comparison of triazolam with a combination of SC and relaxation training, triazolam had an immediate effect whereas the nonpharmacological treatment took 3 weeks to have an equivalent effect (McClusky, Milby, Switzer, Williams, & Wooten, 1991). At a 1-month follow-up, however, the nonpharmacological treatment was more effective than triazolam at maintaining improvement.

The differential course and effects of pharmacological and behavioral treatments for insomnia suggests that it might be possible to use them together. To examine this hypothesis, the investigators assigned 15 insomniacs to either triazolam with behavioral therapy or triazolam with sleep-related information (Milby et al., 1993). At follow-up, triazolam plus behavioral therapy produced greater improvement in total sleep and restedness in the morning than did triazolam plus sleep-related information. These results indicate that hypnotics and behavior therapy are more effective than pharmacotherapy alone and might be combined effectively.

The previous studies did not focus primarily on the elderly. An evaluation of the effectiveness of hypnotics and cognitive-behavioral treatment with the elderly was conducted by Morin, Colecchi, Stone, Sood, and Brink (1999). Seventy-eight community-resident older adults (average age of 64.5 years) with chronic insomnia were randomly assigned to temazepam pharmacotherapy, cognitive-behavioral therapy, combined pharmacotherapy and cognitive-behavioral therapy, and a medication placebo group. All treatments lasted 8 weeks. The cognitive-behavioral treatment was a multicomponent treatment including SC, sleep restriction, and cognitive therapy. The cognitive-behavioral and pharmacological therapies, either alone or in combination, were about equally effective in the short-term treatment of insomnia. Results at the 12-month and 24-month follow-ups found that PWI who received cognitive-behavioral treatment alone were best able to maintain their gains over time. PWI who received either pharmacotherapy or placebo showed the most relapse, and the combined treatment was intermediate.

The results of the Morin, Colecchi, et al. (1999) study raise the possibility that the use of hypnotics undermines the effectiveness of cognitive-behavioral treatments. It may be wise to use behavioral treatments, including SC, as the first stage of treatment, before pharmacotherapy is considered. Behavioral treatments typically have been found to be most effective with patients who are not currently taking hypnotics (Murtagh & Greenwood, 1995).

Countercontrol

SC sometimes presents a challenge with regard to compliance. PWI often find it difficult to follow the instruction to get out of bed if they are not sleeping. This can be a particular problem for the elderly, who may have physical difficulty getting in and out of bed, may be vulnerable to falls, and may not be prepared to leave the warmth of the bed during winter. For these reasons, an alternative stimulus control procedure has been suggested in which individuals are instructed that if they do not fall asleep within about 10 minutes, they are to sit up in bed and engage in other activities such as reading, watching TV, or listening to the radio until they are ready to go to sleep again (Davies, Lacks, Storandt, & Bertelson, 1986).

On the face of it, these instructions appear to be exactly the opposite of instructions 2 and 3 of SC (see Figure 7.1). Indeed, the countercontrol instruction was first used as a control condition in a study with college students having sleep onset insomnia (Zwart & Lisman, 1979). Zwart and Lisman (1979) found that both SC and the countercontrol instruction produced about the same amount of improvement by the end of the treatment period.

A possible explanation for the effectiveness of countercontrol is that it, like SC, also disrupts the usual learned associations between the cues of the bed and bedroom with the arousal and frustration associated with going to sleep. In countercontrol, insomniacs are instructed to do something different from what they ordinarily do. Instead of tossing and turning, they are specifically instructed to sit up and engage in alternative activities until they are ready to sleep again. This can be conceptualized as a stimulus control intervention in which the usual stimulus-response connections are being disrupted.

The practical question is whether staying in bed and engaging in alternative activities is as effective at facilitating new learning as is the traditional stimulus control instructions to not engage in activities that are incompatible with sleep in bed and to get out of bed if not falling asleep. In an evaluation of countercontrol with sleep maintenance insomnia in which elderly as well as younger adults were enrolled, Davies et al. (1986) found that countercontrol was of only moderate effectiveness, reducing the amount of time PWI were awake after sleep onset by about 30% and the number of awakenings about 20%. The researchers did not compare countercontrol directly to SC, but the magnitude of the effects for countercontrol were less than what is typically seen with SC (Morin, Mimeault, et al., 1999).

Although this is weak evidence for the superiority of getting out of bed, it matches our clinical experience. The instruction to get out of bed serves multiple purposes. It reduces the overall time in bed that the person is awake, helping to consolidate sleep. Getting out of bed is an easily understood instruction strengthening the cues of the bed for sleep. Consequently, we do not recommend countercontrol except for individuals who are so physically incapacitated that they are unable to get out of bed by themselves.

Practical Suggestions

To utilize the SC approach, a 1- to 2-week prospective, baseline self-report of the PWI's sleep is helpful. The night-to-night variability of the sleep of the PWI is best portrayed through this method. A daily sleep diary (DSD) (e.g., Morin, 1993) contains information on naps, sleep medication use, sleep onset, awakenings during the night, final awakening, and ratings of sleep. This data can assist the clinician in planning SC treatment. With elderly patients, many of whom may have vision problems, it is wise to use enlarged type for all questionnaires, forms, and diaries.

An important component of the treatment of insomnia is to provide accurate information about sleep and about developmental changes in sleep that occur with aging (see Bootzin, Epstein, Engle-Friedman, & Salvio, 1996). A portion of the first session is spent emphasizing that there is individual variability in the amount of sleep needed by each individual and in describing the changes that occur as individuals age. Although sleep education is not a formal part of SC, it is important in helping to set treatment goals.

To monitor the PWI's progress, daily sleep diaries should be completed during treatment. One note of caution when using DSDs is that patients may not complete the diary each morning and may retrospectively estimate their sleep for the time period just prior to their treatment sessions. In research, we have subjects telephone in their responses each morning to a voicemail service. This may not be feasible in clinical practice. An emphasis on the importance of completion upon awakening is useful. The typical DSD reveals the number of awakenings during the night and their duration; it can be modified to ask if the patient got out of bed if the awakenings were longer than 15 to 20 minutes. Problems complying with SC can be discussed, strategies to increase compliance developed, and modification of the treatment plan made.

Although at first glance SC appears simple, its actual implementation in the home environment can be difficult for PWI. Patients and research subjects often state they tried to follow the instructions "but they didn't work." In fact, SC and their modifications have been widely published in the lay literature, so PWI may have had some exposure to them. In our clinical practice and research, however, we have found that PWI tend to try only portions of the instructions and may do so irregularly.

Many individuals are skeptical that getting out of bed will actually help them get better sleep in the long run. They are more likely to believe that if they are in bed, even if not sleeping, at least their bodies are getting needed rest. What they may not realize is that by staying in bed for long periods of time during which they are not sleeping, they not only are associating the bed with not sleeping but also are likely to be increasing the amount of light, poor quality, transitional sleep. SC and sleep restriction both share the feature of limiting the amount of time in bed as a means of strengthening and consolidating sleep.

There are two keys to the successful delivery and implementation of SC. First, the therapist must review each instruction in detail and provide the rationale. Second, the PWI must fastidiously follow the entire set of instructions. Before embarking on the treatment, we find it useful to explain SC briefly, discuss the strong possibility that the PWI will feel worse before they feel better, and explore their willingness and commitment to trying it. We often point out that nothing has worked so far for them and that they should try following SC as an experiment for 4 weeks.

SC is based on both internal and external cues or stimuli. In the process of following the instructions, PWI learn to strengthen cues associated with sleep and weaken the cues that are incompatible with sleep.

At this point, just prior to beginning an explanation of each instruction, it is useful to review the behavioral nature of the insomnia problem. This provides a foundation for understanding SC and why the instructions work as a whole set. The desired sleep sequence is often well illustrated by first describing the process of getting sleepy and going to bed that is experienced by the good sleeper. This also helps to establish how different their sleep is from the good sleeper. The PWI may offer observations such as that many people read in bed and sleep well. The therapist can point out that the comparison is not with a good sleeper because they don't have a problem sleeping. Rather, the good sleeper provides an example of how well-established behavior develops and maintains. When good sleepers begin to get sleepy, they may start to follow their typical pre-bedtime routine. This routine is often a cue for more sleepiness because the good sleeper's body knows that sleep will follow the pre-bedtime ritual. When the good sleeper gets in bed, more cues for sleepiness are elicited by the bed and bedroom, a place where sleep easily occurs for that person.

The same process occurs when awakening and falling back to sleep during the night: The bed and bedroom are cues for sleepiness for the good sleeper regardless of the time of night. Poor sleepers or PWI have learned over time that sleep does not happen at bedtime or when awakening and trying to fall back to sleep. Long struggles with insomnia, tossing and turning in bed, trying harder to sleep, and worrying about falling asleep and lack of sleep are just some examples of how the bed and bedroom become associated with arousal rather than sleepiness.

PWI will often state that they feel sleepy when going to bed, but when they "hit the pillow," it is like someone turns on a light switch in their mind. Using this analogy can help PWI relate to the experience of arousal cues from the bed and bedroom. This analogy works with older adults as well. The context is different in that they may experience this more when they try to fall back to sleep. An additional point to make prior to beginning the implementation of SC is a reemphasis on the difficulty PWI will encounter at the beginning of treatment. Treatment compliance may be improved by forewarning PWI of these factors.

Some specific issues should be discussed in conjunction with each instruction.

Instruction 1. The first instruction teaches PWI to focus on internal cues for sleep. An inability to detect a feeling of sleepiness can be a barrier to the effective implementation of SC. Persons with insomnia need to learn to become aware of cues for sleepiness. It is helpful to have PWI describe the period prior to going to bed. What cues are PWI using to determine when to go to bed? Often the cues used are external, such as clock time or the end of the nightly news broadcast. Sometimes PWI confuse being fatigued with being sleepy and go to bed too early. A PWI must be taught at this point how to recognize when he or she is sleepy. Does he or she yawn or rub his or her eyes? Does his or her head begin to droop? It is important to emphasize the defeating nature of falling asleep in a place other than bed. The goal is to associate the bed and bedroom with sleepiness. If PWI fall asleep outside of bed, sleepiness does not become cued to the bed.

Instruction 2. The second instruction is the core of SC. Once again, the emphasis is on reserving the bed and bedroom for sleep only so as to learn to associate them with sleepiness. We make an exception only for sexual activity. PWI are told to follow the SC after sexual activity, when ready to go to sleep. Often PWI have developed habits that center around the bed and bedroom such as reading in bed or eating dinner in bed while watching television. The clinician should determine what activities other than sleep and sex are occurring in bed. PWI often cherish these rituals, and trying to eliminate them without an adequate substitute could impede the success of treatment.

Instruction 3. The third instruction is intended to further weaken the bed and bedroom as cues for arousal. PWI must not spend excessive time trying to fall asleep or back to sleep. We point out that a good sleeper probably doesn't take longer than about 10 minutes to fall asleep; therefore, we use 10 minutes as the amount of time PWI should allow to fall asleep. For the older adult, we lengthen the period to about 15 minutes or 20 minutes because older adults usually take longer to fall asleep than younger persons. PWI should get out of bed, go to another room, and engage in a sedentary activity. Persons with sleep maintenance insomnia should follow this instruction when they awaken during the night and can't fall back to sleep. Those who find themselves worrying and planning during the night should be encouraged to set aside some time prior to bedtime to make plans or list worries and possible solutions.

Other obstacles to implementing the third instruction should be considered. Older adults living in cold climates may want to anticipate getting out of bed by arranging their robe and slippers at the bedside as well as a blanket in the room they will use. The therapist and PWI should discuss what type of sedentary activities will be employed when unable to sleep. The materials needed to perform the sedentary activities upon awakening should be prepared before bedtime. It is more likely that this important instruction will be followed if PWI are prepared. Once again, PWI must attend to internal cues of sleepiness so they don't fall asleep in a room other than the bedroom. When PWI begin to feel sleepy, they should return to the bedroom to try and sleep. It is crucial that they capture this sleepy moment and don't allow it to progress into a nighttime nap in the easy chair.

It is important to discourage clock-watching. This practice only stimulates arousal, the antithesis of the SC goal. Practical strategies should be offered such as turning the clock so the time is out of sight and learning how to estimate the passage of 15 to 20 minutes. Often when keeping a daily sleep diary, PWI will complain that the clock is needed to keep track of awakenings. A review of how to complete a diary is called for at this point.

Instruction 4. In the fourth instruction, the importance of repeating this process throughout the night as needed should be emphasized. We explain to persons with insomnia that they may be up several times during the first few nights. They are building up sleepiness, and this will begin to work to their advantage as they find themselves falling asleep or back to sleep after awakening, thereby strengthening the bed and bedroom as a cue for sleepiness. It is possible to gain compliance through simple explanations and reminders of why they are following the instructions and where the instructions are leading them.

Instruction 5. The fifth instruction is focused on establishing a consistent sleep rhythm. Once again, this may cause some sleep deprivation but will facilitate falling asleep the next night. PWI often have substantial night-to-night variability in their sleep. If they don't sleep well one night, they may try to catch up by sleeping later the next day, or they may try going to bed earlier or take a nap. These ineffectual strategies only make sleep less predictable and do not allow the body to establish regular cues for sleep. Even in young adults, keeping a regular sleep schedule and having sufficient time for sleep was more effective at reducing daytime sleepiness than having sufficient time for sleep but in an irregular schedule (Manber, Bootzin, Acebo, & Carskadon, 1996). In the elderly, there is often less adaptability to changing sleep schedules, and regularity of sleep/wake patterns takes on increasing importance.

We try to build in some flexibility to the wake time by allowing PWI to sleep no more than 1 hour longer on the weekends. This is usually not an issue, however, for older adults. In fact, we find that although older persons may have an inconsistent wake time due to futile attempts at gaining sleep, it is often easier for them to establish consistency than it is for the younger adult.

Finally, SC should be followed at the time of the final awakening (i.e., get out of bed for the day no later than 15 to 20 minutes after awakening). At the start of treatment, this extension of the instructions is often overlooked, and PWI may lie in bed for long periods after awakening.

Instruction 6. The rationale for the instruction not to nap is to ensure that the PWI uses the sleep deprivation from the prior night to increase the likelihood of falling asleep quickly. A nap meets some of the sleep need and, consequently, makes it less likely that the PWI will fall asleep quickly.

As individuals age, however, it becomes more difficult to sustain energy throughout the day, and a nap may be desirable (Lacks, 1987). Because irregular napping will disrupt sleep circadian patterns, older persons who nap are instructed to incorporate a brief nap (less than an hour) into their daily schedule. They are encouraged to nap at about the same time of the day, every day. In our experience, late afternoon naps work best. Naps at this time are early enough to have minimal impact on the night's sleep and have the additional benefit of providing the older adult with increased energy during the evening.

Older adults may desire a nap at the beginning of SC treatment because they may feel more tired than usual. If they haven't been consistent nappers, however, they should be encouraged to use the nap only for the first few days to get over the difficult beginning stage of treatment.

Naps should be taken in bed. SC should be followed during naps (i.e., if PWI are not able to fall asleep for the nap within 15 to 20 minutes, they should get out of bed just as they would at night). PWI may use sedentary activities such as rest, relaxation, meditation, or listening to music as a nap substitute, but they should be sure to do these activities in places other than the bed and bedroom. PWI should be careful when relaxing or meditating in a chair or on the couch to avoid falling asleep in a place other than the bed. PWI can also use exposure to bright light and arousing activities such as social interaction, walking, or other light exercise to counteract daytime drowsiness.

Often PWI are not aware of their improvement despite the changes in their daily sleep diary reports. The clinician should take time to shape PWI's awareness of the changes in their sleep-wake patterns. This can be done by a detailed review of the weekly diaries, including comparisons with previous weeks' data. It is also helpful to portray the change pictorially for the patient through a graph of the weekly changes.

The duration and intensity of SC therapy varies from study to study. In our experience, SC usually can be delivered over a 4-week period using weekly sessions. The instructions themselves can be taught easily in one session, but PWI need an opportunity to discuss any problems they have encountered in the implementation of SC in their home environment. Time can be spent problem solving and developing strategies to enhance treatment compliance with the SC. The clinician should plan a 60-minute session to deliver the intervention. The following sessions may be less than 60 minutes depending on the problems encountered by the patient in the implementation process. Follow-up sessions can be implemented by telephone, but there are no published studies supporting this approach. SC has been implemented successfully by nurse therapists (Childs-Clarke, 1990) and by primary care physicians (Baillargeon, Demers, & Ladouceur, 1998).

When feasible, we prefer the group approach to deliver SC because it offers both support and accountability, factors that appear to be strong therapeutic elements (Lacks & Powlishta, 1989). SC has been delivered in both group and individual formats. In a meta-analysis (Morin, Culbert, et al., 1994), individual treatment fared better than the group approach for one variable, number of awakenings. For older adults, this may have implications because sleep maintenance insomnia is their primary insomnia problem. We tell older patients and subjects, however, that the number of awakenings may not change after treatment, and we focus on the length of awakenings as the target of treatment.

The use of SC with cognitive intervention should not require modification of the treatment; however, their use with sleep restriction therapy and relaxation interventions necessitates some adjustment. The point of SC is to avoid spending time in bed awake, so PWI are told not to go to bed until they are sleepy. Sleep restriction therapy prescribes a set bedtime for PWI. The first instruction of SC should be changed to "Lie down intending to go to sleep only when you are sleepy and not before the specified bedtime." This modification is made to accommodate the sleep restriction therapy guidelines while maintaining the important components of both therapies. Relaxation therapy for insomnia is usually practiced in bed; therefore, the second stimulus control instruction must be modified when combining SC and relaxation. Patients should follow SC after performing the relaxation treatment. When combining SC with other behavioral treatments, a longer initial session will be needed to implement the intervention. The duration of therapy may need to be increased because recommendations for implementation of sleep restriction therapy and cognitive therapy range from 6 to 8 weeks (Glovinsky & Spielman, 1991; Morin et al., 1993; Rubinstein, Rothenberg, Maheswaran, Tsai, Zozula, & Spielman, 1990).

SC is compatible with other treatment elements for insomnia. SC does not specifically address issues that are important in treating the older adult such as the need to encourage daytime activity. PWI lead more sedentary lifestyles than other adults (Marchini, Coates, Magistad, & Waldum, 1983). Increased physical activity has been found to improve sleep patterns in older adults (Edinger et al., 1993; Hoch et al., 1987; Stevenson & Topp, 1990; Vitiello et al., 1992). Similarly, there has been increased interest in the use of exposure to bright light as a means of changing circadian rhythms in older adults with sleep problems (Bliwise, 1994). Evening bright light has been found to shift the sleep-wake rhythm and improve the sleep of individuals with sleep maintenance insomnia (Lack & Wright, 1993).

Another important strategy to ensure a successful outcome is to engage the PWI's significant others in the treatment process. As can be seen in the SC, the treatment can disrupt the sleep of bed partners. Their support and encouragement is helpful. One way to secure the significant others' assistance is to include them in the assessment and outcome process by eliciting their perspective of the insomnia problem.

Conclusion

SC has been found to be a highly effective treatment for older, as well as younger, adults and for sleep maintenance, as well as sleep onset, insomnia. Because SC is one of the most effective single-component treatments, multicomponent treatments typically include SC as a critical component. Practical recommendations made in this chapter increase

SC's effectiveness by helping PWI understand the rationale of the treatment and by identifying and providing possible solutions to barriers to compliance.

References

Baillargeon, L., Demers, M., & Ladouceur, R. (1998). Stimulus control: Nonpharmacologic treatment for insomnia. *Canadian Family Physician, 44*, 73-79.

Bliwise, D. L. (1994). Normal aging. In M. H. Kryger, T. Roth, & W. C. Dement (Eds.), *Principles and practice of sleep medicine* (2nd ed., pp. 26-39). Philadelphia: W. B. Saunders.

Bonnet, M. H., & Arand, D. L. (1995). 24-hour metabolic rate in insomniacs and matched normal sleepers. *Sleep, 18*, 581-588.

Bootzin, R. R. (1972). A stimulus control treatment for insomnia. *Proceedings of the American Psychological Association*, 395-396.

Bootzin, R. R. (1973, August). A stimulus control treatment of insomnia. In P. Hauri (Chair), *The treatment of sleep disorders*. Symposium presented at the American Psychological Association Convention, Montreal.

Bootzin, R. R. (1975). *Behavior modification and therapy: An introduction*. Cambridge, MA: Winthrop.

Bootzin, R. R., Epstein, D., Engle-Friedman, M., & Salvio, M. (1996). Sleep disturbances. In L. Carstensen, B. Edelstein, & L. Dornband (Eds.), *The practical handbook of clinical gerontology* (pp. 398-420). Thousand Oaks, CA: Sage.

Bootzin, R. R., Epstein, D., & Wood, J. M. (1991). Stimulus control instructions. In P. J. Hauri (Ed.), *Case studies in insomnia* (pp. 19-28). New York: Plenum.

Bootzin, R. R., Lack, L., & Wright, H. (1999). Efficacy of bright light and stimulus control instructions for sleep onset insomnia. *Sleep, 22*(Suppl.), S153-S154.

Bootzin, R. R., & Nicassio, P. (1978). Behavioral treatments for insomnia. In M. Hersen, R. M. Eisler, & P. M. Miller (Eds.), *Progress in behavior modification* (Vol. 6, pp. 1-45). New York: Academic Press.

Chambers, M. J., & Alexander, S. D. (1992). Assessment and prediction of outcome for a brief behavioral insomnia treatment program. *Journal of Behavior Therapy and Experimental Psychiatry, 23*, 289-297.

Childs-Clarke, A. (1990). Stimulus control techniques for sleep onset insomnia. *Nursing Times, 86*(35), 52-53.

Davies, R., Lacks, P., Storandt, M., & Bertelson, A. D. (1986). Countercontrol treatment of sleep-maintenance insomnia in relation to age. *Psychology and Aging, 1*, 233-238.

Edinger, J. D., Hoelscher, T. J., Marsh, G. R., Lipper, S., & Ionescu-Pioggia, M. (1992). A cognitive-behavioral therapy for sleep-maintenance insomnia. *Psychology and Aging, 7*, 282-289.

Edinger, J. D., Morey, M. C., Sullivan, R. J., Higginbotham, M. B., Marsh, G. R., Dailey, D. S., & McCall, W. V. (1993). Aerobic fitness, acute exercise and sleep in older men. *Sleep, 16*, 351-359.

Engle-Friedman, M., Bootzin, R. R., Hazlewood, L., & Tsao, C. (1992). An evaluation of behavioral treatments for insomnia in the older adult. *Journal of Clinical Psychology, 48*, 77-90.

Epstein, D. R. (1994). *A behavioral intervention to enhance the sleep-wake patterns of older adults with insomnia*. Unpublished doctoral dissertation, University of Arizona, Tucson.

Espie, C. A., Lindsay, W. R., & Brooks, D. N. (1988). Substituting behavioural treatment for drugs in the treatment of insomnia: An exploratory study. *Journal of Behavior Therapy and Experimental Psychiatry, 19,* 51-56.

Espie, C. A., Lindsay, W. R., Brooks, D. N., Hood, E. M., & Turvey, T. (1989). A controlled comparative investigation of psychological treatments for chronic sleep-onset insomnia. *Behavior Research and Therapy, 27,* 79-88.

Ferster, C. B., Nurnberger, J. I., & Levitt, E. B. (1962). The control of eating. *Journal of Mathetics, 1,* 87-110.

Freedman, R. R., & Sattler, H. L. (1982). Physiological and psychological factors in sleep-onset insomnia. *Journal of Abnormal Psychology, 91,* 380-389.

Glovinsky, P. B., & Spielman, A. J. (1991). Sleep restriction therapy. In P. J. Hauri (Ed.), *Case studies in insomnia* (pp. 49-63). New York: Plenum.

Hoch, C. C., Reynolds, C. F., Kupfer, D. J., Houck, P. R., Berman, S. R., & Stack, J. A. (1987). The superior sleep of healthy elderly nuns. *International Journal of Aging and Human Development, 25,* 1-9.

Hoelscher, T. J., & Edinger, J. D. (1988). Treatment of sleep-maintenance insomnia in older adults: Sleep period reduction, sleep education, and modified stimulus control. *Psychology and Aging, 3,* 258-263.

Lack, L., & Wright, H. (1993). The effect of evening bright light in delaying the circadian rhythms and lengthening the sleep of early morning awakening insomniacs. *Sleep, 16,* 436-443.

Lacks, P. (1987). *Behavioral treatment for persistent insomnia.* New York: Pergamon.

Lacks, P., & Morin, C. M. (1992). Recent advances in the assessment and treatment of insomnia. *Journal of Consulting and Clinical Psychology, 60,* 586-594.

Lacks, P., & Powlishta, K. (1989). Improvement following behavioral treatment for insomnia: Clinical significance, long-term maintenance, and predictors of outcome. *Behavior Therapy, 20,* 117-134.

Loewy, D. H., & Bootzin, R. R. (1998). Event-related potential measures of information processing in insomniacs at bedtime and during sleep. *Sleep, 21*(Suppl.), 98.

Manber, R., Bootzin, R. R., Acebo, C., & Carskadon, M. A. (1996). Reducing daytime sleepiness by regularizing sleep-wake schedules of college students. *Sleep, 19,* 432-441.

Marchini, E. J., Coates, T. J., Magistad, J. G., & Waldum, S. J. (1983). What do insomniacs do, think, and feel during the day? A preliminary study. *Sleep, 6,* 147-155.

McClusky, H. Y., Milby, J. B., Switzer, P. K., Williams, V., & Wooten, V. (1991). Efficacy of behavioral versus triazolam treatment in persistent sleep-onset insomnia. *American Journal of Psychiatry, 148,* 121-126.

McCurry, S. M., Logsdon, R. G., Vitiello, M. V., & Teri, L. (1998). Successful behavioral treatment for reported sleep problems in elderly caregivers of dementia patients: A controlled study. *Journal of Gerontology: Psychological Sciences, 538,* P122-P129.

Milby, J. B., Williams, V., Hall, W. V., Khuder, S., McGill, T., & Wooten, V. (1993). Effectiveness of combined triazolam-behavioral therapy for primary insomnia. *American Journal of Psychiatry, 150,* 1259-1260.

Monroe, L. J. (1967). Psychological and physiological differences between good and poor sleepers. *Journal of Abnormal Psychology, 72,* 255-264.

Morin, C. M. (1993). *Insomnia: Psychological assessment and management.* New York: Guilford.

Morin, C. M., & Azrin, N. H. (1987). Stimulus control and imagery training in treating sleep-maintenance insomnia. *Journal of Consulting and Clinical Psychology, 2,* 260-262.

Morin, C. M., & Azrin, N. H. (1988). Behavioral and cognitive treatments of geriatric insomnia. *Journal of Consulting and Clinical Psychology, 56,* 748-753.

Morin, C. M., Colecchi, C., Stone, J., Sood, R., & Brink, D. (1999). Behavioral and pharmacological therapies for late-life insomnia. *Journal of the American Medical Association, 281,* 991-999.

Morin, C. M., Culbert, J. P., & Schwartz, M. S. (1994). Nonpharmacological interventions for insomnia: A meta-analysis of treatment efficacy. *American Journal of Psychiatry, 151,* 1172-1180.

Morin, C. M., Kowatch, R., Berry, T., & Walton, E. (1993). Cognitive-behavior therapy for late-life insomnia. *Journal of Consulting and Clinical Psychology, 61,* 137-146.

Morin, C. M., Mimeault, V., & Gagne, A. (1999). Nonpharmacological treatment of late-life insomnia. *Journal of Psychosomatic Research, 46,* 103-116.

Morin, C. M., Stone, J., McDonald, K., & Jones, S. (1994). Psychological management of insomnia: A clinical replication series with 100 patients. *Behavior Therapy, 25,* 291-309.

Murtagh, D.R.R., & Greenwood, K. M. (1995). Identifying effective psychological treatments for insomnia: A meta-analysis. *Journal of Consulting and Clinical Psychology, 63,* 79-89.

Oosterhuis, A., & Klip, E. C. (1997). The treatment of insomnia through mass media, the results of a televised behavioural training programme. *Social Science and Medicine, 45,* 1223-1229.

Puder, R., Lacks, P., Bertelson, A. D., & Storandt, M. (1983). Short-term stimulus control treatment of insomnia in older adults. *Behavior Therapy, 14,* 424-429.

Rickels, K., Schweizer, E., Case, W. G., & Greenblatt, D. J. (1990). Long-term therapeutic use of benzodiazepines: I. Effects of abrupt discontinuation. *Archives of General Psychiatry, 47,* 899-907.

Riedel, B. W., Lichstein, K. L., Peterson, B. A., Epperson, M. T., Means, M. K., & Aguillard, R. N. (1998). A comparison of the efficacy of stimulus control for medicated and nonmedicated insomniacs. *Behavior Modification, 22,* 3-28.

Rubinstein, M. L., Rothenberg, S. A., Maheswaran, S., Tsai, J. S., Zozula, R., & Spielman, A. J. (1990). Modified sleep restriction therapy in middle-aged and elderly chronic insomniacs. *Sleep Research, 19,* 276.

Stevenson, J. S., & Topp, R. (1990). Effects of moderate and low intensity long-term exercise by older adults. *Research in Nursing and Health, 13,* 209-213.

Stuart, R. B. (1967). Behavioral control of overeating. *Behavior Research and Therapy, 5,* 357-365.

Vitiello, M. V., Schwartz, R. S., Davis, M. W., Ward, R. R., Ralph, D. D., & Prinz, P. N. (1992). Sleep quality and increased aerobic fitness in healthy aged men: Preliminary findings. *Journal of Sleep Research, 1*(Suppl.), 245.

Zwart, C. A., & Lisman, S. A. (1979). An analysis of stimulus control treatment of sleep-onset insomnia. *Journal of Consulting and Clinical Psychology, 47,* 113-118.

8

Relaxation

KENNETH L. LICHSTEIN

R elaxation is the most frequently used psychological method of insomnia treatment in the pub-
lished research (Morin, Culbert, & Schwartz, 1994). Qualitative reviews
(Lacks & Morin, 1992; Lichstein & Riedel, 1994) and meta-analyses
(Morin et al., 1994; Murtagh & Greenwood, 1995) agree that the several types of relaxation are moderately to highly effective treatments for
insomnia.

Relaxation refers to a collection of methods including muscular relaxation (also known as progressive relaxation), passive methods of body
focusing, soothing imagery techniques, and the various methods of
meditation. Perhaps Benson (1975) best captured the essence of relaxation that defines the common threads connecting the numerous methods. He identified four essential elements of relaxation: (a) quiet envi-

AUTHOR'S NOTE: The preparation of this chapter was supported in part by grant
AG12136 from the National Institute on Aging, by the H. W. Durham Foundation, by Meth-
odist Healthcare, and by the Department of Psychology's Center for Applied Psychological
Research, part of the state of Tennessee's Center of Excellence Grant program.

ronment; (b) attending to a repetitive, benign stimulus; (c) passive attitude; and (d) comfortable position.

Any method that produces these four conditions is likely to evoke the relaxation response comprising experiential and physiological calm, and it is the reliable elicitation of this response that determines if a procedure is deemed relaxation (Lichstein, 1988a). Cognitive and/or physiological arousal are the core instigators of insomnia (Morin, 1993), and relaxation works by abating these obstacles to sleep.

Although the usefulness of relaxation with middle-aged adults is well established, efficacy with older adults with insomnia (OAWI) is less clear. This caution originated with early studies that employed progressive relaxation with mixed-age samples. These studies found that the treatment response to progressive relaxation declined on some sleep measures with the advancing age of the subject but left open the question if progressive relaxation could be more effectively delivered to OAWI or if other methods of relaxation would be more effective (see further discussion below). This review will attempt to clarify the current status of relaxation for OAWI and will describe relaxation methods that appear to maximize the likelihood of effectiveness with OAWI.

Types of Relaxation

Following are brief descriptions of the most common methods of relaxation used with OAWI. More extensive descriptions of clinical procedures are available elsewhere (Lichstein, 1988a). In addition, a verbatim account of a hybrid passive relaxation induction is given later in this chapter. We have been using this method with good success in our older adult studies.

All the following procedures require the client to assume a comfortable position (often reclined), close the eyes, and adopt a passive, relaxed attitude. Inductions are delivered in a soothing voice and usually take 10-20 minutes. Home practice is thought to be critical. For purposes of insomnia treatment, practice must occur at bedtime or during awakenings during the night. In addition, some clinicians recommend a second daily practice at a time removed from bedtime.

Progressive relaxation refers to alternately tensing for a short time (5-10 seconds) and relaxing (about 1 minute) about 15 major muscle groups covering the whole body. During the procedure, the client is to notice the contrast between feelings of tension and relaxation and is asked to dwell on comfortable sensations during the relaxation phases.

Passive relaxation generally refers to a variant of progressive relaxation that eliminates the tensing phase. The client sequentially imagines sections of the body and dwells on comforting sensations in each.

Autogenic training combines imagery and focusing on bodily sensations. In insomnia work, an abbreviated version of this procedure is used most often. It consists of slowly repeating self-statements focusing on heaviness and warmth in one's arms and legs.

Imagery requires the client to form a mental image of an object or situation that is presumed to have relaxing effects. Pleasant imagery comprising a serene nature scene is typical, but neutral imagery (as a distracter) has been used as well.

Meditation refers to a family of methods that derive from ancient Asian influences. Examples are the popular Transcendental Meditation, secular versions of the same, and passive varieties of yoga. Meditation procedures typically require focusing on a repetitive stimulus, such as a word, an object, or one's respiration.

Clinical Outcome Studies

Studies of relaxation for OAWI may be divided into three categories: mixed-age studies that conducted correlational analyses between age and treatment outcome that shed some light on treatment response of older adults, studies that employed treatment packages for insomnia in which relaxation was a component, and studies that tested relaxation as a unitary treatment. The third category is the most informative of the efficacy of relaxation.

Mixed-Age Studies

These studies are distinguished by the range of ages of the participants. To qualify for inclusion in this section, the range must extend from young or middle-aged adulthood (age 50 or younger) to older adulthood (at least age 65). Conclusions on treatment effectiveness with older adults are based on correlations between age and pre- to posttreatment sleep improvement: (a) negative correlations suggest diminishing effectiveness with advancing age, (b) positive correlations suggest increased effectiveness with advancing age, and (c) the absence of significant correlation is interpreted to mean that treatment response was constant across the age span. Correlations of the latter two types support the conclusion that insomnia treatment is no less effective with older adults.

Two of the earlier studies of progressive relaxation for insomnia observed negative age-outcome correlations that set a pessimistic tone for managing OAWI. Lick and Heffler (1977) evaluated progressive relaxation and reported a negative correlation between age and two of their sleep measures, latency to sleep and rated feelings on awakening. No significant correlations were found for the remaining measures: hours slept, number of awakenings, rated quality of sleep, and percentage of days taking sleep medication. Despite no decrease of effect associated with age for most of the measures, this study is often cited as evidence that progressive relaxation is less effective for OAWI. Similar findings were reported by Nicassio and Bootzin (1974), who tested progressive relaxation and autogenic training. Significant treatment gains were made only for latency to sleep in the two treated conditions. The remaining four measures—hours slept, number of awakenings, rated feeling on awakening, and rated quality of sleep—did not change. The correlation with age was reported only for latency to sleep, and advancing age was associated with diminished gains. Presumably, however, older adults had no less a treatment response than younger participants on the remaining four measures.

Alperson and Biglan (1979) tested the joint effects of Benson's (1975) method of secular meditation and stimulus control. Treatments were delivered by self-administered manuals. This study comprised separate young and old groups who received the same treatment package so that comparisons of age-dependent treatment response were easily made. At posttreatment, the young group was significantly lower than the old group on latency to sleep. Differences were nonsignificant on the remaining four sleep measures: sleep time, number of awakenings, rated quality of sleep, and rated worrying about sleep. Within-group changes showed that both groups significantly improved on one sleep pattern measure each: total sleep time for the old group and latency to sleep for the young group. In addition, the young group improved on ratings of sleep quality and worry. It is also possible that OAWI are less responsive to self-administered formats. In my opinion, the authors were too quick to conclude that these treatments were "not as effective with older persons as they are with younger persons" (p. 355).

The above three studies provided some of the earliest insights into treating OAWI. Their results were generally viewed as discouraging, though the majority of sleep measures showed no therapeutic decline with advancing age, and they likely delayed active clinical research with this population. More recent mixed-age studies testing relaxation have not observed a substantial decline in treatment response associated with age. Woolfolk and McNulty (1983) contrasted four types of relaxation comprising combinations of neutral imagery, somatic focusing, and muscle tension-release. They found no correlation between sleep outcome and age. Lichstein et al. (1999) employed progressive relaxation to treat sleep-medicated and unmedicated people with insomnia. Age was correlated with 10 outcome measures: 5 sleep measures and 5 measures of daytime functioning (e.g., rated daytime sleepiness, anxiety, and depression). Only one significant correlation was found: Increased number of awakenings was associated with advancing age.

Overall, it does appear that progressive relaxation consistently loses effectiveness with older adults, but this usually affects only some aspects of sleep, and the magnitude of this drop-off appears to be small. We certainly could not conclude from this group of studies that progressive relaxation is ineffective with older adults, nor do they inform us of the effectiveness of other relaxation approaches with OAWI.

Treatment Packages

Chapter 4 of this volume discusses the nature and advantages of package treatments. For purposes of this chapter, studies were selected that addressed OAWI and included relaxation in the treatment package.

Although package treatments tend to be more clinically powerful than unitary interventions for insomnia, for purposes of scientific inquiry a major drawback of such approaches is they preclude distinguishing between effective and ineffective components. We cannot claim, in most cases, that relaxation, or any other particular component, made an important clinical contribution to the outcome. Nevertheless, the frequent inclusion of relaxation in such packages suggests that it is a worthwhile component in the clinical judgment of investigators, and this endorsement deserves recognition. Six studies of package treatments for OAWI have included a relaxation component, and all reported successful outcomes.

Morin, Colecchi, Ling, and Sood (1995) employed a very full package intervention to treat five OAWI who were dependent on sleep medication. Treatment comprised 10 sessions of progressive relaxation, stimulus control, sleep restriction, cognitive therapy for dysfunctional beliefs relating to sleep, sleep hygiene instruction, and sleep education. Each patient was also given an individually tailored, gradual medication withdrawal schedule. By the end of the treatment period, all patients greatly reduced sleep medication consumption, but sleep generally worsened as well. By 3-month follow-up, sleep variables had improved to be comparable to or better than baseline, while medication consumption remained low. This study collected polysomnography (PSG) data as well, but only on four participants at posttreatment and three at follow-up. The PSG data generally corroborated the self-report data, but PSG changes were usually of a smaller magnitude.

Lichstein, Wilson, and Johnson (in press) offered relaxation, stimulus control, and sleep hygiene instruction to older adults exhibiting insomnia secondary to a medical or psychiatric disorder. The method of relaxation was the hybrid passive relaxation procedure described below. To qualify as secondary insomnia, the origin of the insomnia had to follow closely the appearance of a primary condition that would plausibly cause insomnia, such as depression or chronic pain, or variations in severity of a preexisting insomnia had to track closely variations in the primary disorder. Forty-four volunteers qualified and were randomized to the package treatment or a no-treatment control group. By 3-month follow-up, wake time during the night, sleep efficiency percent, and rated quality of sleep all showed significantly greater gains for the treated group.

McCurry, Logsdon, and Teri (1996) employed a pre-post design to treat four older adults who were also caregivers to spouses with Alzheimer's disease. The stress associated with the caregiver role and the practical difficulties of managing an Alzheimer's patient (e.g., agitated nighttime behaviors also known as sundowning) may have contributed to the caregivers' insomnia. Treatment consisted of secular meditation, stimulus control, sleep compression, sleep education, and sleep hygiene instruction. All four participants exhibited substantial self-reported sleep improvement that was well-maintained to 3-month follow-up. More recently, this same group reported a larger trial with the same population (McCurry, Logsdon, Vitiello, & Teri, 1998). Thirty-six volunteers were randomized to treatment or no-treatment groups. The same treatment package was administered to the treatment group, and these individuals showed significantly greater improvement than the control group on rated quality of sleep and sleep efficiency percentage.

Jones (1990) treated medicated OAWI in a primary care setting. Patients were randomized to a treatment group consisting of an unspecified method of relaxation, personal counseling, and an individualized drug withdrawal plan or to a no-treatment control group. Sleep was not an outcome measure, but 39% of treated subjects reported reducing or discontinuing their sleep medication compared to 20% in the control group. Of those that did stop or reduce hypnotics, 81% reported generally feeling the same or better.

The last study in this section was a case study of a 61-year-old woman who exhibited sleep maintenance insomnia and features of narcolepsy (Kolko, 1984). Progressive relaxation was combined with fluid restriction to control nocturia and snapping a rubber band on her wrist to arrest daytime sleepiness. Substantial improvement in nighttime sleep and daytime sleepiness was observed over the course of a year.

Unitary Relaxation Studies

Progressive Relaxation (PR)

Johnson (1993) studied a large sample, 176 OAWI, but used a case study design. The group showed significant improvement after PR training on five sleep variables (e.g., latency to sleep and number of arousals). One interesting finding was the response of the oldest participants. Nearly half the sample was older than 85 years, making this one of the largest samples of the very old. Correlations revealed a diminished treatment response with advancing age with respect to movement during sleep, awakenings, latency to sleep, rated calmness at bedtime, and rated soundness of sleep.

De Berry (1981-1982) recruited 10 women, aged 69-84, who exhibited both elevated anxiety and insomnia, and who were widowed within the past 5 years. Participants were randomized to a treatment group given PR supplemented by unspecified visual imagery or to a control group given self-instructed relaxation. Only sketchy details of the control group were provided. Table 8.1 codes this control group as no treatment because it did not satisfy the definition of either a legitimate alternate treatment or placebo. The treated group outperformed the control group on several self-report measures: latency to sleep and awakenings, headache activity, and state anxiety.

Other recent trials with PR have found modest therapeutic outcomes. These data are consistent with the view that OAWI are less responsive to PR than younger adults.

Bliwise, Friedman, Nekich, and Yesavage (1995) reported a comparison of sleep restriction and PR with 32 OAWI. This same study was reported earlier with preliminary data by Friedman, Bliwise, Yesavage, and Salom (1991). The PR group exhibited significant improvement on total sleep time by 3-month follow-up but did not improve as much as the sleep restriction group. Both groups showed significant and comparable improvement in latency to sleep.

Engle-Friedman, Bootzin, Hazlewood, and Tsao (1992) compared four treatment groups: no treatment, social support and sleep hygiene, PR, and stimulus control. The latter two groups also received social support and sleep hygiene. All groups improved on most self-report sleep measures at posttreatment. About half the participants supplied 2-year follow-up data. At this point, the stimulus control group did best on latency to sleep. Pre-post PSG data were collected on about half the participants, and these showed no treatment effects.

Edinger, Hoelscher, Marsh, Lipper, and Ionescu-Pioggia (1992) employed a multiple baseline design with seven OAWI complaining of sleep maintenance insomnia. Participants were administered four sessions of PR, followed by four sessions of a package comprising sleep education, stimulus control, and sleep restriction. Following PR, most of the participants showed little change in wake time during the night, the primary dependent variable, but substantial improvement in this measure occurred after the package treatment. Gains were well maintained at 3-month follow-up. A sleep assessment device, an objective measure of sleep that reconstructs the sleep pattern based on verbal responses to fixed interval cues during the night, corroborated self-report sleep data at posttreatment.

TABLE 8.1 Studies of Relaxation Interventions for OAWI

Study	Relaxation Method[a]	Number of Sessions[b]	Design[c]	Relaxation Role[d]	Other Treatment (O)	No Treatment (N)	Placebo (P)
Bliwise et al. (1995)	PR	4	R	P	PR < O		
De Berry (1981-1982)	PR	8	R	P		PR > N	
Edinger et al. (1992)	PR	4	S	P	PR < O		
Engle-Friedman et al. (1992)	PR	4	R	P	PR = O		
Gilbert et al. (1993)	PA	8	NR	P		PA > N	
Johnson (1993)	PR	5	C	P		PR > N	
Jones (1990)[f]			R	C		R > N	
Kolko (1984)	PR	2	C	C		PR > N	
Lichstein (1988b)	OR	7	C	P	OR < O		
Lichstein & Johnson (1993)	PA	3	NR	P		PA > N	
Lichstein et al. (in press)	PA	4	R	C		PA > N	
McCurry et al. (1996)	MED	2	C	C		MED > N	
McCurry et al. (1998)	MED	4-6	R	C		MED > N	
Morin et al. (1995)	PR	9	S	C		PR > N	

Column group header: *Outcome in Relaxation Condition Compared to[e]* spans the last three columns (Other Treatment (O), No Treatment (N), Placebo (P)).

a. The relaxation methods used were progressive relaxation (PR), passive relaxation (PA), ocular relaxation (OR), and meditation (MED).
b. The number of relaxation treatment sessions is given. In the case of package treatments, I determined the number of sessions in which relaxation was included.
c. The design of the study is designated as a case study (C), single subject design (S), nonrandomized groups design (NR), or randomized groups design (R).
d. The role of relaxation in the study is rated as primary (P) if it was the sole or main treatment for at least one group, or component (C) if there was more than one treatment in the group.
e. The reported comparisons are based on statistically significant differences between groups. For example, PR > N means that progressive relaxation outcome was significantly better than no treatment.
f. The method of relaxation and the number of treatment sessions were not specified.

193

Passive Relaxation (PA)

Gilbert, Innes, Owen, and Sansom (1993) employed an unspecified form of PA in a residential care facility. A second similar facility served as the control group. Benzodiazepine use was the primary dependent variable. Most residents used these medications as hypnotics (91%), but some used them as anxiolytics (9%). Benzodiazepine consumption decreased by half in the treated group but was unchanged in the untreated group. These investigators did not collect sleep data. Rated sleep satisfaction did not differentiate the two groups, suggesting that hypnotic reduction did not provoke sleep deterioration.

Lichstein and Johnson (1993) treated sleep-medicated and nonmedicated OAWI. A group of noncomplaining sleepers was also included. The same treatment was applied to all groups, the hybrid passive relaxation method presented below. Medicated OAWI reduced consumption of sleep medication by 47% to 6-week follow-up. Their sleep changed little over this period. Nonmedicated OAWI showed significant improvement on number of awakenings during the night and total wake time during the night. By follow-up, the nonmedicated OAWI were equivalent to the baseline sleep level of the noncomplaining sleepers on these two measures.

Ocular Relaxation

This is a little known method first introduced by Jacobson (1929). It consists of tensing the eye muscles, much as you would skeletal muscles in progressive relaxation, to relax the eyes and calm cognitions (described in Lichstein, 1988a). This procedure was applied in a case of severe, lifetime insomnia (Lichstein, 1988b). Neither it nor stimulus control that followed produced a positive treatment response. Finally, sleep compression, which is our version of sleep restriction, did bring substantial insomnia relief.

Summary of
Relaxation Treatments

Table 8.1 presents studies of OAWI that employed relaxation treatments. Omitted from this table are the several studies of mixed-age individuals reviewed above, because these studies preclude comparison of relaxation with other treatments just for older adults. Judgments of comparative efficacy of groups are complicated by the presence of multiple dependent measures, as most sleep studies monitor half a dozen sleep variables. For purposes of Table 8.1, one group was judged superior to another if most of the sleep measures or the main ones were significantly better.

Some of the studies had noteworthy characteristics that are not communicated in the table. Five studies addressed difficult-to-treat subtypes: OAWI taking sleep medication (Gilbert et al., 1993; Jones, 1990; Lichstein & Johnson, 1993; Morin et al., 1995) and older adults with secondary insomnia (Lichstein et al., in press). All-night sleep evaluations (PSG) are expensive but are nevertheless the gold standard of sleep assessment. Only two studies conducted PSG (Engle-Friedman et al., 1992; Morin et al., 1995), and in both studies PSG data were not collected from the full sample.

Patterns evident in Table 8.1 reveal some general conclusions about the 14 studies. First, there is not a single placebo-controlled study of relaxation for OAWI. The placebo column was left in the table for emphasis. Second, when relaxation was compared with no treatment, it was superior in every case. In three of four studies comparing it to other treatments, however, it did not perform as well as sleep restriction (Bliwise et al., 1995; Lichstein, 1988b) or a treatment package that included sleep restriction (Edinger et al., 1992). These data suggest that sleep restriction with OAWI is consistently superior to relaxation. Further, two of these studies used progressive relaxation, and the third used ocular relaxation, an infrequently used procedure. Perhaps progressive relaxation is not well tolerated by older adults. Third, the mean number of relaxation treatment sessions was 5.0, which is not a particularly large number. Three of the studies with the weakest results had fewer sessions than this (Bliwise et al., 1995; Edinger et al., 1992; Engle-Friedman et al., 1992). This matter of treatment exposure is complex. Different types of treatments may require differing minimum numbers of sessions to be effective. Similarly, studies that share the same number of treatment sessions may have in actuality delivered differing levels of quality of treatment exposure. Although it is premature to conclude that these clinical outcomes for relaxation suffered from insufficient treatment exposure, this possibility cannot be ruled out. Fourth, the most methodologically rigorous method of evaluating treatments is by randomized studies.

There are only three such studies that tested relaxation as a unitary treatment (Bliwise et al., 1995; De Berry, 1981-1982; Engle-Friedman et al., 1992); they all evaluated progressive relaxation, and relaxation performed strongly in only one of them (De Berry, 1981-1982).

A Detailed
Relaxation Induction

Progressive relaxation is the most common method of relaxation used for insomnia, and this is true in treating older adults as well (see Table 8.1). As pointed out above, however, a number of progressive relaxation studies with OAWI have yielded disappointing results. Progressive relaxation is a procedurally complex, physically demanding procedure. Although it has never been proven, perhaps these features have compromised its effectiveness with older adults. For example, arthritis may make it difficult for some OAWI to tolerate the muscle tensing.

Our studies with older adults have relied on a hybrid method comprising several passive forms of relaxation. In contrast to progressive relaxation, this is a procedurally simple, physically gentle procedure. This method also has the advantage of providing a relaxation menu. The components are (a) fostering a relaxed attitude, (b) slow deep breathing, (c) passive relaxation, and (d) autogenic phrases. The components sample a variety of relaxation approaches, are procedurally distinct, and are functionally independent. Clients may adopt the whole method intact, or they may only retain one or more components should some parts be preferred over others. By offering several components, we increase the likelihood that we will present at least one method that is pleasing to the client.

This relaxation procedure takes about 10 minutes. The script is read by the therapist. We employ line numbers in the script to aid the therapist in keeping his or her place during pauses.

Hybrid Passive Relaxation

1   **Verbatim text is given in regular print, instructions to the therapist in bold.**
2   **If the client is wearing contact lenses, glasses, or distracting jewelry, ask if he or**

3   **she would like to remove them. Proceed at a slow pace with a soothing voice.**

4   I will help you achieve a deeper level of relaxation. Most people find this is a

5   pleasant experience. It is not hypnosis. You will not lose consciousness and you

6   will not lose control. You will simply begin to feel more relaxed, more comfortable.

7   We will use a combination of several different proven breathing and focusing

8   methods.

9   Please close your eyes and find a comfortable position. Keep your eyes

10   closed throughout the procedure and focus your attention on my instructions.

11   **If the client's arms or legs are crossed, ask the client to uncross them.**

12   **Relaxed Attitude**

13   To begin, you should adopt an attitude of relaxation. A relaxed . . . patient . . .

14   passive . . . attitude. If there are distracting noises, that's OK. Just let them pass.

15   If your mind wanders away from relaxation to other matters, that's OK. Don't

16   force it to come back. Allow your mind to wander and in time it will wander

17   back to relaxation. Maintain a relaxed attitude about your mind wandering.

18   You cannot hurry or force relaxation. Just allow yourself to gradually slip into

19   relaxation and allow it to happen at its own pace.

20   **Deep Breaths**

21   I want you to take a deep breath, hold it for 5 seconds and say "relax" softly

22   as you slowly exhale. You may go ahead and do this now. **If the timing is off**

23   **or the client is rushing, insert a reminder like "next time hold the breath a little**

24   **longer" or "next time take a longer, slower exhale."**

25   Go ahead and take four more deep breaths, hold each one for 5 seconds, and

26   say "relax" softly as you slowly exhale. **Pause about a minute while the subject**

27   **takes breaths. Give further hints if timing is off.**

28   **Passive Relaxation**

29   I'm going to help you focus attention on different parts of your body. And when

30   you focus on a part of your body, I want you to let go . . . relax. Release whatever

31   tension you find in that part of your body and seek out comfortable feelings of

32   relaxation in its place.

33   Let's begin with your right arm. Your hand . . . forearm . . . and upper arm.

34   Let the tension drain from your arm. In your mind seek out sensations in your

35   arm that are peaceful and comfortable . . . tranquil and soothing. Let the relaxation

36   in your right arm grow deeper and deeper. **The focus on the right arm should**

37   **take about 45 seconds.**

38   Let's continue with your left arm. The left hand . . . forearm . . . and upper arm.

39   Just let them go loose and limp . . . soft and calm. . . . Let the comfortable feelings

40   of tranquillity grow deeper and deeper . . . deeper and deeper. **The focus on the**

41   **left arm should take about 45 seconds.**

42   Focus your attention on your face and your neck. Let all those muscles go.

43   Forehead . . . jaw . . . tongue . . . and the many muscles in your neck. Let the

44   tension in those muscles melt away. Dwell on the comfortable feelings of

45   relaxation that are growing there. . . . The peaceful, tranquil feelings of relaxation
46   are growing deeper and deeper. **The focus on the face and neck should take about**
47   **45 seconds.**
48   Now I want you to focus on your chest, your back, and your abdomen. Let go
49   of those muscles. Allow your breathing to slow down and relax. Feel the muscles
50   becoming soft and loose . . . soft and loose. . . . Focus on calm, soothing sensations
51   in your chest . . . your back . . . and your abdomen. **The focus on the chest, back,**
52   **and abdomen should take about 45 seconds.**
53   Now focus on your right leg. Your right foot . . . calf . . . thigh. Let go . . . let the
54   tension drain away and focus on the pleasant relaxing sensations, growing deeper
55   and deeper. . . . Let the warm, comfortable feelings of relaxation grow in your
56   right leg . . . deeper and deeper. **The focus on the right leg should take about 45**
57   **seconds.**
58   Let's continue with your left leg. Your left foot . . . calf . . . thigh. Just let them
59   go loose and limp . . . soft and calm. . . . Let the comfortable feelings of tranquillity
60   grow deeper and deeper . . . deeper and deeper. **The focus on the left leg should**
61   **take about 45 seconds.**
62   **Autogenic Phrases**
63   Now I want to suggest some phrases that you can repeat slowly in your mind to
64   help expand the sensations of relaxation. The phrases go:
65   I am at peace . . . my arms and legs are heavy and warm . . . I am at peace . . . my
66   arms and legs are heavy and warm . . . I am at peace . . . my arms and legs are
67   heavy and warm.
68   Repeat this slowly in your mind and try to *feel* the peacefulness . . . the
69   heaviness . . . and the warmth in your arms and legs.
70   **Repeat one last time for the subject.** I am at peace . . . my arms and legs are
71   heavy and warm. Go ahead and repeat this slowly in your mind and *feel* those
72   sensations.
73   **Pause 1 minute.** Okay. This relaxation session is concluded. You can open your
74   eyes whenever you are ready and sit up.

Comments on Hybrid
Passive Relaxation

Typically, the client will not communicate with the therapist during
the relaxation induction, but the therapist will be responsive if the client
volunteers comments in the midst of the procedure. At the conclusion of
the procedure, we always conduct a careful debriefing, particularly in
the first couple of treatment sessions.

We want to know what worked and what didn't, and we will tailor the
procedure to maximize its effectiveness with each client. For example,

clients with a history of respiratory illness may find deep breathing distressing, and we will omit this portion for such individuals. Alternatively, individuals with discomfort in particular parts of their body may experience the somatic focusing on that part as soothing. We will delete or expand parts of the procedure to achieve the strongest relaxation effect.

An important part of the debriefing, estimating the magnitude of the relaxation response, is initiated at the outset of the induction. We ask the client to rate his or her level of relaxation using the relaxation rating scale given in the Relaxation Log (see Figure 8.1). The first rating, prescore, is taken just before asking the client to close his or her eyes or shortly thereafter. The second rating, postscore, is solicited immediately upon completing the relaxation induction. The magnitude of this change is highly dependent on the prescore level. If the client is already relaxed, there may not be room for much change. Pre-post rating improvement of 3 points is common. Should the postscore be at or below the prescore, this is highly instructive and should alert the therapist to explore, identify, and defeat obstacles to relaxation. Heart rate, estimated by a 20-second pulse rate, is a simple and convincing measure of relaxation impact as well and can be used along with or instead of the relaxation rating score.

We have encountered a number of older adults in our insomnia studies with hearing loss, and therapists should be alert to this possibility. Some individuals may be reluctant to admit this, may attempt to conceal this handicap, and may deprive themselves of hearing the full induction. If hearing loss is suspected or confirmed, the following steps may prove helpful. The therapist may have to increase the volume of his or her "soft, soothing" manner of speaking during the induction. The therapist may situate him- or herself closer to the client and on the "good" side if there is differential hearing loss. The client should be told to ask for repeated instructions during the induction when these are not clearly heard, or to employ a prearranged signal, such as raising the index finger, to prompt the therapist to repeat a segment.

If the client asks for a relaxation tape, we will tape-record the induction and allow the client to practice with the tape at home. We have not found that the tape produces a therapeutic increment, and our research on relaxation for hypertension bolsters this impression (Hoelscher, Lichstein, Fischer, & Hegarty, 1987). We will provide a tape only on request.

RELAXATION LOG   Name_____

Day 1	Date	Time	Relaxation Rating		Pulse Rate		Duration
			Before	After	Before	After	
EXAMPLE →	9/15/98	1:30 pm	4	7	74	69	9 min

Day 2	Date	Time	Relaxation Rating		Pulse Rate		Duration
			Before	After	Before	After	

Day 3	Date	Time	Relaxation Rating		Pulse Rate		Duration
			Before	After	Before	After	

Day 4	Date	Time	Relaxation Rating		Pulse Rate		Duration
			Before	After	Before	After	

Day 5	Date	Time	Relaxation Rating		Pulse Rate		Duration
			Before	After	Before	After	

Day 6	Date	Time	Relaxation Rating		Pulse Rate		Duration
			Before	After	Before	After	

Day 7	Date	Time	Relaxation Rating		Pulse Rate		Duration
			Before	After	Before	After	

relaxation rating:

very aroused				normal			completely and	
and upset				calm			deeply relaxed	
1	2	3	4	5	6	7	8	9	10

Figure 8.1. Form to Log Home Relaxation Practice Frequency, Duration, Rating of Degree of Relaxation, and Pulse Rate

We usually ask the client to self-administer the procedure during the third or fourth treatment session. The therapist can observe the timing of breaths and of the overall procedure. The therapist can also observe body movement and evidence of tension, either of which can detract from the relaxation effect and may escape the awareness of the client. The therapist will offer feedback to correct serious procedural shortcomings. Minor deviations from the protocol are tolerated in the interest of not disturbing the client's relaxed attitude. The most common problem we encounter is rushing the procedure.

Home practice of the procedure is critical. Clients are instructed to practice nightly at bedtime, during the night if they awaken, and one other time during the day. The daytime practice is important because it is a nonstressful opportunity for skill development. If the client is anxious at bedtime and that is the main practice time, then that anxiety will compete with relaxation, and if the relaxation skill is not well developed, then the anxiety will diminish the relaxation effect, rather than the reverse. We ask clients to pick a time of day when stress, distraction, and hurriedness are minimal, so they can focus on mastering relaxation. We discuss the scheduling of relaxation practice and carefully explain its importance to the client.

Unobtrusive, empirical measures of home relaxation practice have shown that self-reported practice levels reliably overestimate actual practice (Lichstein & Hoelscher, 1986). Indeed, empirical monitoring of home relaxation practice is conducted in only a small percentage of clinical settings (Lichstein, 1988a), leaving the question of how much relaxation practice actually occurred indeterminate. This ambiguity creates greater pressure on the therapist to convince the client of the importance of home practice.

Much like the disruptive effects of clock watching in stimulus control (see Chapter 7 of this volume), a perfectionistic attitude in performing relaxation may degrade the experience. Clients should not perceive pressure to duplicate all the details of the induction in their home practice. Sustaining a relaxed attitude is most important for the client, and this often means sacrificing perfect procedure. It is preferable that the client settle into a procedure that flows smoothly and feels comfortable, rather than fostering tension because the client is striving to relax just right. We deemphasize details such as procedural sequence and even content. If the client fashions a procedural variation that is relaxing for him or her, we encourage its use. When assigning home practice, these matters should be discussed with the client. Pace is about the only procedural detail that we work to preserve. We have found that if relaxation is rushed, the relaxation effect suffers.

We supply the client with two forms to encourage home practice and to monitor its progress. The Relaxation Procedure form (Figure 8.2) is a brief outline that defeats forgetfulness of the procedure. The Relaxation Log (Figure 8.1) serves as a further practice reminder and is used to collect adherence data. The log provides space for two practices a day for a week. For those clients who practice more often than this, we ask them to divide the boxes to record more than one practice per row or to give the additional information on the back.

We train clients to take their own pulse either by their wrist or by their neck. Pulse rate provides valuable, objective data that usually show a drop from pre to post due to some combination of relaxation effect and adaptation, and clients often draw encouragement from these data. We do not want clients collecting pulse rate data at bedtime; therefore, pulse rate data boxes for the second practice of the day are omitted from the Relaxation Log. Many clients find it disruptive to collect these data at bedtime, and it may interfere with the sleep induction effects of the treatment. Indeed, we advise clients that all the data for the bedtime session (i.e., relaxation ratings, duration, etc.) may be recorded in the morning if they feel it would be alerting to record them at bedtime.

Further generic details on conducting relaxation therapy are given elsewhere (Lichstein, 1988a). These include training therapists, tailoring strategies, assessing relaxation effects, and managing obstacles to therapeutic progress.

Discussion

There is insufficient high-quality data to determine the status of relaxation for OAWI. Based on the 14 available studies (Table 8.1), preliminary conclusions would include that (a) relaxation is superior to no treatment; (b) relaxation is not as effective as other psychological treatments, particularly sleep restriction; (c) relaxation is a common and possibly valuable component in effective package treatments; and (d) passive relaxation may be more effective than progressive relaxation. These conclusions are consistent with the existing data, but the strength, clarity,

Relaxation Procedure

1. Close your eyes and get as comfortable as possible.
2. Assume a passive, relaxed attitude; do not try to hurry or force relaxation.
3. Take 5 deep breaths and hold each breath for 5 seconds before exhaling slowly. Say "relax" each time you exhale.
4. Relax the following areas of your body. Concentrate on each area for about 45 seconds, let go of tension in each area, and concentrate on feelings of relaxation and calmness.

   a. Right arm
   b. Left arm
   c. Face and neck
   d. Chest, back, and abdomen
   e. Right leg
   f. Left leg

5. Repeat this phrase slowly to yourself for about a minute, and try to feel these sensations: "I am at peace, my arms and legs are heavy and warm."
6. Continue to concentrate on feelings of relaxation.

It is important to practice this procedure at least twice daily, with one practice occurring at bedtime. Relaxation should also be used if you awaken during the night. Repeated practice is necessary to become skilled at relaxing yourself. The procedure should take about 10 minutes. If you are taking less than 10 minutes to complete the procedure, you should slow down your pace.

Figure 8.2. Handout to Clients to Guide Home Relaxation Practice

and consistency of the existing data do not provide high assurance of the validity of these conclusions. More confident conclusions must await placebo-controlled trials, more carefully conducted comparisons with other treatments, more carefully conducted comparisons among the variety of forms of relaxation, and the greater availability of PSG evaluations.

The question of the efficacy of passive relaxation can serve to illustrate the kind of data needed to elevate the scientific merits of this domain. Passive relaxation has performed very well in our studies (Lichstein & Johnson, 1993; Lichstein et al., in press), but it has not received a rigorous test in comparison to other treatments or placebo groups. Still unanswered is the question of passive relaxation vs. progressive relaxation effectiveness with different age groups. We conclude, therefore, that studies with OAWI comparing progressive relaxation with passive relaxation would be worthwhile. Further, the relaxation factor could be crossed with an age factor comprising young and old adults with insomnia. This study would help clarify which method is superior with which age group. If this study also included a placebo group and PSG data, it could potentially achieve an important advance in the literature.

Many of the relaxation treatments for OAWI are underpowered. The majority of the studies are degraded by one or more of the following: few treatment sessions, small number of participants, and underemphasized home relaxation practice. Assuming relaxation for OAWI was effective, it would still labor to yield strong clinical outcomes hampered by these weaknesses. To illustrate, a recent meta-analysis of progressive relaxation training across a wide range of target disorders found that outcome was correlated with the number of treatment sessions (Carlson & Hoyle, 1993). In relaxation applications with OAWI, the number of treatment sessions is minimal on the average and dips below the average in several of the studies exhibiting weak results. These studies leave to conjecture the estimates of clinical outcome were a satisfactory level of treatment presented. A satisfactory number of sessions would probably be in the 6-10 range.

If the therapist presents relaxation once a week and the client is to practice at least once daily between sessions, then at least six-sevenths of treatment exposure is self-administered, and the therapist's knowledge of this practice is usually reliant on client self-report. There can be no doubt (see discussion above) that (a) many if not most clients are going to exaggerate reports of practice levels, (b) the discrepancy between actual and reported practice may be large, and (c) disappointing clinical outcomes sometimes result from the treatment not being practiced even when robust practice levels are reported. Fair tests of relaxation treatments for OAWI require demonstration that adequate practice occurred (Lichstein, Riedel, & Grieve, 1994), and the existing literature does not provide such assurance (see Chapter 4 of this volume for an extended discussion of this and other aspects of treatment implementation). Minimally, therapists must exhort their clients to practice. Recruiting the help of a spouse may prove useful. Soliciting independent confirmation of practice from a spouse is a simple, helpful way of elevating the quality of data and creating added pressure for the client to practice.

Psychological treatment for OAWI in general is a young area, and perhaps results from clinical trials of relaxation applications are among the most preliminary. The ambiguity that shrouds relaxation for OAWI is to me inspiring rather than discouraging. There is enough data to suggest that reasonable efficacy exists in this area, but not enough to assert strong claims. The relaxation domain is ripe for the application of rigorous methodologies that will provide more fair and robust tests of treatments and that will exalt the confidence due their findings.

References

Alperson, J., & Biglan, A. (1979). Self-administered treatment of sleep onset insomnia and the importance of age. *Behavior Therapy, 10*, 347-356.

Benson, H. B. (1975). *The relaxation response.* New York: William Morrow.

Bliwise, D. L., Friedman, L., Nekich, J. C., & Yesavage, J. A. (1995). Prediction of outcome in behaviorally based insomnia treatments. *Journal of Behavior Therapy and Experimental Psychiatry, 26*, 17-23.

Carlson, C. R., & Hoyle, R. H. (1993). Efficacy of abbreviated progressive muscle relaxation training: A quantitative review of behavioral medicine research. *Journal of Consulting and Clinical Psychology, 61*, 1059-1067.

De Berry, S. (1981-1982). An evaluation of progressive muscle relaxation on stress related symptoms in a geriatric population. *International Journal of Aging and Human Development, 14*, 255-269.

Edinger, J. D., Hoelscher, T. J., Marsh, G. R., Lipper, S., & Ionescu-Pioggia, M. (1992). A cognitive-behavioral therapy for sleep-maintenance insomnia in older adults. *Psychology and Aging, 7*, 282-289.

Engle-Friedman, M., Bootzin, R. R., Hazlewood, L., & Tsao, C. (1992). An evaluation of behavioral treatments for insomnia in the older adult. *Journal of Clinical Psychology, 48*, 77-90.

Friedman, L., Bliwise, D. L., Yesavage, J. A., & Salom, S. R. (1991). A preliminary study comparing sleep restriction and relaxation treatments for insomnia in older adults. *Journal of Gerontology: Psychological Sciences, 46*, P1-P8.

Gilbert, A., Innes, J. M., Owen, N., & Sansom, L. (1993). Trial of an intervention to reduce chronic benzodiazepine use among residents of aged-care accommodation. *Australian and New Zealand Journal of Medicine, 23*, 343-347.

Hoelscher, T. J., Lichstein, K. L., Fischer, S., & Hegarty, T. B. (1987). Relaxation treatment of hypertension: Do home relaxation tapes enhance treatment outcome? *Behavior Therapy, 18*, 33-37.

Jacobson, E. (1929). *Progressive relaxation.* Chicago: University of Chicago Press.

Johnson, J. E. (1993). Progressive relaxation and the sleep of older men and women. *Journal of Community Health Nursing, 10*, 31-38.

Jones, D. (1990). Weaning elderly patients off psychotropic drugs in general practice: A randomized controlled trial. *Health Trends, 22*, 164-166.

Kolko, D. J. (1984). Behavioral treatment of excessive daytime sleepiness in an elderly woman with multiple medical problems. *Journal of Behavior Therapy and Experimental Psychiatry, 15,* 341-345.

Lacks, P., & Morin, C. M. (1992). Recent advances in the assessment and treatment of insomnia. *Journal of Consulting and Clinical Psychology, 60,* 586-594.

Lichstein, K. L. (1988a). *Clinical relaxation strategies.* New York: Wiley.

Lichstein, K. L. (1988b). Sleep compression treatment of an insomnoid. *Behavior Therapy, 19,* 625-632.

Lichstein, K. L., & Hoelscher, T. J. (1986). A device for unobtrusive surveillance of home relaxation practice. *Behavior Modification, 10,* 219-233.

Lichstein, K. L., & Johnson, R. S. (1993). Relaxation for insomnia and hypnotic medication use in older women. *Psychology and Aging, 8,* 103-111.

Lichstein, K. L., Peterson, B. A., Riedel, B. W., Means, M. K., Epperson, M. T., & Aguillard, R. N. (1999). Relaxation to assist sleep medication withdrawal. *Behavior Modification, 23,* 379-402.

Lichstein, K. L., & Riedel, B. W. (1994). Behavioral assessment and treatment of insomnia: A review with an emphasis on clinical application. *Behavior Therapy, 25,* 659-688.

Lichstein, K. L., Riedel, B. W., & Grieve, R. (1994). Fair tests of clinical trials: A treatment implementation model. *Advances in Behaviour Research and Therapy, 16,* 1-29.

Lichstein, K. L., Wilson, N. M., & Johnson, C. T. (in press). Psychological treatment of secondary insomnia. *Psychology and Aging.*

Lick, J. R., & Heffler, D. (1977). Relaxation training and attention placebo in the treatment of severe insomnia. *Journal of Consulting and Clinical Psychology, 45,* 153-161.

McCurry, S. M., Logsdon, R. G., & Teri, L. (1996). Behavioral treatment of sleep disturbance in elderly dementia caregivers. *Clinical Gerontologist, 17*(2), 35-50.

McCurry, S. M., Logsdon, R. G., Vitiello, M. V., & Teri, L. (1998). Successful behavioral treatment for reported sleep problems in elderly caregivers of dementia patients: A controlled study. *Journal of Gerontology: Psychological Sciences, 53B,* P122-P129.

Morin, C. M. (1993). *Insomnia: Psychological assessment and management.* New York: Guilford.

Morin, C. M., Colecchi, C. A., Ling, W. D., & Sood, R. K. (1995). Cognitive behavior therapy to facilitate benzodiazepine discontinuation among hypnotic-dependent patients with insomnia. *Behavior Therapy, 26,* 733-745.

Morin, C. M., Culbert, J. P., & Schwartz, S. M. (1994). Nonpharmacological interventions for insomnia: A meta-analysis of treatment efficacy. *American Journal of Psychiatry, 151,* 1172-1180.

Murtagh, D.R.R., & Greenwood, K. M. (1995). Identifying effective psychological treatments for insomnia: A meta-analysis. *Journal of Consulting and Clinical Psychology, 63,* 79-89.

Nicassio, P., & Bootzin, R. (1974). A comparison of progressive relaxation and autogenic training as treatments for insomnia. *Journal of Abnormal Psychology, 83,* 253-260.

Woolfolk, R. L., & McNulty, T. F. (1983). Relaxation treatment for insomnia: A component analysis. *Journal of Consulting and Clinical Psychology, 51,* 495-503.

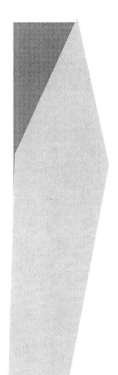

9

Cognitive Therapy

CHARLES M. MORIN
JOSÉE SAVARD
FRANCE C. BLAIS

Cognitive therapy has gained much popularity and growth in the last 20 years. Since its initial formulation for depression (Beck, Rush, Shaw, & Emery, 1979), it has been adapted to a variety of clinical problems including anxiety, substance abuse, eating disorders, marital problems, and personality disorders (Freeman, Pretzer, Fleming, & Simon, 1990). It is only recently, however, that cognitive therapy has been integrated into the clinical management of insomnia. This chapter will discuss the application of cognitive therapy to late-life insomnia, with special reference to older adults' sleep requirements expectations, causal attributions of insomnia, and perceived consequences of sleep loss. After providing examples of dysfunctional beliefs and attitudes about sleep and discussing their role in insomnia, cognitive restructuring procedures are described. A summary of the evidence supporting the use of these clinical procedures concludes this chapter.

AUTHORS' NOTE: Preparation of this chapter was supported in part by grants from the National Institute of Mental Health (#MH55409) and by the Medical Research Council of Canada (MT-14039).

The Role of Dysfunctional Beliefs
and Attitudes in Insomnia

Insomnia often begins in reaction to stressful events such as medical illness, bereavement, occupational stress, or a separation. In situational or
short-term insomnia, sleep usually normalizes after the stressor has
faded away or the person has adapted to it. In many cases, however, insomnia may develop a chronic course. The individual's responses to the
initial sleep difficulties, mainly his or her behaviors and thoughts, determine in large part whether the sleep disturbance will cease or become
chronic. When insomnia persists over time, most people develop some
maladaptive habits (e.g., daytime napping, excessive time spent in bed)
and entertain some dysfunctional cognitions (e.g., worries about sleep
loss, ruminations about its consequences). Although these behavioral
and cognitive responses are fairly normal reactions initially, they often
become maladaptive over time and feed on the vicious cycle of insomnia
(see Figure 9.1). Both types of factors exert their negative effects by increasing arousal (i.e., physiological, cognitive, and emotional arousal)
and performance anxiety, which are literally opposite to the relaxation
state required to sleep. Both the influence of maladaptive behaviors on
the development of chronic insomnia and the behavioral strategies that
may be used to treat insomnia are described in other chapters. The focus
of the present chapter is on the cognitive aspects and the use of cognitive
strategies to treat older adults with insomnia.

Common Faulty Beliefs Entertained
by Poor Sleepers

Before describing typical dysfunctional sleep cognitions, it is useful to
distinguish among several levels of cognitions. Automatic thoughts are
the immediate and spontaneous responses to events. They are called automatic because an individual tends to interpret similar situations auto-
matically in the same way. Automatic thoughts, which are the most con-
scious level of cognitions, are shaped by underlying, more deeply
ingrained, dysfunctional beliefs and attitudes or schemas. Schemas remain silent until a given situation activates them and gives rise to specific automatic thoughts. Finally, negative thoughts can be grouped into

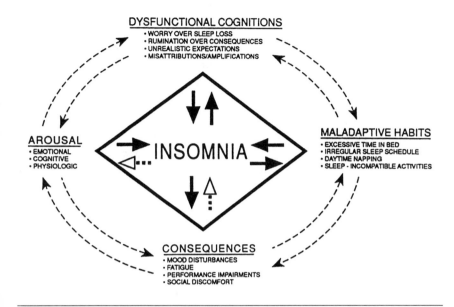

Figure 9.1. A Micro-Analytic Model of Chronic Insomnia
SOURCE: From *Insomnia: Psychological Assessment and Management* (p. 57), Morin. © Copyright 1993 by Guilford Press. Reprinted with permission.

a number of specific cognitive errors or filters (e.g., catastrophization, overgeneralization, dichotomous thinking).

Most individuals with sleep difficulties, including elderly persons, entertain a number of faulty beliefs and attitudes about sleep and sleeplessness that may contribute to maintaining their problem over time. Those sleep cognitions usually can be grouped in one of the following categories: (a) unrealistic sleep requirements expectations, (b) faulty appraisals of sleep difficulties, (c) misattributions of daytime impairments, and (d) misconceptions about the causes of insomnia (Morin, 1993).

Unrealistic expectations regarding sleep requirements. People with insomnia often believe that they absolutely need 8 hours of sleep each night to feel refreshed and function well during the day. Although the average duration of sleep in noncomplaining good sleepers varies between 7 and 8.5 hours per night, there are individual differences in sleep needs, and the total amount of nocturnal sleep generally decrease with aging (see Morgan, Chapter 1, this volume). Trying too hard to achieve sleep standards (i.e., 8 hours of uninterrupted sleep) that are unrealistic for one's age group can cause performance anxiety, which in turn increases arousal and exacerbates the underlying sleep problem.

Faulty appraisals of sleep difficulties. A common reaction to the occurrence of insomnia is for the individual to worry over sleep loss and to ruminate about its consequences (e.g., "Insomnia can seriously affect my physical health"). Insomnia is also commonly perceived as a loss of personal control (e.g., "I lost control over my ability to sleep") rather than as a consequence of situational or extenuating factors (e.g., illness). Such faulty appraisals can increase physiological and emotional arousal, as well as performance anxiety, and turn what would have been a temporary sleep problem into a chronic one.

Misattributions of daytime impairments. Many individuals with insomnia tend to blame their sleep problem for everything that goes wrong during the day. Fatigue, performance decrements, and mood disturbances are often attributed exclusively to poor sleep. Lack of energy is a common complaint among older adults, and it is often attributed to disrupted or lack of sleep. Although some of these consequences may result from poor sleep, the exclusive attribution of all daytime impairments to insomnia is erroneous and, ultimately, perpetuates the insomnia course.

Misconceptions about the causes of insomnia. Another possible scenario is for the older person to attribute his or her sleep problem to aging or pain. Although such factors may contribute to sleep problems, the exclusive attribution of insomnia to such external factors is likely to reinforce a person's belief that nothing can be done to improve sleep, that one is condemned to live with sleep problems the rest of his or her life or until the pain has been eliminated.

Aside from these beliefs and attitudes specific to insomnia, other types of cognitive errors or distortions that are involved in other psychological problems can also play a role in insomnia (Beck, Emery, & Greenberg, 1985; Beck et al., 1979; Freeman et al., 1990). These cognitive errors include excessive ruminations or even obsessions about sleep (e.g., "I must have some sleep tonight"), magnification (e.g., "I will never be able to get through the day after such a miserable night"), catastrophizing (e.g., "Insomnia is destroying my entire life"), overgeneralization (e.g., "I have always slept poorly and I will always do so"), dichotomous thinking (e.g., "Because my spouse falls asleep in minutes, I should be able to do the same"), selective recall (e.g., "Every time I sleep poorly, I can't function during the day"), and even fortune-telling (e.g., "What's the use of going to bed tonight when I know I won't be able to sleep?"). The following vignette illustrates some examples of dysfunctional sleep cognitions.

> Mary, a 67-year-old woman, has had trouble maintaining sleep for more than 2 years. She is very concerned about the potential consequences of insomnia on daytime functioning and on her health. Last night she awoke at 2:00 a.m. and became obsessed with self-statements such as "Another poor night's sleep. I'll be so tired that I won't be able to play bridge tomorrow. God! If this sleep problem persists, I'll get seriously sick!" As a result of those self-statements and her fear of insomnia, she became increasingly anxious and could not fall back to sleep before 5:00 a.m.

Evidence Supporting the Role of Cognitive Factors in Insomnia

Two separate lines of investigation have examined the role of cognitive factors in insomnia. Some studies have focused on intrusive thoughts at bedtime, and others have concentrated on the underlying and perhaps more affectively laden beliefs and attitudes about sleeplessness. As might be expected, individuals with insomnia tend to report more negative thoughts about sleep during nocturnal awakenings than good sleepers (Kuisk, Bertelson, & Walsh, 1989; Watts, Coyle, & East, 1994). Among older adults, highly distressed poor sleepers also endorse more negative thoughts about insomnia and other themes (e.g., worries about health, work, and family) during nocturnal awakenings compared to good sleepers and low-distressed poor sleepers (Fichten et al., 1998). Negative cognitions about sleep (e.g., thoughts about not falling asleep) during the period preceding sleep onset are associated with a longer subjective sleep latency (Van Egeren, Haynes, Franzen, & Hamilton, 1983). Overall, the evidence from those studies and several others (Lichstein & Fanning, 1990; Lichstein & Rosenthal, 1980) indicate that poor sleepers report more intrusive thoughts at night than good sleepers and that cognitive arousal in the form of excessive mentation is generally more strongly associated with sleep disturbances than is somatic arousal. What remains unclear, however, is whether this cognitive activity causes insomnia or simply represents an epiphenomenon of nighttime wakefulness.

Another line of evidence indicates that the content and affective tone of sleep-related cognitions may play a greater role in mediating insomnia than the rate of cognitive activity alone. For instance, individuals with insomnia tend to endorse state (presleep) and trait (daytime) measures reflecting an anxious, worrisome cognitive style, as well as low self-efficacy (Edinger, Stout, & Hoelscher, 1988; Kales & Kales, 1984; Van Egeren et al., 1983; Watts, East, & Coyle, 1995), and these features are associated with more sleep difficulties. In addition, recent studies with older adults have shown that dysfunctional beliefs and attitudes about sleep (such as those described earlier), which are probably more stable and deeply ingrained than automatic thoughts, play an important role in insomnia. For example, one study showed that older adults with chronic insomnia endorse more frequent and stronger dysfunctional beliefs and attitudes about sleep than self-defined good sleepers (Morin, Stone, Trinkle, Mercer, & Remsberg, 1993). Specifically, poor sleepers held more unrealistic expectations about their sleep requirements, held stronger beliefs about the consequences of insomnia (e.g., on physical and mental health), and worried more about losing control and about the unpredictability of sleep (e.g., hopelessness) than normal controls. Furthermore, these dysfunctional cognitions were associated with greater emotional distress and more severe sleep disturbances. Another study found that those same dysfunctional sleep cognitions were significantly related to insomnia complaints in older adults (Fins et al., 1996). Collectively, these findings tend to support clinical observations that erroneous beliefs and maladaptive attitudes about sleep are instrumental in producing emotional arousal and in exacerbating sleep disturbances.

Following these two lines of evidence on the role of cognitive factors in insomnia, researchers have used several forms of cognitive interventions for insomnia. Some have focused on controlling intrusive thoughts with clinical procedures such as imagery training, worry control, and thought stopping (see Espie, 1991), whereas others have used formal cognitive restructuring therapy to alter dysfunctional beliefs and attitudes about sleep. The next section will focus on the latter approach, which targets primarily affectively laden cognitions rather than automatic-intrusive thoughts.

Cognitive Therapy: Goals, Rationale, and Basic Principles

Cognitive therapy is a structured, directive, and psychoeducational intervention. It is based on the assumption that negative emotions, maladaptive behaviors, and physiological symptoms associated with psychological disorders are largely the result of dysfunctional cognitions (i.e., unrealistic, distorted, or faulty beliefs, expectations, or appraisals) (Freeman et al., 1990). The goal of cognitive therapy is to guide patients to reevaluate the accuracy of their thinking and to reinterpret events and situations they experience in a more realistic and rational way. The basic premise is that, by modifying their cognitions, patients will feel better and behave more adaptively.

In the context of insomnia treatment, cognitive therapy seeks to alter dysfunctional beliefs and attitudes (both automatic thoughts and schemas) about sleep. This is accomplished by training and guiding the patient to identify maladaptive sleep cognitions, challenge their validity, and reframe them into more adaptive substitutes. Specifically, cognitive therapy of insomnia is directed at correcting unrealistic sleep expectations, revising false attributions about the causes of insomnia, and reappraising perceptions of its consequences. The issue is not to deny the presence of sleep difficulties or their impact on a person's life; rather, the main objective is to bring the patient to view insomnia and its consequences from a more realistic and rational perspective. Because patients often perceive themselves as victims of insomnia, an important goal of treatment is to strengthen their sense of control in coping with the sleep problem. In turn, this process should alleviate psychological distress and improve sleep patterns.

Cognitive therapy relies on the same clinical procedures used in the cognitive management of other disorders such as anxiety and depression (e.g., reappraisal, reattribution, decatastrophizing, attention shifting, hypothesis testing). As a preliminary step to implementing those procedures, it is particularly important to provide patients with a conceptual framework of insomnia, that is, an explanation of the role of cognitive processes on emotions, physiological arousal, and behavior (i.e., cognitive theory of emotions). This process is facilitated by starting off with examples, unrelated to insomnia, that can trigger various negative emotions (e.g., being stuck in a traffic jam, not being selected for a job). The important point here is to illustrate how a person's interpretation of a given situation may modulate the types of emotional reaction to that situation. Collaboratively, the therapist and the patient elicit several examples to illustrate this relationship among thoughts, emotions, and behaviors. Once the cognitive model is understood and the importance of targeting beliefs and attitudes about sleep is integrated, the next steps are to (a) identify patient-specific dysfunctional sleep cognitions, (b) challenge their validity, and (c) replace them with more rational substitutes.

Identifying Dysfunctional Sleep Cognitions and Underlying Beliefs

An important task is to identify the patient's dysfunctional thoughts about sleep. Many patients are unaware of these thoughts and of their influence on the development of anxious or dysphoric emotions fueling their sleep disturbances. Thus, increasing awareness of those cognitions is a crucial component of treatment. Self-monitoring is usually the most effective strategy to achieve this goal. Because of the automatic quality and inconspicuous nature of thoughts, beliefs, and expectations, training is often essential to help patients obtain adequate records of them. It is important to point out to patients that these self-statements continually flow through their mind in response to external events (e.g., a bad night's sleep, poor work performance). Although not everyone engages in this process to the same extent, virtually every person who experience sleep disturbance entertains some thoughts about the causes and consequences of poor sleep.

Starting from a recent example when the patient had trouble sleeping, the therapist guides the patient, through verbal questioning, to identify the underlying automatic thoughts and the associated emotions. The therapist can use questions such as "What was running through your mind when you were unable to sleep?" and "How did you feel at that time?" To facilitate recollection, the patient may also be asked to imagine himself or herself in a distressing situation and to report thoughts and emotions triggered by that situation.

Therapist: Close your eyes and listen carefully to this. It's 4:00 a.m., and you have been lying wide awake in bed since 2:00 a.m. You have been tossing and turning for the past 2 hours, but nothing seems to help you get back to sleep. You keep wondering whether you'll ever go back to sleep. You keep thinking about the children and grandchildren coming over for the weekend. Now, I would like you to tell me what goes through your mind right at this moment.

Patient: Well, I feel that I'm getting uptight and tense. No matter how hard I try to go back to sleep, nothing seems to work. I have to get back to sleep pretty soon; otherwise, I'll be a mess tomorrow. I've got only a couple hours left before getting up. If I don't get back to sleep soon, I know I won't be able to do housekeeping, cooking, and fully enjoy their presence.

Along with verbal questioning and imagery recollection, it is most helpful to use a daily record of automatic thoughts about sleep and insomnia. Table 9.1 presents an example of this daily record with the standard three-column format. The patient is asked to identify (a) the situation or activating event, which may involve a stream of thoughts, daydreams, or recollections that led to the unpleasant emotion; (b) the automatic thoughts and/or image(s) that went through his or her mind at that time; and (c) the emotional reactions (e.g., helplessness/anxiety/anger). The intensity of emotional reactions can also be rated on a scale from 0 to 100. Patients should keep this record on a daily basis and pay particular attention to their automatic thoughts when they worry about insomnia or when they have trouble sleeping at night or functioning during the day. The more consistent a patient is in keeping this record, the easier it will be to identify his or her faulty thinking about sleep, and the easier it may be to correct it during therapy sessions.

The Dysfunctional Beliefs and Attitudes About Sleep Scale (DBAS) (Morin, 1994) is another useful assessment tool to identify the patient's sleep cognitions. The DBAS is a 30-item self-report scale designed to assess sleep-related beliefs and attitudes. The patient indicates to what extent he or she agrees or disagrees with the statement on a visual analogue scale ranging from 0 (strongly disagree) to 100 (strongly agree). Other re-

TABLE 9.1 Example of an Automatic Thought Record

Situation	Automatic Thoughts	Emotions
Watching TV in the evening	"I must have some sleep tonight, I have so much to do tomorrow."	Anxious 80%
Lying in bed awake at 4:00 a.m.	"I'll never get over this sleep problem"	Helpless 90%

sponse formats (e.g., Likert-type scale) also can be used to facilitate its comprehension. There are no right or wrong answers; rather, the dysfunctional nature of those beliefs is reflected by the degree with which patients endorse a particular item. The content of those items reflects several themes, such as causal attributions and perceived consequences of insomnia, sleep requirements expectations, control and predictability of sleep, and beliefs about sleep-promoting practices (see Table 9.2). Although initially designed as an assessment device to evaluate the severity of dysfunctional sleep cognitions, the DBAS is also a useful tool for clinicians to select relevant targets for cognitive therapy sessions.

Challenging the Validity of Cognitions

After patient-specific sleep cognitions are identified, their validity should be explored. The main task is to guide the patient in viewing his or her thoughts as only one of many possible interpretations, rather than as absolute truths. A variety of probing questions are suggested to encourage the patient to check the validity of those cognitions (see Table 9.3).

Exchanging Dysfunctional Sleep Cognitions for More Adaptive and Rational Substitutes

The third step of therapy consists of finding alternatives to the dysfunctional sleep cognitions by using cognitive restructuring techniques

---

TABLE 9.2 Examples of Items From the Dysfunctional Beliefs and Attitudes About Sleep Scale

---

Causal attributions of insomnia
I feel that insomnia is basically the result of aging, and there isn't much that can be done about this problem.
I believe insomnia is essentially the result of a chemical imbalance.

Perceived consequences of insomnia
I am concerned that chronic insomnia may have serious consequences for my physical health.
After a poor night's sleep, I know that it will interfere with my daily activities on the next day.
When I feel irritable, depressed, or anxious during the day, it is mostly because I did not sleep well the night before.

Sleep requirements expectations
I need 8 hours of sleep to feel refreshed and function well during the day.
Because my bed partner falls asleep as soon as his or her head hits the pillow and stays asleep through the night, I should be able to do so too.

Control and predictability of sleep
I can't ever predict whether I'll have a good or poor night's sleep.
I am worried that I may lose control over my abilities to sleep.
My sleep problem is getting worse all the time and I don't believe anyone can help.

Beliefs about sleep-promoting practices
Because I am getting older, I should go to bed earlier in the evening.
A "nightcap" before bedtime is a good solution to sleep problems.
When I have trouble getting to sleep, I should stay in bed and try harder.

---

such as reattribution, decatastrophizing, reappraisal, and attention shifting (Beck et al., 1985; Beck et al., 1979; Freeman et al., 1990). Self-monitoring is still extremely useful at this stage to help the patient modify his or her thinking about sleep and realize how much the emotional reaction changes depending on the nature of the thoughts entertained. For that purpose, two columns are added to the daily record of automatic thoughts. First, more rational and realistic thoughts are identified, and second, the associated emotions are reassessed as a function of this alternative thinking (see Table 9.4).

TABLE 9.3 Examples of Probing Questions

1. What is the evidence that supports this idea?
2. What is the evidence against this idea?
3. Is there an alternative explanation?
4. What is the worst that could happen? Could I live through it?
5. What is the best that could happen?
6. What is the most realistic outcome?
7. What would I tell _____ (a friend) if he or she were in the same situation?
8. How would someone else interpret the same situation?

SOURCE: From *Cognitive Therapy: Basics and Beyond*, Beck. © Copyright 1995 by Guilford Press. Reprinted with permission.

TABLE 9.4 Example of Utilization of an Automatic Thought Record for Cognitive Restructuring

Situation	Automatic Thoughts	Emotions	Alternative Thoughts	Emotions
Awake in bed in the middle of the night	"I won't be able to function to-morrow"	Anxious 90%	"There is no point in worry-ing about this now. Some-times I can still function after a poor night's sleep."	Anxious 15%

Decatastrophizing. As explained earlier, individuals suffering from insomnia have a tendency to amplify the consequences of insomnia. Providing accurate information about the objective consequences of insomnia is often very reassuring. Sometimes, it is necessary to use more directive methods to bring the patient to see that his or her subjective complaints about daytime impairments are magnified and disproportionate in relation to objective deficits. One verbal intervention that is particularly helpful to decatastrophize insomnia consists of asking the patient "What is the worst that could happen if you did not sleep to-night"; the patient is then encouraged to imagine the worst scenario and also to imagine that the most certain consequence of sleeplessness is sleepiness. Another intervention could be something like "Insomnia can have unpleasant consequences, but in itself, insomnia is not dangerous." When implemented properly, these interventions often bring some relief in terms of reducing the fear of insomnia.

Reattribution. Older adults with insomnia tend to attribute their sleep problem to external factors such as aging or pain. Unfortunately, such external attribution is often accompanied by the underlying belief that nothing can be done to overcome insomnia, that, because of growing older or because of pain, one is condemned to suffer sleep disturbance indefinitely. Causal reattribution can be accomplished by explaining the multidimensional aspects of insomnia and the influence of the individual's behaviors and cognitions in the perpetuation of insomnia. It is important to emphasize that behavioral and cognitive factors are always involved in maintaining chronic insomnia, regardless of the primary etiological factors (e.g., aging, pain). The patient can then be taught how to change some of those factors over which he or she has some control (e.g., reducing time spent in bed). Thus, even if insomnia is secondary to pain, some portion of the sleep disturbances may be independent of pain and receptive to psychological interventions (see Lichstein, Chapter 12, this volume, for a discussion of the concept of partial secondary insomnia).

Reappraisal. Older adults with insomnia often entertain unrealistic expectations about their sleep requirements (e.g., "I must have 8 hours of sleep every night") and their daytime energy level (e.g., "I should always arise in the morning feeling well rested"). An important goal of cognitive therapy is to bring those patients to realize that changes in sleep and daytime energy are not always pathological. As such, they may benefit from reappraising their expectations and adjusting them to age-appropriate norms. It is important to distinguish between normal changes in sleep patterns that accompany aging (e.g., waking up once or twice for 10 or 15 min each time) from changes that require clinical attention (e.g., spending 1 hour awake in the middle of the night most of the nights). Some older adults think that using a sleeping pill will make them sleep as well as when they were younger. It is important to correct such false expectations.

Attention shifting. Some seniors have reduced their activity level significantly because of poor sleep and lack of energy. They believe that insomnia is the worst thing that can happen and feel that it is preventing them from enjoying life. Unless sleep improves, they feel they can no longer do their household chores or even participate in leisure activities (e.g., playing bridge). Although it is important for the clinician to show empathy for those people, it is equally important to bring them to stop viewing themselves as victims of something over which they have no control. They are encouraged to deemphasize the importance of sleep loss or to avoid giving it more importance than it deserves, and to resume their daily activities. In this attention-shifting process, it is often necessary to challenge some of the reasons for reducing activities or social contacts with friends and family members. Sometimes, boredom or even depression may become an additional focus of treatment.

Clinical Vignettes

This section presents narratives of therapy sessions with our patient, Mary, to illustrate how cognitive restructuring techniques (reattribution, decatastrophizing, and reappraisal) are used to alter dysfunctional cognitions about sleep in an older adult.

In the first script, the therapist is attempting to **decatastrophize the perceived impact of insomnia on daytime functioning and health.**

> **Therapist:** We have seen that you worry a great deal about the consequences of insomnia. For example, you're afraid you won't be able to function during the day after a poor night's sleep and that you might eventually get sick because of insomnia. Is that right?
>
> **Patient:** Yes, it is.
>
> **Therapist:** Now, let's look at the first concern, that you're not able to function during the day after a poor night's sleep. Have there been times when this has happened?
>
> **Patient:** Of course, there have!
>
> **Therapist:** Would you say that every time you had a poor night's sleep you were unable to function the next day?

Patient: Well, maybe not every time.

Therapist: Can you remember times when you were able to function fairly well during the day despite having slept poorly the preceding night?

Patient: Oh yes! I guess it has happened many times.

Therapist: On the contrary, have there been times when you had difficulties functioning or had no energy during the day even though you had slept well the night before?

Patient: Yes, that has happened several times as well.

Therapist: So, it sounds like your appraisal is not entirely accurate and that your level of functioning is not entirely dependent on the quality of your sleep. Would you agree with that assessment?

Patient: Yes. I never realized that before.

Therapist: Good! Now, how could we reformulate this thought in a more realistic way?

Patient: Well, that could be something like: "Insomnia is not the only cause of poor functioning during the day. Although I may feel more tired during the day after a poor night's sleep, most of the time I can still function pretty well."

Therapist: Very good! And you might even add that the more you worry about those daytime impairments, the greater the chance it will affect your sleep the next night. This is like a self-fulfilling prophecy.... Now, let's look at the other thought, that you could get sick because of insomnia. Have you ever read in the newspaper that someone died because of insomnia?

Patient: (Laughs). No, I haven't.

Therapist: Would you say that poor sleepers are all sicker than good sleepers?

Patient: Probably not. I know good sleepers who are sicker than me.

Therapist: And there are probably older people with insomnia who are healthier than good sleepers, right?

Patient: Right.

Therapist: So, again, what alternative, more realistic, thoughts can we identify?

Patient: Hmm ... something like: "There is no evidence that anyone died from lack of sleep alone" and "Insomnia is not the main cause of poor health."

Therapist: Excellent! How about adding this one: "Excessive worrying about insomnia may be more detrimental to health than sleep loss itself," or "Insomnia is not dangerous; it may be very unpleasant, but it isn't dangerous to my health."

Patient: Yes, that's probably right as well!

In the second example, the therapist uses **reattribution techniques to modify some misconceptions about the causes of insomnia.**

Therapist: You said that your sleep problem has gotten worse with time. What does that mean to you?

Patient: It means that insomnia is an inevitable consequence of aging, and I can't do anything about it.

Therapist: How do you feel about that?

Patient: I feel discouraged and hopeless.

Therapist: How old are you?

Patient: I am 67 years old.

Therapist: Do all people of your age you know have sleep disturbances?

Patient: No. I guess not, but there are a few.

Therapist: So, you're telling me that not all older people suffer from insomnia. Is it possible that factors other than age are involved?

Patient: Hum. . . . I guess so, but I don't know which ones.

Therapist: Are there any events or activities you do during the day that affect your sleep negatively?

Patient: Yes, for example, when I have an appointment with my doctor . . . I never know what to expect and . . . I worry days in advance of my scheduled appointment and I have more trouble sleeping then.

Therapist: Good. Do you have another example of a situation that has a negative impact on your sleep?

Patient: I don't sleep well after I've had a fight with my husband.

Therapist: Okay. Now, is there any event or activities you do during the day that improves your sleep?

Patient: Hum . . . I noticed lately that when I am physically active during the day or when I go to bed later in the evening, I sleep more soundly.

Therapist: Good! So, do you think that other factors than age can affect your sleep?

Patient: I guess so.

Therapist: Does that mean that something can be done to improve your sleep?

Patient: I guess so too.

Therapist: Now, how could we reformulate your belief that insomnia is an inevitable consequence of aging?

Patient: Well, I'd say that age is not the only cause of insomnia and that some of the causal factors can be changed.

Therapist: Great! How do you feel about that now?

Patient: I feel reassured and more confident that I can do something to improve my sleep!

In the following example, the therapist uses **reappraisal to modify unrealistic sleep expectations.**

Therapist: You said that when you see your husband sleeping like a log for a solid 7 hours, you feel very anxious and even angry. What is typically going through your mind at that moment?

Patient: Well, I think, "Why am I sleeping only 6 hours and always spending over 2 hours awake in the middle of the night? What's wrong with me? There is no reason why I shouldn't sleep like him. It's abnormal to sleep so little and to be awake for so long."

Therapist: Do all people you know have the same height?

Patient: Of course not!

Therapist: What is the normal height for an adult?

Patient: Well, there is no norm really. People have different heights.

Therapist: Right. You know, sleep and height have that in common, that they are fairly variable across individuals. Beyond some normative range, there is wide variability among individuals in terms of how fast they fall asleep, how often they wake up, and the overall quality and duration of sleep.

Patient: Really? Are you telling me that I have to consider my sleep as normal and that I should accept that?

Therapist: Not necessarily. To be awake for 2 hours in the middle of the night is not right. However, your total sleep time of about 6 hours may not be that far from what you really need. At any rate, it is simply better to avoid comparing yourself with other people, since there will always be someone who sleeps better than you, the same way there will always be someone smarter, healthier, stronger, and taller than you. It's also better to have realistic goals regarding sleep.

Patient: Oh! I see what you mean now. This is very typical to compare myself with people who are better than me. No wonder why I feel so anxious!

Therapist: Exactly, pursuing an unrealistic goal is counterproductive because it makes us more anxious and, as a consequence, aggravates the underlying sleep problem.

Patient: It's difficult to fall asleep when you feel anxious, hey? (Laughs).

Therapist: I would say that it's even impossible. Then, what alternative thoughts should you entertain next time you see your husband sleeping soundly?

Patient: That I shouldn't necessarily aim at sleeping as long as he does; that he doesn't represent a norm to attain. That there are individual differences on that respect. I guess I should also accept that some days it will be easier to sleep than others and that I'm not abnormal for that.

Therapist: Very good!

These scripts illustrate how the clinician can reframe some erroneous sleep cognitions with formal cognitive restructuring techniques. There are times, however, when simple didactic education may be sufficient to correct misconceptions or faulty beliefs about sleep and insomnia. In those instances, providing accurate information about normal sleep in aging (see Morgan, Chapter 1, this volume) and about the objective consequences of insomnia may be sufficient to alleviate distress and insomnia.

Evidence Supporting the Use of Cognitive Therapy

The efficacy of cognitive therapy for insomnia, as a single treatment modality, has not yet been evaluated in a controlled study. Several investigators, however, have incorporated cognitive interventions as part of multicomponent treatment protocols for both younger (Jacobs, Benson, & Friedman, 1996; Morin, Stone, McDonald, & Jones, 1994; Sanavio, 1988; Sanavio, Vidotto, Bettinardi, Rolletto, & Zorzi, 1990) and older individuals (Edinger, Hoelscher, Marsh, Lipper, & Ionescu-Pioggia, 1992; Morin, Colecchi, Stone, Sood, & Brink, 1999; Morin, Kowatch, Barry, & Walton, 1993). The nature of those interventions has ranged from formal cognitive restructuring therapy to a variety of clinical procedures (e.g., thought stopping, imagery training, time out for worry, paradoxical intention) aimed at reducing cognitive arousal at night (Espie & Lindsay, 1987; Mitchell, 1979; Thoresen, Coates, Kirmil-Gray, & Rosekin, 1981; Woolfolk & McNulty, 1983), or psychoeducational interventions designed to teach age-appropriate sleep expectations/norms in older adults (Edinger et al., 1992; Riedel, Lichstein, & Dwyer, 1995).

Sanavio and his colleagues conducted two elegant studies in which they examined the clinical benefits of a combination of cognitive procedures (e.g., thought stopping, paradoxical intention, and cognitive restructuring of irrational beliefs about sleep requirements). In the first study (Sanavio, 1988), 24 individuals (aged 23 to 59) with sleep onset insomnia were treated with cognitive therapy or EMG biofeedback training. All subjects completed a measure of presleep cognitive intrusions and physical tension before treatment. Patients treated with cognitive therapy showed greater reductions of cognitive intrusions, but there was no differential outcome on sleep measures between patients with high levels of cognitive intrusion who were treated with cognitive therapy and those who received biofeedback. The average sleep latency was reduced by about 32 min, and total sleep time was increased by 52 min. In a second study with 40 adults (mean age 39.6) who had mixed sleep onset and maintenance insomnia (Sanavio et al., 1990), this same cognitive intervention was compared to biofeedback and to stimulus control combined with progressive relaxation training. All three treatment conditions were superior to a wait-list control condition, but there was no significant difference among the three active treatments in the amount or stability of the clinical benefits. In the cognitive therapy condition, sleep onset latency was reduced from an average of 48 min at baseline to 31 min at posttreatment, and wake after sleep onset was reduced from 62 min to 28 min for the same period.

In a study conduced with older adults, Edinger and his colleagues (1992) examined the added benefits of cognitive-behavior therapy (CBT) (stimulus control, sleep restriction, and sleep education) to relaxation training in seven older adults (aged 55 to 68 years) with sleep maintenance insomnia. The cognitive/educational component provided information about the effects of aging on sleep and age-appropriate sleep norms, the influence of circadian rhythms, and the impact of excessive worrying about the effects of sleep loss. The findings showed that the addition of CBT yielded significant reductions of time awake after sleep onset over those obtained initially by relaxation training alone. Because of the multifaceted nature of CBT, it was not possible to determine the relative contribution of the educational intervention relative to stimulus control and sleep restriction. The authors noted, however, that patients reported a greater sense of control over their sleep after treatment, something that we have also noted frequently when using formal cognitive restructuring therapy for insomnia in older adults.

Lichstein and his colleagues have also integrated a standard sleep education program into their behavioral interventions for insomnia in older adults (Riedel et al., 1995). The primary goal of this educational program is to bring seniors to adjust their sleep expectations with age-appropriate norms. This self-help educational intervention, combined with sleep restriction, has proved particularly useful for improving sleep continuity and sleep satisfaction, although treatment outcome was enhanced with the addition of therapist guidance.

Formal cognitive therapy, as outlined in the first section of this chapter, has been an integral component of our multifaceted CBT program for insomnia. It has been used with several patient populations including those with primary or secondary insomnia (Morin et al., 1994), older adults who were dependent on hypnotic medications (Morin, Colecchi, Ling, & Sood, 1995), and unmedicated older adults (Morin, Kowatch, et al., 1993). Because it has always been combined with behavioral and educational interventions, it is not possible to determine the specific contribution of cognitive therapy to the overall therapeutic outcome. Clinical evidence suggests, however, that cognitive therapy is particularly useful in assisting older adults in distinguishing normal changes in sleep patterns with aging from clinical insomnia and also in decatastrophizing the impact of insomnia on one's health and daytime functioning. Cognitive therapy also appears to be a key ingredient in facilitating the process, for seniors, of attempting to discontinue hypnotic medications. It is instrumental in alleviating excessive apprehensions about drug discontinuation and in guiding patients to reinterpret withdrawal symptoms (rebound insomnia) as temporary and manageable (Morin et al., 1995; Pat-Horenczyk et al., 1994).

Cognitive therapy may also play an important role in mediating and maintaining therapeutic changes over time. For example, in a secondary analysis of a study of late-life insomnia with 78 older adults (Morin et al., 1999), patients who were treated with CBT, alone or in combination with pharmacotherapy, showed significant reductions of dysfunctional beliefs and attitudes in sleep at posttreatment (as measured by the DBAS), and these changes were correlated with improved sleep efficiency (Morin, Blais, & Mimeault, 1996). It is interesting that a low score on the DBAS at posttreatment, indicating few dysfunctional sleep cognitions, was predictive of better sleep patterns at follow-ups across all treatment conditions (i.e., CBT alone, pharmacotherapy alone, or combined treatment). This finding suggests that attitudinal changes may be essential to maintain treatment gains over time, regardless of whether the initial treatment is behavioral or pharmacological in nature.

Clinical Observations and Obstacles

A few additional comments derived primarily from clinical observations will highlight some additional benefits of cognitive therapy in the management of insomnia, as well as some potential obstacles in its implementation with older adults. First, patients treated with cognitive therapy often report a greater sense of control (self-efficacy) over their sleep and reduced emotional distress about residual sleep difficulties after completing treatment. Because insomnia is often a recurrent problem, cognitive therapy is particularly useful to teach patients how to cope with those occasional bouts of insomnia. Whether such benefits are also obtained with behavioral interventions alone remains unclear. Second, because cognitive therapy alters irrational thinking, it is not uncommon for patients to derive generalized benefits in addressing other problem areas of their life (e.g., anxiety and depression) that may or may not be related to sleep. Third, formal cognitive therapy may not always be essential to achieve the desired goal. For instance, a simpler educational/didactic approach may be sufficient to educate seniors about normal developmental changes in sleep patterns with aging and about individual differences in sleep duration/requirements (Lichstein & Riedel, 1994). Likewise, accurate information about the objective consequences of insomnia is sometimes sufficient to alleviate emotional distress that is often triggered by the fear of insomnia and its presumed consequences.

Implementation of cognitive therapy may pose special obstacles with older adults. Older adults are facing biological changes in sleep, and most will have a much longer experience with insomnia than younger individuals. Sometimes, their belief system is more strongly engrained, and their thinking pattern may be less flexible than in younger adults, although some of those variations may be due to personality factors rather than age alone. Also, although most healthy seniors will be able to grasp the main concepts of cognitive therapy, those with neuropsychological impairments affecting attention span, memory, and flexibility of thinking may have more difficulties in understanding the principles of cognitive therapy and in adopting new perspectives on their sleep problem. A similar problem is often encountered with older adults who have a lower educational background. The main implication for clinicians is to remain very concrete when implementing cognitive therapy and to provide practical examples to illustrate new concepts.

Conclusion

Despite the extensive evidence supporting the use of behavioral interventions for insomnia, there has been no controlled evaluation of formal cognitive therapy for insomnia. Nevertheless, at least six group studies have incorporated cognitive restructuring therapy, and two more have included sleep education as part of multifaceted interventions. Of those studies, four have been conducted with older adults. All those studies have shown positive results, and none has reported a negative outcome. Thus, when cognitive therapy is combined with behavioral procedures (i.e., stimulus control, sleep restriction, relaxation training), sleep improvements are at least comparable to, if not slightly superior to, those achieved using behavioral treatment alone. The benefits of cognitive therapy extend beyond its initial impact on sleep parameters; some preliminary evidence suggests that this treatment modality may play an important function in mediating and maintaining long-term therapeutic outcome.

Although insomnia is a very prevalent complaint in late life, there is a widespread assumption among individuals who suffer from this condition, and even among health care professionals, that sleep disturbance is an inevitable consequence of aging. It may be no surprise, then, that the complaint of insomnia in late life is often overlooked and remains untreated. Although the specific contribution of cognitive therapy to the overall outcome has yet to be documented, clinical evidence suggests that this treatment modality is a useful strategy in the management of late-life insomnia, particularly to alter faulty beliefs and attitudes that often contribute to perpetuating emotional distress and sleep disturbances.

References

Beck, A. T., Emery, G., & Greenberg, R. L. (1985). *Anxiety disorders and phobias: A cognitive perspective.* New York: Basic Books.

Beck, A. T., Rush, A. J., Shaw, B. F., & Emery, G. (1979). *Cognitive therapy of depression.* New York: Guilford.

Beck, J. A. (1995). *Cognitive therapy: Basics and beyond.* New York: Guilford.

Edinger, J. D., Hoelscher, T. J., Marsh, G. R., Lipper, S., & Ionescu-Pioggia, M. (1992). A cognitive-behavioral therapy for sleep-maintenance insomnia in older adults. *Psychology and Aging, 7,* 282-289.

Edinger, J. D., Stout, A. L., & Hoelscher, T. J. (1988). Cluster analysis of insomniacs' MMPI profiles: Relation of subtypes to sleep history and treatment outcome. *Psychosomatic Medicine, 50,* 77-87.

Espie, C. A. (1991). *The psychological treatment of insomnia.* Chichester, UK: Wiley.

Espie, C. A., & Lindsay, W. R. (1987). Cognitive strategies for the management of severe sleep-maintenance insomnia: A preliminary investigation. *Behavioral Psychotherapy, 15,* 388-395.

Fichten, C., Libman, E., Creti, L., Amsel, R., Tagalakis, V., & Brender, W. (1998). Thoughts during awake times in older good and poor sleepers: The self-statement test 60+. *Cognitive Therapy and Research, 22,* 1-20.

Fins, A. I., Edinger, J. D., Sullivan, R. J., Marsh, G. R., Dailey, D., Hope, T. V., Young, M., Shaw, E., & Vasilas, D. (1996). Dysfunctional cognitions about sleep among older adults and their relationship to objective sleep findings. *Sleep Research, 25,* 242.

Freeman, A., Pretzer, J., Fleming, B., & Simon, K. M. (1990). *Clinical applications of cognitive therapy.* New York: Plenum.

Jacobs, G. D., Benson, H., & Friedman, R. (1996). Perceived benefits in a behavioral medicine insomnia program: A clinical report. *The American Journal of Medicine, 100,* 212-216.

Kales, A., & Kales, J. D. (1984). *Evaluation and treatment of insomnia.* New York: Oxford University Press.

Kuisk, L. A., Bertelson, A. D., & Walsh, J. K. (1989). Presleep cognitive hyperarousal and affect as factors in objective and subjective insomnia. *Perceptual and Motor Skills, 69,* 1219-1225.

Lichstein, K. L., & Fanning, J. (1990). Cognitive anxiety in insomnia: An analogue test. *Stress Medicine, 6*, 47-51.

Lichstein, K. L., & Riedel, B. W. (1994). Behavioral assessment and treatment of insomnia: A review with an emphasis on clinical application. *Behavior Therapy, 25*, 659-688.

Lichstein, K. L., & Rosenthal, T. L. (1980). Insomniacs' perceptions of cognitive versus somatic determinants of sleep disturbances. *Journal of Abnormal Psychology, 89*, 105-107.

Mitchell, K. R. (1979). Behavioral treatment of presleep tension and intrusive cognitions in patients with severe predormital insomnia. *Journal of Behavioral Medicine, 2*, 57-69.

Morin, C. M. (1993). *Insomnia: Psychological assessment and management*. New York: Guilford.

Morin, C. M. (1994). Dysfunctional beliefs and attitudes about sleep: Preliminary scale development and description. *The Behavior Therapist, 17*, 163-164.

Morin, C. M., Blais, F. C., & Mimeault, V. (1996). Changes in beliefs and attitudes about sleep among insomnia patients treated with cognitive-behavior therapy and pharmacotherapy. *Sleep Research, 25*, 169.

Morin, C. M., Colecchi, C. A., Ling, W. D., & Sood, R. K. (1995). Cognitive behavior therapy to facilitate benzodiazepine discontinuation among hypnotic-dependant patients with insomnia. *Behavior Therapy, 26*, 733-745.

Morin, C. M., Colecchi, C. A., Stone, J., Sood, R. K., & Brink, D. (1999). Behavioral and pharmacological therapies for late-life insomnia: A randomized clinical trial. *Journal of the American Medical Association, 281*, 991-999.

Morin, C. M., Kowatch, R. A., Barry, T., & Walton, E. (1993). Cognitive behavior therapy for late-life insomnia. *Journal of Consulting and Clinical Psychology, 61*, 137-146.

Morin, C. M., Stone, J., McDonald, K., & Jones, S. (1994). Psychological management of insomnia: A clinical replication series with 100 patients. *Behavior Therapy, 25*, 291-309.

Morin, C. M., Stone, J., Trinkle, D., Mercer, J., & Remsberg, S. (1993). Dysfunctional beliefs and attitudes about sleep among older adults with and without insomnia complaints. *Psychology and Aging, 8*, 463-467.

Pat-Horenczyk, R., Hocohen, D., Steinbuk, M., Peled, R., Zomer, J., & Lavie, P. (1994). Changes in attitudes toward insomnia following cognitive intervention as part of a withdrawal treatment from hypnotics. *Sleep Research, 23*, 184.

Riedel, B. W., Lichstein, K. L., & Dwyer, W. O. (1995). Sleep compression and sleep education for older insomniacs: Self-help versus therapist guidance. *Psychology and Aging, 10*, 54-63.

Sanavio, E. (1988). Pre-sleep cognitive intrusions and treatment of onset-insomnia. *Behaviour Research and Therapy, 26*, 451-459.

Sanavio, E., Vidotto, G., Bettinardi, O., Rolletto, T., & Zorzi, M. (1990). Behavior therapy for DIMS: Comparison of three treatment procedures with follow-up. *Behavioural Psychotherapy, 18*, 151-167.

Thoresen, C. E., Coates, T. J., Kirmil-Gray, K., & Rosekin, M. (1981). Behavioral self-management in treating sleep-maintenance insomnia. *Journal of Behavioral Medicine, 4*, 41-52.

Van Egeren, L., Haynes, S. N., Franzen, M., & Hamilton, J. (1983). Presleep cognitions and attributions in sleep-onset insomnia. *Journal of Behavioral Medicine, 6*, 217-232.

Watts, F. N., Coyle, K., & East, M. P. (1994). The contribution of worry to insomnia. *British Journal of Clinical Psychology, 33*, 211-220.

Watts, F. N., East, M. P., & Coyle, K. (1995). Insomniacs' perceived lack of control over sleep. *Psychology and Health, 10*, 81-95.

Woolfolk, R. L., & McNulty, T. F. (1983). Relaxation treatment for insomnia: A component analysis. *Journal of Consulting and Clinical Psychology, 51*, 495-503.

10

Pharmacologic Treatment

DANIEL J. BUYSSE
CHARLES F. REYNOLDS III

Increasing age is associated with an increase in insomnia complaints and insomnia disorders. Epide-
miological studies over a range of times and countries indicate that significant insomnia complaints are present in 25-35% of adults over age 65
(e.g., Dodge, Cline, & Quan, 1995; Mellinger, Balter, & Uhlenhuth, 1985;
Middelkoop, Smilde-van den Doel, Neven, Kamphuisen, & Springer,
1996). Among elderly individuals with insomnia, 75-85% have persistent complaints for 2 or more years (Ganguli, Reynolds, & Gilby, 1996;
Morgan & Clarke, 1997). The presence of insomnia complaints and disorders is associated with significant costs and morbidity. Individuals with
insomnia complaints have more work-related problems, greater health
care costs, more absenteeism, and greater functional impairment than

AUTHORS' NOTE: Preparation of this chapter was supported in part by grants
AG15138, MH52247, and MH00295 from the National Institutes of Health.

those without such complaints (Kuppermann et al., 1995; Simon & VonKorff, 1997). Insomnia complaints are also related to the subsequent development of psychiatric disorders including major depression, panic disorder, and substance abuse (Breslau, Roth, Rosenthal, & Andreski, 1996; Ford & Kamerow, 1989; Weissman, Greenwald, Nino-Murcia, & Dement, 1997). Thus, insomnia represents a common and significant health problem among the elderly.

A wide variety of behavioral and medication treatments are available for the treatment of insomnia. Although many individuals prefer to use behavioral treatments for their insomnia, some may have limited access to such treatments or may be unable to comply with the sessions and training needed to establish an effective behavioral treatment. On the other hand, the ready availability of prescription medications and their relative ease of use make it very likely that such medications will remain a major element of treatment in the elderly.

Understanding the types of pharmacologic treatments available and their beneficial and adverse effects in the elderly can be important for several other reasons. First, the elderly have a much higher use of hypnotic medications than younger individuals with insomnia. Second, the elderly are at increased risk for toxicity and adverse effects from medications of all sorts. Third, the elderly have a greater potential for drug interactions because of concurrent treatment for other health problems.

Patterns of Hypnotic Use in the Elderly

Approximately 5-10% of the adult population in Europe and North America has used a benzodiazepine hypnotic in the previous year (Mellinger et al., 1985; Olfson & Pincus, 1994; Swartz et al., 1991). The use of hypnotic medications increases dramatically with age: 10-20% of community-dwelling individuals over age 65 and up to 40% of institutionalized individuals have recently used some form of sleep medication (Henderson et al., 1995; Seppälä, Hyyppä, Impivaara, Knuts, & Sourander, 1997). The prevalence of continuous or long-term benzodiazepine use is more variable, ranging from 10-25% in some studies (Balter & Uhlenhuth, 1992; Simon, VonKorff, Barlow, Pabiniak, & Wagner, 1996) to 50-80% in others (Ohayon, 1997; Seppälä et al., 1997). Despite some important differences among specific populations, hypnotic use is consistently associated with female sex, poor physical health, and psychiatric symptoms.

Benzodiazepine Receptor Agonists

Benzodiazepines and related drugs are the most commonly prescribed hypnotics across all age groups. These drugs replaced barbiturates and related compounds (e.g., methyprylon, meprobamate) as the drugs of choice for treatment of insomnia because of their more favorable side effect profile, wide therapeutic index, and safety in overdose.

Pharmacology

All benzodiazepine and related drugs have hypnotic, anxiolytic, muscle relaxant, and anticonvulsant properties. Benzodiazepines work by binding a specific receptor site in the benzodiazepine-gamma aminobutyric acid (GABA)-chloride ion channel macromolecular complex in neuronal membranes. GABA is the major inhibitory neurotransmitter throughout the nervous system. When benzodiazepines bind at their specific recognition site, they increase GABA binding affinity. GABA binding in turn promotes chloride ion influx, resulting in hyperpolarization of the cell membrane and inhibition of neuronal activity (Tallman, Paul, Skolnick, & Gallagher, 1980). Newer non-benzodiazepine drugs such as zolpidem, zopiclone, and zaleplon bind at the same recognition site and have similar actions on the brain, or *pharmacodynamics*. These drugs may have fewer anticonvulsant, mylorelaxant, and anxiolytic properties than true benzodiazepines.

Although all benzodiazepines and related drugs have similar mechanisms of action, they have very different *pharmacokinetic* characteristics. Pharmacokinetic properties refer to the actions of the body on a drug's disposition and include rate of gastrointestinal (GI) absorption, extent of distribution in fatty tissues such as the central nervous system, and rate of elimination. Although all benzodiazepine drugs are metabolized in the liver, their specific routes of metabolism differ. Drugs that are metabolized by oxidation may compete with the metabolism of other drugs and thereby have important drug-drug interactions. Other benzodiazepines metabolized by conjugation are less likely to show drug interactions. As a result of their metabolism, some hypnotics produce active metabolites that may contribute to the drug's sleep-inducing properties. The rate at which various drugs are metabolized by the liver is typically described by the elimination half-life ($t_{1/2}$), the amount of time necessary to eliminate one-half of the drug from plasma. Benzodiazepine drugs have elimination half-life periods ranging from a few hours to several days. The total duration of a drug's action results from the combination of its pharmacokinetic properties, rather than half-life alone.

Pharmacokinetic properties can help to inform the clinician about specific drug indications. For instance, a patient who has primarily sleep onset difficulty should be prescribed a drug with a rapid onset of action and short duration of action. On the other hand, a patient with awakenings in the middle of the night or early morning may benefit from a longer-acting drug. Table 10.1 summarizes the relevant pharmacokinetic profiles for benzodiazepine receptor drugs commonly used as hypnotics.

Pharmacodynamic and pharmacokinetic properties may be affected by age. A given dose of a benzodiazepine drug often has a more potent action in elderly than younger subjects, even when plasma concentration is taken into effect; this effect may be related to changes in receptor sensitivity or density (Cook, 1986). Factors that influence pharmacokinetic changes in the elderly include lower plasma protein levels, which may lead to a greater amount of free drug in plasma. The elderly also have an increased volume of distribution (space into which a drug can be distributed) because of their higher percentage of body fat. Finally, the elimination half-life of several benzodiazepine drugs, including temazepam, oxazepam, and flurazepam, may lengthen in the elderly (Dreyfuss, Shader, Harmatz, & Greenblatt, 1986; Greenblatt, Divoll, Harmatz, MacLaughlin, & Shader, 1981). Elimination half-life periods may also be longer for some drugs in women than in men (Smith, Divoll, Gillespie, & Greenblatt, 1983). The clinical relevance of pharmacodynamic and pharmacokinetic changes is that elderly individuals may require lower doses to achieve the same sedative effect as younger individuals.

Efficacy

Numerous clinical trials have demonstrated the efficacy of benzodiazepine receptor agonists for the treatment of insomnia in the elderly, as

TABLE 10.1 Pharmacokinetic Properties of Benzodiazepine Receptor Agonists

Medication	Usual Geriatric Therapeutic Dose (mg)	Time for Onset (minutes)	$T_{1/2}$ (hr)[a]	Active Metabolite
Clonazepam[b]	0.25-1	20-60	19-60	No
Estazolam	0.5-1	15-30	8-24	No
Flurazepam	15	30-60	2-5[c] 47-100[d]	Yes
Lorazepam[b]	0.25-1	30-60	8-24	No
Oxazepam	10-15	30-60	2.8-5.7	No
Quazepam	7.5	20-45	15-40[c] 39-120[d]	Yes
Temazepam	7.5-15	45-60	3-25	No
Triazolam	0.125	15-30	1.5-5	No
Zolpidem	5	15	1.5-4.5	No
Zaleplon	5	15	1.0	No

SOURCE: Adapted from "Treatment of Insomnia in the Elderly" (Table 15.1), Reynolds, Regestein, Nowell, & Neylan. © Copyright 1998 by Williams & Wilkins. Reprinted with permission.
a. Terminal elimination half-life.
b. Used as hypnotic not indicated by Food and Drug Administration (FDA).
c. Parent compound.
d. Active metabolite.

summarized in Table 10.2. Several points about these studies deserve mention. First, most have involved a relatively small number of subjects. Second, selection criteria have not always been clearly specified, and selection criteria can vary widely from one study to the next. Third, most of these studies were short in duration, ranging from several days to 3 weeks, and therefore do not adequately reflect actual patterns of benzodiazepine use in the community. Finally, most studies of insomnia have focused exclusively on subjective or laboratory measures of sleep quantity or quality. Although these are clearly important outcomes, patients with insomnia also complain of daytime difficulties with concentration,

(Text continued on page 240)

TABLE 10.2 Controlled Studies of Benzodiazepines for Chronic Insomnia in the Elderly

Source	n	Age	Agent/Dose	Duration	Measurement	Result
Frost & DeLucchi (1979)	6	range 67-82	Flurazepam 15 mg	15 nights	PSG	Increased TST, sleep continuity
Piccione et al. (1980)	27	70 range 60-94	Chloral hydrate 250-500 mg Triazolam 0.25-0.50 mg	5 nights	Patient self-report	Both doses of triazolam, but not chloral hydrate, better than placebo
Caldwell (1982)	57	range 60-81	Quazepam 15 mg	5 nights	Questionnaire, physician global evaluation	Quazepam better than placebo for sleep quantity and quality; no serious adverse effects
Carskadon et al. (1982)	13	range 64-79	Triazolam 0.25 mg Flurazepam 15 mg	3 nights	PSG, MSLT, POMS	Increased TST, worsened MSLT with flurazepam; improved MSLT with triazolam; improved POMS with flurazepam; worsened POMS with triazolam
Fillingim (1982)	75 convalescent home residents	81	Temazepam 30 mg Flurazepam 30 mg	4 nights	Patient self-report	Comparable efficacy for both drugs; less drug hangover with temazepam
Martinez & Serna (1982)	41	65	Quazepam 15 mg	5 nights	Questionnaire, PSG	Quazepam better than placebo in increasing quantity and quality of sleep

Study	N	Age	Drug/dose	Duration	Measures	Results
Elie & Deschenes (1983)	30	75 (1.8) range 60-93	Zopiclone 5, 7.5, 10 mg Flurazepam 15 mg	3 weeks	Self-report	Zopiclone 7.5-10 mg comparable to flurazepam; no clinically significant side effects
Viukari & Miettinen (1984)	20	76 (1.3)	Diazepam 5 mg Promethazine 25 mg Propiomazine 25 mg	3 weeks	Staff observation, psychomotor tests	Both diazepam and propiomazine prolonged sleep; no rebound insomnia; no effect on psychomotor skills
Roehrs et al. (1985)	22	67 (6.6) range 60-85	Triazolam 0.125 mg	2 nights	PSG, MSLT	Increased TST, improved MSLT
Meuleman et al. (1987)	17 nursing home residents	78.1 (11) range 56-97	Temazepam 15 mg Diphenhydramine 50 mg	5 nights	Self-report, observe sleep diary, psychomotor tests	Shortened sleep latency and longer sleep duration with diphenhydramine; poorer performance on psychomotor tests with both agents
Mamelak et al. (1989)	36	range 60-72	Flurazepam 15 mg Brotizolam 0.25 mg	2 weeks	Questionnaire, MSLT, neuropsychological tests	Rebound insomnia with brotizolam; both drugs increased daytime sleepiness; only placebo-treated group sleeping better than baseline at end of treatment

TABLE 10.2 Continued

Source	n	Age	Agent/Dose	Duration	Measurement	Result
Elie et al. (1990)	44	76 (1.3) range 60-90	Zopiclone 5, 7.5 mg Triazolam 0.125, 0.25 mg Placebo	21 nights	Self-report sleep questionnaire	Improved sleep latency and sleep soundness, but not sleep quality, for both drugs vs. placebo; no withdrawal or rebound
Mouret et al. (1990)	10	68.1 (10)	Triazolam .25 mg Zopiclone 7.5 mg	15 nights	PSG	Improved sleep with both drugs; slow-wave sleep decreased with triazolam, increased with zopiclone
Schlich et al. (1991)	107	63.2 (1.1) range 40-86	Zolpidem 10-20 mg	6 months	Observer and patient report	Improved sleep latency, sleep duration, sleep quality
Shaw et al. (1992)	119	74.5 (0.9)	Zolpidem 10-20 mg	3 weeks	Nursing observation	Zolpidem 10 mg and 20 mg dose improved total sleep duration, reduced wakefulness; no withdrawal symptoms
Kummer et al. (1993)	14	67.8 (2.2) range 59-85	Zolpidem 20 mg	179 nights	PSG	Improved sleep efficiency and total sleep time

Study	N	Age	Medication	Duration	Measure	Results
Roger et al. (1993)	221	81 (58-98)	Zolpidem 5 mg	3 weeks	Sleep quality visual analog scale, clinician global impression	All measures of sleep quality improved for all treatments vs. baseline; no rebound insomnia
Vgontzas et al. (1994)	8	67 (1.4)	Temazepam 7.5 mg	7 nights	PSG	Decreased total wake time
Dehlin et al. (1995)	102	79 range 60-95	Zopiclone 5 mg Flunitrazepam 1 mg	14 nights	Sleep diary	Improved sleep quality, decreased wakefulness in both groups vs. baseline
Roth et al. (1997)	30	65.9 (4.6)	Quazepam 7.5 mg Quazepam 15 mg Placebo	7 nights	PSG	Increased total sleep time, decreased sleep latency for both doses vs. placebo

SOURCE: Adapted from "Treatment of Insomnia in the Elderly" (Table 15.2), Reynolds, Regestein, Nowell, & Neylan. © Copyright 1998 by Williams & Wilkins. Reprinted with permission.

irritability, and minor mood changes, which are infrequently reflected in clinical studies.

In a meta-analysis of treatment efficacy of benzodiazepines for insomnia in middle-aged adults, Nowell and colleagues (Nowell et al., 1997) identified 22 clinical studies that met the criteria of studying chronic insomnia patients in a randomized placebo-controlled double-blind trial. The median treatment duration was 7 days, and the longest was 35 days. Combined effect sizes across studies ranged from 0.56 to 0.71 for subjective outcomes of sleep onset latency, total sleep time, number of awakenings, and sleep quality. By convention, these effect sizes are considered moderately large and substantiate the efficacy of benzodiazepines for chronic insomnia. Although no comparable quantitative analysis has been conducted for older subjects, a qualitative review of benzodiazepines in the elderly yielded similar results: Patients reported moderate improvements in subjective measures of sleep latency, total sleep time, and awakenings per night (Grad, 1995). Our own summary in Table 10.2 supports this assessment.

As noted above, most studies of benzodiazepine drugs have not considered a wide range of patient outcomes. Leger and colleagues (Leger, Quera-Salva, & Philip, 1996) reported that treatment with zopiclone, a benzodiazepine receptor agonist, was associated with greater improvements in quality of life measures, social activities, and professional activities compared to placebo after both 14 days and 8 weeks of treatment. Another study showed that treated patients reported fewer symptoms of feeling blue, down in the dumps, or depressed, as well as fewer symptoms of being easily upset or irritated compared to those with untreated insomnia (Balter & Uhlenhuth, 1991).

The effects of benzodiazepines and related medications on polysomnographic sleep measures have been well documented (for review, see Parrino & Terzano, 1996; Riemann et al., 1994). These effects are summarized in Table 10.3. In addition to consistent changes in sleep latency and wakefulness during the night, benzodiazepines decrease the number of periodic limb movements and associated arousals in patients with periodic limb movement disorder (Hening, Allen, Walters, & Chokroverty, 1999). Benzodiazepines can also decrease oxyhemoglobin saturations during the night and may theoretically worsen sleep apnea. Such effects may be important in the elderly, given the increased prevalence of sleep apnea and other sleep-related breathing disturbances in the elderly. In patients with mild to moderate degrees of sleep apnea, however, the change in oxyhemoglobin saturation and number of apneas usually is neither large in magnitude nor clinically significant (Berry, Kouchi, & Bower, 1995; Quera-Salva, McCann, & Boudet, 1994).

The efficacy and polysomnographic effects of benzodiazepines have been studied primarily during short-term administration, but as indicated above, many patients take these drugs chronically. Available data yield conflicting results regarding the efficacy of chronic benzodiazepine administration. Several early polysomnographic studies suggested that tolerance develops to their hypnotic effects over several weeks (e.g., Kales, Kales, Bixler, Scharf, & Russek, 1976). Other laboratory studies, however, have shown continued efficacy of these drugs. For instance, triazolam had continued efficacy when administered over a period of 5 weeks in one study (Mitler, Seidel, Van Den Hoed, Greenblatt, & Dement, 1984). Other studies have shown continued efficacy for zolpidem versus placebo over 5 weeks and in a single-blind study for 6 months (Kummer et al., 1993; Scharf, Roth, Vogel, & Walsh, 1994). Studies using self- or observer-rated assessments have suggested efficacy for benzodiazepines and related compounds for even longer amounts of time. Continued efficacy for benzodiazepines such as nitrazepam, lormatazepam, midazolam, and temazepam has been demonstrated for 12 to 24 weeks with no evidence of tolerance (Allen, Mendels, Nevins, Chernik, & Hoddes, 1987; Oswald, French, Adam, & Gilham, 1982). Single-blind studies of patients with mean ages from 58 to 63 showed reduced sleep latency and increased total sleep time for as long as 1 year of treatment with zolpidem (Maarek, Cramer, Attali, Coquelin, & Morselli, 1992; Schlich, L'Heritier, Coquelin, Attali, & Kryrein, 1991). In epidemiological studies, as many as two-thirds of patients taking benzodiazepines chronically report satisfaction with their sleep (Ohayon, 1996).

Adverse Effects

The most common adverse effect of benzodiazepines and related hypnotics is a direct extension of their intended therapeutic effect, sedation. Daytime sleepiness arises when the duration of action of the hypnotic medication is longer than the nocturnal sleep. Studies using the

TABLE 10.3 Effects of Hypnotic Drugs on Polysomnographic Sleep

Drug Class	Sleep Continuity	Slow-Wave Sleep	REM Sleep	Other Effects
Benzodiazepine receptor agonists	↓ sleep latency, awakenings ↑ sleep time, sleep efficiency	→ to ↓	↓ REM time (true benzodiazepines) → REM time (other benzodiazepine receptor agonists) → phasic REM activity	• Respiratory suppression (increased apnea, reduced oxyhemoglobin saturation) • Reduced periodic limb movements • Increased sleep spindles and activity
Tricyclic antidepressants	Variable effects from ↓ sleep latency, awakenings; ↑ sleep time, sleep efficiency (e.g., trimipramine, amitriptyline, doxepin) to ↑ sleep latency, awakenings; ↓ sleep time, sleep efficiency (e.g., clomipramine, protriptyline, desipramine)	→ to ↓ for most agents; ↑ for some (e.g., doxepin)	↓ to ↓↓ REM time (→ for trimipramine), ↑ phasic REM activity	• Slight reduction in apnea • May worsen periodic limb movements or restless legs (especially clomipramine)
SSRI antidepressants	→ to ↑ sleep latency, awakenings; → to ↓ sleep time, sleep efficiency	→ to ↓	↓ to ↓↓ REM time ↑ phasic REM activity	• Slight reduction in apnea • May worsen periodic limb movements or restless legs • Eye movements during NREM sleep

Trazodone, nefazodone	↓ sleep latency, awakenings; ↑ sleep time, sleep efficiency	→ (nefazodone); → to ↑ (trazodone)	REM time → to ↑ (nefazodone), → (trazodone)	• Nefazodone less sedating
Bupropion	↑ sleep latency, awakenings; ↓sleep time, sleep efficiency	→ to ↓	↑ REM time; ↑ phasic REM activity	
Melatonin	↓ sleep latency, → to ↓ awakenings; → to ↑ sleep time, sleep efficiency	↑	→ REM time and phasic activity	
Antihistamines (diphenhydramine)	↓ sleep latency, awakenings; ↑ sleep time, sleep efficiency	→	→ to ↓ REM time; → phasic REM activity	

multiple sleep latency test have documented an increase in daytime sleepiness during the administration of long-acting benzodiazepines such as flurazepam (Carskadon, Seidel, Greenblatt, & Dement, 1982; Mitler et al., 1984), although there is also some evidence that this effect may diminish over time. By contrast, short-acting benzodiazepines are not associated with a consistent increase in daytime sleepiness. Concerns regarding daytime sedation are heightened in the elderly because of the possibility of longer elimination half-life periods and greater sensitivity to drug effects.

Benzodiazepine drugs also cause dose-related anterograde amnesia (for review, see Buysse, 1991). In fact, some investigators have suggested that this property may be responsible for benzodiazepines' positive subjective effects (Perlis, Giles, Mendelson, Bootzin, & Wyatt, 1997; Roth, Roehrs, Wittig, & Zorick, 1984). Nevertheless, these amnestic properties may be clinically significant, particularly in the elderly and in those with coexisting medical problems. Studies in long-term users of benzodiazepines, including nursing home residents, indicate cognitive impairment across a range of neuropsychological tests, including tests of attention, motor performance, and recall. With discontinuation of the drug, improvements in test performance have been noted in some studies (Salzman et al., 1992; Tönne et al., 1995) but not in others (Tata, Rollings, Collins, Pickering, & Jacobson, 1994).

Benzodiazepine medications have also been related to an increased risk of injurious falls and hip fracture in the elderly. Increased risk is associated with new prescriptions or recent dose increases, use of long-acting benzodiazepines, higher doses, multiple benzodiazepines, and use in institutionalized individuals (Herings, Stricker, deBoer, Bakker, & Sturmans, 1995; Mustard & Mayer, 1997; Neutel, Hirdes, Maxwell, & Patten, 1996; Ray, Griffin, & Downey, 1989). Data regarding another potential source of morbidity, automobile crashes, are mixed. One case-control study of older individuals involved or not involved in injurious crashes showed an elevated risk associated with cyclic antidepressants and opiate analgesics, but not with benzodiazepines (Leveille et al., 1994). Another study showed an elevated rate ratio of injurious crashes within the first week and during continuous use of long half-life benzodiazepines, but not short half-life benzodiazepines (Hemmelgarn, Suissa, Huang, Boivin, & Pinard, 1997).

In a population-based study, daily use of hypnotics in general—but not with benzodiazepine hypnotics in particular—was associated with increased all-cause mortality among the elderly, even after controlling for symptoms of insomnia (Kripke et al., 1998). Most studies examining the risk of benzodiazepines for falls and motor vehicle accidents, however, have not concurrently examined the risks of untreated insomnia. One such study found that, among independent-living elderly, insomnia—but not use of long-acting benzodiazepines—was associated with an increased risk of major injurious falls (Koski, Luukinen, Laippala, & Kivelä, 1998).

Finally, the use of benzodiazepines also raises the sometimes contentious issues of abuse and discontinuance syndromes. Benzodiazepines were used by 0.5-3.0% of the population for nonmedical purposes in a previous year (Woods & Winger, 1995), but random population surveys have shown that fewer than 10% of patients increased the dose of their prescription benzodiazepine during a previous year (Balter & Uhlenhuth, 1992). Even among patients who wish to discontinue their chronic use of benzodiazepine medication, their patterns of use suggest stability or declining doses over time as well as a tendency toward intermittent rather than consistent dosing (Romach, Busto, Somer, Kaplan, & Sellers, 1995). Thus, true abuse of benzodiazepines appears to be uncommon.

Benzodiazepines can be associated with three different types of discontinuance syndromes (American Psychiatric Association, 1990). *Rebound* refers to an increase in the original symptom beyond the baseline level. There have been inconsistent reports of rebound insomnia with short-acting benzodiazepine medications. Population surveys and results from large treatment effectiveness studies show rebound insomnia in 14-20% of patients treated with benzodiazepines, a rate indistinguishable from that seen with over-the-counter drugs or placebo (Balter & Uhlenhuth, 1991; Hajak et al., 1998). *Withdrawal* refers to the appearance of new symptoms, not originally present, upon discontinuance of the drug. Withdrawal symptoms occur in up to 40-100% of patients treated chronically with benzodiazepines, can persist for days or weeks following discontinuance of the medication, and can be severe enough to require rigorous treatment (Busto, Sellers, & Naranjo, 1986; Lader, 1994; Noyes, Garvey, Cook, & Suelzer, 1991). Typical withdrawal symptoms include dizziness, confusion, depression, and feelings of unreality. Cognitive and behavioral treatment can help patients discontinue chronic benzodiazepine use, although an increase in sleep disturbance is typical during these interventions (Habraken et al., 1997; Morin, Colecchi, Ling,

& Sood, 1995). Finally, *recurrence* is another potential discontinuance syndrome, one that has received little attention. As discussed in the introduction, insomnia tends to be a chronic problem, and it should not be surprising that some patients show a return of insomnia symptoms after they discontinue their medication. This may simply reflect a return of the original syndrome, however, rather than a failure of benzodiazepine treatment per se. Among younger adults treated for anxiety disorders, symptoms of anxiety persist after benzodiazepine discontinuance, and approximately 25-35% of patients who discontinue medications return to benzodiazepines or other medications (Rickels, Case, Schweizer, Garcia-Espana, & Fridman, 1991). A similar situation often occurs in recurrent mood disorders, where chronic medication treatment is used as a maintenance form of therapy.

Antidepressants

Antidepressants frequently are used as an alternative to benzodiazepine hypnotics. This may relate to their lower abuse potential, even though physiologic dependence clearly results from the continued use of antidepressants. A wealth of data has been accumulated regarding the EEG sleep effects of antidepressant medications. Fewer data have been designed to specifically address their efficacy in primary insomnia, and none of these have specifically focused on the elderly. The absence of data in this area is unfortunate because the elderly may be more sensitive to some side effects of antidepressant medications. A survey of the National Disease and Therapeutic Index between 1987 and 1996 showed an overall decline in the prescription of benzodiazepine hypnotics of about 50% at the same time that use of antidepressants for insomnia increased by 100% (Walsh & Schweitzer, 1999). These trends were evident in patients between 50 and 69 years of age and in those over 70 years of age; however, the exact prevalence of antidepressant use for insomnia in the elderly is difficult to ascertain. Survey data suggest that less than 10% of hypnotic prescriptions in the elderly are for antidepressants (Englert & Linden, 1998; Ohayon & Caulet, 1996; Seppälä et al., 1997), and among residents in long-term care facilities, 10-12% are using tricyclic antidepressants for depression or insomnia (Conn & Goldman, 1992).

Pharmacology

Antidepressants are a diverse group of drugs with a wide range of activities on central neurotransmission. In general, antidepressant drugs are thought to exert their therapeutic effect through alterations in serotenergic and noradrenergic neurotransmission. The net effect of antidepressant treatment is often a down-regulation of post-synaptic receptors; however, the specific mechanisms of action and side effect profiles differ widely among individual agents. Several antidepressant side effects, and their sedative potential, are related to specific receptor effects including antagonism of histamine, alpha$_1$ adrenergic, and serotonin 5-HT$_2$ receptors. The efficacy of all antidepressant agents appears to be equivalent in the treatment of depression, but their specific side effect profiles may make one particular agent better suited to a patient with particular symptoms. Antidepressant classes, typical therapeutic doses, mechanisms of action, and side effect profiles have been summarized by Richelson (1996).

Antidepressant effects on sleep also vary considerably among different agents, as discussed in Sharpley and Cowen (1995) and Thase (1998), and as summarized in Table 10.3. Although earlier studies suggested that the sleep effects of antidepressants may directly mediate their therapeutic effects, more recent studies have cast doubt on the theory that either slow-wave sleep or REM sleep effects of antidepressants are responsible for their antidepressant activity (vanBemmel, 1997).

Efficacy Data

Studies of sleep changes during antidepressant administration in depressed patients show that drugs such as doxepin, trazodone, and amitriptyline decrease insomnia complaints, increase polysomnographic sleep continuity measures, and (in the case of trazodone) increase slow-wave sleep (e.g., Casper et al., 1994; Parrino, Spaggiari, Boselli, Di Giovanni, & Terzano, 1994; Scharf & Sachais, 1990). Perhaps more surprising, even "activating" drugs such as fluoxetine can improve insomnia complaints in depressed patients relative to placebo (Satterlee & Faries, 1995). Fluoxetine is associated with symptoms of agitation, anxiety, or insomnia in as many as 40% of patients, but sedating events occur in as many as 20% (Beasley, Sayler, Weiss, & Potvin, 1992). The apparent discrepancy in these findings may be explained by methodological differences among studies. Improvements in insomnia are seen when changes in mean symptom levels are examined, but insomnia or hypersomnia complaints are noted in studies that tabulate the discrete occurrence of specific side effects in specific individuals.

Specific antidepressant drugs have different effects on EEG and subjectively reported sleep disturbance in patients with depression. For instance, fluvoxamine is more alerting than desipramine, which in turn is more alerting than amitriptyline (Kupfer et al., 1991; Shipley et al., 1985). Trimipramine and imipramine both improve sleep quality, but trimipramine improves polysomnographic sleep continuity to a greater extent (Ware, Brown, Moorad, Pittard, & Cobert, 1989). A series of comparisons between fluoxetine and nefazodone have consistently shown that both drugs improve subjective sleep disturbance in depressed patients, although nefazodone improved both subjective and polysomnographic measures of sleep disturbance to a greater degree (Armitage, Yonkers, Cole, & Rush, 1997; Gillin, Rapaport, Erman, Winokur, & Albala, 1997; Rush et al., 1998). A longitudinal study in elderly depressed patients treated with nortriptyline showed that both subjective and objective measures of sleep quality and continuity were maintained over a 12-month period (Buysse et al., 1996).

Very few studies have examined the efficacy of antidepressants in patients with primary insomnia. A study of nine "poor sleepers" (mean age 61) showed increased total sleep time, decreased wakefulness, and improved sleep quality over a 3-week trial of trazodone, with rebound insomnia during drug withdrawal (Montgomery, Oswald, Morgan, & Adam, 1983). In middle-aged patients with insomnia, doxepin improved polysomnographic measures of sleep continuity (Hajak et al., 1996), and trimipramine improved both polysomnographic sleep efficiency and subjective sleep quality (Hohagen et al., 1994). Finally, an open-label pilot study of paroxetine in middle-aged and older subjects with primary insomnia showed improvement in a multivariate measure of sleep quantity based on both diary and PSG measures (Nowell, Reynolds, Buysse, Dew, & Kupfer, 1999). Small improvements were also noted in diary-based measures of sleep quality and in both diary-based and polysomnographic measures of sleep efficiency. Thus, the small amount of available evidence suggests that antidepressants may have beneficial effects on subjective and objective sleep measures in patients with major depression, as well as in patients with primary insomnia.

Combination Treatments

Although antidepressant drugs may have beneficial effects on insomnia for the majority of patients, some patients complain of continued or worsened insomnia. It has become common practice to use sedating tricyclic drugs, trazodone, or benzodiazepine hypnotics among patients treated with selective serotonin reuptake inhibitors (SSRIs). A retrospective drug utilization review showed that 35% of patients prescribed SSRIs were also prescribed medications for anxiety or insomnia and that 15% of the total were receiving once daily dosing of such medications, which suggests treatment for insomnia (Rascati, 1995). Available data suggest that these approaches are likely to be effective. Open-label and placebo-controlled trials of trazodone in patients with antidepressant-associated insomnia showed that trazodone significantly improved subjective sleep measures (Jacobsen, 1990; Nierenberg, Adler, Peselow, Zornberg, & Rosenthal, 1994), and a smaller case series suggests that this approach may also lead to improvements in depression (Nierenberg, Cole, & Glass, 1992). Approximately 20% of patients may experience excessive sedation when taking a trazodone-fluoxetine combination (Metz & Shader, 1990), and the potential for a "serotonin syndrome" also exists.

Combinations of benzodiazepines with tricyclic antidepressants or nefazodone are also effective for treating insomnia in depression (Dominguez, Jacobson, Goldstein, & Steinbook, 1984; Rickels, 1988; Scharf, Hirschowitz, Zemlan, Lichstein, & Woods, 1986). Concurrent treatment with benzodiazepines does not impair the antidepressant response to tricyclic drugs and may be associated with improved tolerance and retention in treatment for some patients (Buysse et al., 1997; Nolen, Haffmans, Bouvy, & Duivenvoorden, 1993).

Adverse Effects

Side effects associated with specific antidepressants can range from "nuisance" side effects such as dry mouth, constipation, and GI upset to potentially serious complications such as cardiac conduction delays, hypotension, and lethal overdoses. Rebound insomnia can follow discontinuation of antidepressants. A number of studies involving tricyclic drugs have also demonstrated significant psychomotor performance deficits (reviewed in Buysse, 1991). A longitudinal study of cognitive decline among older men and women found that non-benzodiazepine psychotropic drug use, which included antidepressant drug use, was associated with cognitive decline (Dealberto, McAvay, Seeman, & Berkman, 1997). Epidemiologic data also suggest that cyclic antidepressants are associated with an elevated risk of injurious motor vehicle collisions (Leveille et al., 1994).

Melatonin

Melatonin has gained widespread use as a sleep-promoting substance over the past several years, but its use was not preceded by properly conducted empirical clinical trials. There are few data regarding the effectiveness of melatonin for primary insomnia, particularly among the elderly. Published studies have used widely different study designs, subjects, and methodologies (Mendelson, 1997).

Pharmacology

Melatonin is a hormone produced by the pineal gland in a strong circadian pattern, with secretion being maximal during darkness and essentially absent during light in both nocturnal and diurnal species. Because it is secreted primarily at night, which corresponds to the timing of the major sleep period in humans, melatonin has been implicated as a sleep-promoting substance. The issue may be particularly salient in the elderly, who frequently have reduced melatonin secretion (Reiter, 1995). Melatonin is distributed and eliminated rapidly, its chief metabolic route being hydroxylation in the liver. A variety of preparations are available, some with rapid absorption and short bio-availability and others with sustained actions (Brzezinski, 1997). The elimination half-life for various melatonin preparations ranges from several minutes to approximately 8 hours. Doses of melatonin administered for sleep-promoting effects have varied from 0.1 mg to as much as 80 mg in clinical trials. Doses above 1 mg are likely to produce supra-physiologic concentrations. Although melatonin's precise mechanism of action is not known, it is likely to act through interaction with melatonin receptors in the suprachiasmatic nucleus (SCN) of the hypothalamus, which is the pacemaker of the human biological clock. Specifically, melatonin may dampen the alerting signals typically produced by the SCN during light hours (Sack, Hughes, Edgar, & Lewy, 1997). In addition, melatonin shifts circadian rhythms according to a phase response curve (Deacon & Arendt, 1995; Lewy, Ahmed, Jackson, & Sack, 1992).

Efficacy

Melatonin has been used to shift circadian rhythms in blind people (Sack, Lewy, Blood, Stevenson, & Keith, 1991) and to treat jet lag (Arendt, Aldhous, & Marks, 1986; Petrie, Conaglen, Thompson, & Chamberlain, 1989) and delayed sleep phase syndrome (Dahlitz et al., 1991). In healthy subjects, daytime melatonin administration causes sleepiness and fatigue (Dollins, Zhdanova, Wurtman, Lynch, & Deng, 1994; Tzischinsky & Lavie, 1994). When administered to healthy subjects at night, melatonin decreases sleep latency and the number of awakenings, and it improves sleep efficiency in a noise-induced insomnia paradigm (Waldhauser, Saletu, & Trinchard-Lugan, 1990; Zhdanova, Wurtman, Morabito, Piotrovska, & Lynch, 1996). Not all studies have shown an effect of melatonin, particularly when administered for a single night (James, Mendelson, Sack, Rosenthal, & Wehr, 1987).

Studies in middle-aged insomnia patients have also yielded inconsistent findings. One study of single-night administration did not show any changes in polysomnographic sleep continuity measures (James, Sack, Rosenthal, & Mendelson, 1989). Measures of subjective sleep ratings showed no effect with a dose of 5 mg for 1 week (Ellis, Lemmens, & Parkes, 1996) but an increase in subjective total sleep time with 14 days' administration of 75 mg (MacFarlane, Cleghorn, Brown, & Streiner, 1991). Five studies of melatonin for insomnia in the elderly have been reported. The study with the most rigorous design included 14 elderly subjects treated with placebo or melatonin 0.5 mg in a randomized crossover trial lasting 14 nights for each trial. Although each type of melatonin treatment shortened polysomnographic sleep latency, there were no changes in total sleep time, sleep efficiency, wakefulness after sleep onset, quality, subjective sleep quality, or daytime alertness (Hughes, Sack, & Lewy, 1998). Three other studies used actigraphy as the main outcome measure in elderly individuals with insomnia. These studies showed that melatonin 0.3-2 mg improved sleep efficiency, awakenings, and/or sleep latency (Garfinkel, Laudon, Nof, & Zisapel, 1995; Haimov et al., 1995; Wurtman & Zhdanova, 1995).

Adverse Effects

Careful studies of melatonin side effects have not yet been conducted. Because melatonin is involved in the regulation of seasonal reproductions in some animals, and because pineal tumors may also affect fertility, there are some concerns that melatonin may also affect the reproductive status of young adult women. Other potential side effects include a worsening of sleep apnea (Maksoud, Moore, & Harshkowitz, 1997), impaired cognitive and psychomotor performance during daytime administration (Rogers, Phan, Kennaway, & Dawson, 1997), and disruption of sleep or activity rhythms (Middleton, Stone, & Arendt, 1996).

Antihistamines

Antihistamines frequently are used as over-the-counter sedative agents and are commonly prescribed in nursing homes for this purpose. Despite their widespread use, few controlled studies have been conducted in elderly populations to support their efficacy or safety. On the other hand, considerable evidence suggests that these drugs can impair psychomotor performance.

Antihistamines are a diverse group of drugs with varying pharmacokinetic properties. Diphenhydramine is the prototype of these drugs and is the most commonly available over-the-counter preparation. The elimination half-life ranges from 3 to 4.5 hours in young adults and is as long as 5 hours in the elderly. The sedative effects of diphenhydramine correlate with its plasma levels (Carruthers, Shoeman, Hignite, & Azarnoff, 1978). Antihistamines exert their effect by antagonizing histamine H_1 receptors. Histaminergic neurons in the posterior hypothalamus promote awakening and form important reciprocal connections with GABA-ergic neurons in the ventro-lateral preoptic area of the hypothalamus (Sherin, Shiromani, McCarley, & Saper, 1996). The net effects of histamine antagonism are a decrease in histaminergic activation and an increase in GABA-mediated neural inhibition.

The effects of antihistamines on daytime performance and sleepiness have been well described. Sedating antihistamines clearly impair performance, including sustained attention, vigilance, and other standard performance tests (reviewed in Buysse, 1991), and "non-sedating antihistamines" show fewer effects in this regard. Sleep laboratory tests of daytime sleep tendency in healthy young adults confirm these findings, with drugs such as diphenhydramine causing increased daytime sleepiness and "non-sedating" drugs such as terfenadine, loratadine, and cetirizine causing no significant changes (Gengo & Gabos, 1987; Roehrs, Tietz, Zorick, & Roth, 1984; Roth, Roehrs, Koshorek, Sicklesteel, & Zorick, 1987). Diphenhydramine 50 mg significantly improved subjective ratings of sleep quality, sleep time, sleep latency, and wakefulness after sleep onset in middle-aged adults with insomnia (Rickels et al., 1983). A more recent study examined the effects of the benzodiazepine lorazepam versus a combination drug containing lorazepam plus diphenhydramine (Saletu et al., 1997). Polysomnographic and subjective measures showed a slight advantage for the combination preparation in terms of sleep latency and sleep quality. Alertness was more impaired under the combination medication, although other performance measures were actually somewhat better in the combination preparation.

Few studies have specifically examined sleep effects of antihistamines in the elderly. Three studies have confirmed the expected sedative properties of antihistamines relative to placebo, and comparable in magnitude to benzodiazepines. These effects included increased sleep time, decreased awakening, and shorter sleep latency as judged by self and observer reports, polysomnography, and actigraphy (Adam & Oswald, 1986; Meuleman, Nelson, & Clark, 1987; Viukari & Miettinen, 1984). Study durations ranged from 1 night to 5 weeks, and the studies included outpatients, inpatients, and nursing home residents. In general, cognitive effects were comparable between antihistamines and benzodiazepine drugs.

Clinical Guidelines

Pharmacologic treatment of insomnia in elderly patients can be safe and effective but needs to be considered as one component in a comprehensive treatment plan. As with any other treatment, this entails adequate evaluation, careful implementation and follow-up, and appropriate treatment for specific patients.

Patient Evaluation

As described in Chapter 3 of this volume, a comprehensive assessment is essential prior to treating insomnia in older adults. Several aspects of this evaluation are particularly important with regard to pharmacologic treatment. First, the presence of other primary sleep disorders
must be determined. In particular, sleep apnea is a common problem in
the elderly and constitutes a relative contraindication for drugs such as
benzodiazepines and melatonin. Restless legs syndrome and periodic
limb movement disorder increase with age and also require specialized
treatment. A thorough medical history is critical because specific medical disorders may again constitute relative contraindications to some
forms of treatment. For instance, chronic obstructive pulmonary disease
and waking hypercapnia are relative contraindications benzodiazepines, and some cardiac arrhythmias are a relative contraindication for
tricyclic antidepressants. Liver and kidney disease may impair the elimination of hypnotic drugs, leading to prolonged sedative effects. Patients
with organic brain disease such as dementia and stroke are at increased
risk of cognitive side effects from essentially all hypnotic medications, including benzodiazepines, sedating antidepressants, and antihistamines.

It is also important to consider other concurrent medications prior to
instituting pharmacologic treatments. A wide range of medications are
metabolized by the cytochrome oxidase P450 system in the liver. These
drugs include some benzodiazepines and several antidepressant drugs.
Individuals who are concurrently prescribed several drugs that compete
for the same enzyme system can develop increased side effects and toxicity from elevated blood levels of these medications. Likewise, a careful
substance abuse history is necessary to identify those who are currently
using or abusing sleep active substances such as alcohol, over-the-counter hypnotic drugs, caffeine, and nicotine.

Principles of Treatment in the Elderly

The decision to treat insomnia in the elderly should begin with a careful analysis of behavioral interventions that may help a particular pa-

tient. Many elderly individuals spend excessive time in bed at night, take long daytime or evening naps, and have irregular sleep/wake habits, each of which can disrupt sleep. In addition, elderly patients can benefit from more specific behavioral techniques as described in other chapters of this volume. Pharmacologic treatment of elderly patients usually should be instituted in conjunction with, or after an unsuccessful trial of, behavioral treatment. Even pharmacotherapy has important educational and behavioral elements. For instance, most hypnotic medications are more effective when taken 15 to 30 minutes before bedtime and at later rather than earlier bedtimes. An elderly patient who wishes to take a sleeping pill at 8:00 p.m., go to bed at 9:00 p.m., fall asleep within 30 minutes, and sleep continuously until 9:00 a.m. has unrealistic expectations. A later bedtime and/or earlier awakening time, along with medication dosing close to bedtime, should be recommended.

A second major principle of pharmacologic treatment is to use the lowest effective dose. Doses for many drugs need to be lower in the elderly than in middle-aged subjects because of changes in pharmacokinetics and pharmacodynamics, as discussed above. Because most patients have had insomnia for many years, there is little risk involved in using very low doses initially, then gradually increasing the dose into what might more typically be considered a "therapeutic" range.

A final general principle is that of follow-up. Pharmacotherapy can produce adverse daytime effects, and these need to be monitored carefully through regular follow-up. Because patients' medication regimens and health status change over time, follow-up needs to be continued as long as a patient is receiving medication. The issue of optimal duration of hypnotic treatment is rather contentious. Ideally, hypnotics would be used for a short amount of time, and the Food and Drug Administration (FDA) has approved their use only in this setting. Unfortunately, this recommendation does not conform to our knowledge about the natural history of most insomnia disorders. It is often reasonable to initiate a trial of hypnotic medication for approximately 1 month, then attempt to taper and discontinue the medication. Some patients, however, may require a longer duration of treatment. Under such circumstances, careful monitoring of continued effects and side effects is of paramount importance.

Pharmacologic Treatment in
Specific Clinical Situations

Primary Insomnia

Most of this chapter has focused on treatment of primary insomnia; however, primary insomnia constitutes only approximately 10% of insomnia cases in the population and 25% of cases seen at sleep disorder centers (Buysse et al., 1994; Ohayon, 1997). There is also evidence that primary insomnia is even less common among the elderly. On the other hand, because neither the International Classification of Sleep Disorders nor the *Diagnostic and Statistical Manual of Mental Disorders (DSM-IV)* recognizes a specific category of age-related insomnia, many elderly will by default be diagnosed with primary insomnia. Benzodiazepine hypnotics are the recommended pharmacologic treatment for primary insomnia. The exact role of other agents, such as antidepressants, melatonin, and antihistamines, has not been carefully evaluated, and thus a recommendation for clinical scenarios that support their use is difficult to make. Patients with primary insomnia should have pharmacotherapy in conjunction with or following behavioral treatment.

Insomnia Secondary to Mental Disorder

A majority of patients with chronic insomnia have another diagnosable mental disorder. In these cases, treatment should be directed at the underlying mental disorder, which usually is a depressive or anxiety disorder. There are basically three options for treating the insomnia associated with depressive and anxiety disorders: treatment with a single antidepressant drug, such as an SSRI, tricyclic drug, or newer atypical agent; combined treatment using a relatively less-sedating antidepressant with a low dose of a second and more sedating antidepressant (e.g., an SSRI or bupropion plus a low-dose tricyclic drug or trazodone); or an antidepressant plus a benzodiazepine hypnotic. The efficacy of these strategies is discussed above. A potential fourth strategy, that of benzodiazepines alone, is not recommended for the large majority of patients with depressive and anxiety disorders because benzodiazepines are not effective antidepressant medications. Some individuals with generalized anxiety disorder or panic disorder, however, may benefit from single treatment with benzodiazepines.

Medical Disorders

Insomnia may result from nonspecific features of many medical disorders such as pain, immobility, and stress. Insomnia may also have more specific causes, such as abnormal respiration during congestive heart failure or stroke. For insomnia in these situations, the underlying medical disorder should always be treated aggressively. If the patient's pulmonary and cardiac status permit, low doses of benzodiazepine drugs may be useful. The insomnia and pain associated with fibromyalgia and rheumatoid arthritis may also benefit from antidepressant drugs.

Dementia

Patients with dementia frequently have sleep disturbance, which may include the "sundowning" syndrome characterized by wakefulness and agitation at night along with excessive daytime sleepiness. Unfortunately, patients with dementia are also more susceptible to the cognitive side effects of hypnotics, antihistamines, and antidepressant medications. Trials of melatonin in this population are currently under way. At present, the best recommendations are to improve daytime activity and light exposure, minimize sources of sleep disruption at night, and carefully review medications to minimize those with potential sleep-disrupting effects. Very cautious trials of low-dose, short-acting benzodiazepine drugs may be appropriate in some patients, but careful monitoring of side effects, including confusion, is essential. High-potency antipsychotic drugs such as haloperidol, atypical antipsychotic drugs such as risperidal, and SSRI antidepressants are also used commonly.

Substance Abuse

Patients with a history of abuse of alcohol or other sedatives are not ideal candidates for benzodiazepine hypnotics. Although some alcohol-dependent patients may be able to use benzodiazepines appropriately, other treatments including behavioral management should be sought. Many clinicians prefer to use sedating antidepressant drugs in patients with a substance abuse history, although the effectiveness of this approach has not been demonstrated.

Obstructive Sleep Apnea Syndrome

Some patients with obstructive sleep apnea may have sleep continuity difficulties as a result of their underlying sleep disorder and/or continuous positive airway pressure treatment. Antidepressant drugs do not worsen apnea and may be appropriate in this setting. Low doses of benzodiazepine drugs have also been administered to patients with sleep apnea and seem to have little effect on respiration during sleep. This approach should be used very cautiously, however, and ideally with laboratory monitoring of results.

Restless Legs Syndrome/Periodic Limb Movements

Patients with restless legs syndrome report insomnia, particularly sleep onset problems. Benzodiazepine drugs have been used effectively for patients with periodic limb movement disorder. Dopaminergic drugs such as carbidopa/levodopa, pergolide, and pramipexole are usually the first-line treatments for this disorder (reviewed in Hening et al., 1999).

Summary

Insomnia is a prevalent problem with real consequences in older adults. Several classes of medications are available to treat insomnia in the elderly. Efficacy has been demonstrated for some of these but not for others. All medications can also have clinically significant adverse effects. Further research is needed to define the specific role of specific drugs for the treatment of insomnia in the elderly and to carefully evaluate the benefits of such treatment against the potential risks. Appropriate pharmacotherapy of insomnia in the elderly should be part of a comprehensive treatment plan, including adequate assessment, integration with behavioral treatment, careful selection of a specific agent, and equally careful follow-up of treatment results.

References

Adam, K., & Oswald, I. (1986). The hypnotic effects of an antihistamine: Promethazine. *British Journal of Clinical Pharmacology, 22*(6), 715-717.

Allen, R. P., Mendels, J., Nevins, D. B., Chernik, D. A., & Hoddes, E. (1987). Efficacy without tolerance or rebound insomnia for midazolam and temazepam after use for one to three months. *Journal of Clinical Pharmacology, 27*(10), 768-775.

American Psychiatric Association. (1990). *Benzodiazepine dependence, toxicity, and abuse: A task force report.* Washington, DC: Author.

Arendt, J., Aldhous, M., & Marks, V. (1986). Alleviation of jet lag by melatonin: Preliminary results of controlled double blind trial. *British Medical Journal, 292,* 1170.

Armitage, R., Yonkers, K., Cole, D., & Rush, A. J. (1997). A multi-center, double-blind comparison of the effects of nefazodone and fluoxetine on sleep architecture and quality of sleep in depressed outpatients. *Journal of Clinical Psychopharmacology, 17*(3), 161-168.

Balter, M. B., & Uhlenhuth, E. H. (1991). The beneficial and adverse effects of hypnotics. *Journal of Clinical Psychiatry, 52*(7), 16-23.

Balter, M. B., & Uhlenhuth, E. H. (1992). New epidemiologic findings about insomnia and its treatment. *Journal of Clinical Psychiatry, 53*(12, Suppl.), 34-39.

Beasley, C. M., Sayler, M. E., Weiss, A. M., & Potvin, J. H. (1992). Fluoxetine: Activating and sedating effects at multiple fixed doses. *Journal of Clinical Psychopharmacology, 12,* 328-333.

Berry, R. B., Kouchi, K., & Bower, J. (1995). Triazolam in patients with obstructive sleep apnea. *American Journal of Respiratory and Critical Care Medicine, 151,* 450-454.

Breslau, N., Roth, T., Rosenthal, L., & Andreski, P. (1996). Sleep disturbance and psychiatric disorders: A longitudinal epidemiological study of young adults. *Biological Psychiatry, 39*(6), 411-418.

Brzezinski, A. (1997). Melatonin in humans. *New England Journal of Medicine, 336*(3), 186-195.

Busto, U., Sellers, E. M., & Naranjo, C. A. (1986). Withdrawal reaction after long term therapeutic use of benzodiazepines. *New England Journal of Medicine, 315,* 854-859.

Buysse, D. J. (1991). Drugs affecting sleep, sleepiness and performance. In T. H. Monk (Ed.), *Sleep, sleepiness and performance* (pp. 249-306). London: John Wiley & Sons.

Buysse, D. J., Reynolds, C. F., Hauri, P. J., Roth, T., Stepanski, E. J., Thorpy, M. J., Bixler, E. O., Kales, A., Manfredi, R. L., Vgontzas, A. N., Mesiano, D. A., Houck, P. R., & Kupfer, D. J. (1994). Diagnostic concordance for DSM-IV sleep disorders: A report from the APA/NIMH DSM-IV field trial. *American Journal of Psychiatry, 151*(9), 1351-1360.

Buysse, D. J., Reynolds, C. F., Hoch, C. C., Houck, P. R., Kupfer, D. J., Mazumdar, S., & Frank, E. (1996). Longitudinal effects of nortriptyline on EEG sleep and the likelihood of recurrence in elderly depressed patients. *Neuropsychopharmacology, 14*(4), 243-252.

Buysse, D. J., Reynolds, C. F., Houck, P. R., Perel, J. M., Frank, E., Begley, A. E., Mazumdar, S., & Kupfer, D. J. (1997). Does lorazepam impair the antidepressant response to nortriptyline and psychotherapy? *Journal of Clinical Psychiatry, 58*(10), 426-432.

Caldwell, J. R. (1982). Short-term quazepam treatment of insomnia in geriatric patients. *Pharmatherapeutica, 3*(4), 278-282.

Carruthers, S. G., Shoeman, D. W., Hignite, C. E., & Azarnoff, D. L. (1978). Correlation between plasma diphenhydramine level and sedative and antihistamine effects. *Clinical Pharmacology and Therapeutics, 23*(4), 375-382.

Carskadon, M. A., Seidel, W. F., Greenblatt, D. J., & Dement, W. C. (1982). Daytime carry-over of triazolam and flurazepam in elderly insomniacs. *Sleep, 5*(4), 361-371.

Casper, R. C., Katz, M. M., Bowden, C. L., Davis, J. M., Koslow, S. H., & Hanin, I. (1994). The pattern of physical symptom changes in major depressive disorder following treatment with amitriptyline or imipramine. *Journal of Affective Disorders, 31*(3), 151-164.

Conn, D. K., & Goldman, Z. (1992). Pattern of use of antidepressants in long-term care facilities for the elderly. *Journal of Geriatric Psychiatry and Neurology, 5,* 228-232.

Cook, P. J. (1986). Benzodiazepine hypnotics in the elderly. *Acta Psychiatrica Scandinavica, 74*(Suppl. 332), 149-158.

Dahlitz, M., Alvarez, B., Vignau, J., English, J., Arendt, J., & Parkes, J. D. (1991). Delayed sleep phase syndrome response to melatonin. *Lancet, 337,* 1121-1124.

Deacon, S., & Arendt, J. (1995). Melatonin-induced temperature suppression and its acute phase-shifting effects correlate in a dose-dependent manner in humans. *Brain Research, 688,* 77-85.

Dealberto, M. J., McAvay, G. J., Seeman, T., & Berkman, L. (1997). Psychotropic drug use and cognitive decline among older men and women. *International Journal of Geriatric Psychiatry, 12,* 567-574.

Dehlin, O., Rubin, B., & Rundgren, A. (1995). Double-blind comparison of zopiclone and flunitrazepam in elderly insomniacs with special focus on residual effects. *Current Medical Research and Opinion, 13*(6), 317-324.

Dodge, R., Cline, M. G., & Quan, S. F. (1995). The natural history of insomnia and its relationship to respiratory symptoms. *Archives of Internal Medicine, 155,* 1797-1800.

Dollins, A. B., Zhdanova, I. V., Wurtman, R. J., Lynch, H. J., & Deng, M. H. (1994). Effect of inducing nocturnal serum melatonin concentrations in daytime on sleep, mood, body temperature and performance. *Proceedings of the National Academy of Sciences of the United States of America, 91,* 1824-1828.

Dominguez, R. A., Jacobson, A. F., Goldstein, B. J., & Steinbook, R. M. (1984). Comparison of triazolam and placebo in the treatment of insomnia in depressed patients. *Current Therapeutic Research, 36*(5), 856-865.

Dreyfuss, D., Shader, R. I., Harmatz, J. S., & Greenblatt, D. J. (1986). Kinetics and dynamics of single doses of oxazepam in the elderly: Implications of absorption rate. *Journal of Clinical Psychiatry, 47,* 511-514.

Elie, R., & Deschenes, J. P. (1983). Efficacy and tolerance of zopiclone in insomniac geriatric patients. *Pharmacology, 27*(Suppl. 2), 179-187.

Elie, R., Frenay, M., Le Morvan, P., & Bourgouin, J. (1990). Efficacy and safety of zopiclone and triazolam in the treatment of geriatric insomniacs. *International Clinical Psychopharmacology, 5*(Suppl. 2), 39-46.

Ellis, C. M., Lemmens, G., & Parkes, J. D. (1996). Melatonin and insomnia. *Journal of Sleep Research, 5*(1), 61-65.

Englert, S., & Linden, M. (1998). Differences in self-reported sleep complaints in elderly persons living in the community who do or do not take sleep medication. *Journal of Clinical Psychiatry, 59,* 137-144.

Fillingim, J. M. (1982). Double-blind evaluation of temazepam, flurazepam, and placebo in geriatric insomniacs. *Clinical Therapeutics, 4*(5), 369-380.

Ford, D. E., & Kamerow, D. B. (1989). Epidemiologic study of sleep disturbances and psychiatric disorders. *Journal of the American Medical Association, 262,* 1479-1484.

Frost, J. D., & DeLucchi, M. R. (1979). Insomnia in the elderly. *Journal of the American Geriatrics Society, 27,* 541-546.

Ganguli, M., Reynolds, C. F., & Gilby, J. E. (1996). Prevalence and persistence of sleep complaints in a rural elderly community sample: The MoVIES Project. *Journal of the American Geriatrics Society, 44*, 778-784.

Garfinkel, D., Laudon, M., Nof, D., & Zisapel, N. (1995). Improvement of sleep quality in elderly people by controlled-release melatonin [see comments]. *Lancet, 346*(8974), 541-544.

Gengo, F. M., & Gabos, C. (1987). Antihistamines, drowsiness, and psychomotor impairment: Central nervous system effect of cetirizine. *Annals of Allergy, 59*, 53-57.

Gillin, J. C., Rapaport, M., Erman, M. K., Winokur, A., & Albala, B. J. (1997). A comparison of nefazodone and fluoxetine on mood and on objective, subjective, and clinician-rated measures of sleep in depressed patients: A double-blind, 8-week clinical trial. *Journal of Clinical Psychiatry, 58*(5), 185-192.

Grad, R. M. (1995). Benzodiazepines for insomnia in community-dwelling elderly: A review of benefit and risk. *Journal of Family Practice, 41*(5), 473-481.

Greenblatt, D. J., Divoll, M., Harmatz, J. S., MacLaughlin, D. S., & Shader, R. I. (1981). Kinetics and clinical effects of flurazepam in young and elderly noninsomniacs. *Clinical Pharmacology and Therapeutics, 30*, 475-486.

Habraken, H., Soenen, K., Blondeel, L., VanElsen, J., Bourda, J., Coppens, E., & Willeput, M. (1997). Gradual withdrawal from benzodiazepines in residents of homes for the elderly: Experience and suggestions for future research. *European Journal of Clinical Pharmacology, 51*, 355-358.

Haimov, I., Lavie, P., Laudon, M., Herer, P., Vigder, C., & Zisapel, N. (1995). Melatonin replacement therapy of elderly insomniacs. *Sleep, 18*(7), 598-603.

Hajak, G., Clarenbach, P., Fischer, W., Rodenbeck, A., Bandelow, B., Broocks, A., & Ruther, E. (1998). Rebound insomnia after hypnotic withdrawal in insomniac outpatients. *European Archives of Psychiatry & Clinical Neuroscience, 248*(3), 148-156.

Hajak, G., Rodenbeck, A., Adler, L., Huether, G., Bandelow, B., Herrendorf, G., Staedt, J., & Ruther, E. (1996). Nocturnal melatonin secretion and sleep after doxepin administration in chronic primary insomnia. *Pharmacopsychiatry, 29*, 187-192.

Hemmelgarn, B., Suissa, S., Huang, A., Boivin, J. F., & Pinard, G. (1997). Benzodiazepine use and the risk of motor vehicle crash in the elderly. *Journal of the American Medical Association, 278*, 27-31.

Henderson, S., Jorm, A. F., Scott, L. R., Mackinnon, A. J., Christensen, H., & Korten, A. E. (1995). Insomnia in the elderly: Its prevalence and correlates in the general population. *Medical Journal of Australia, 162*, 22-24.

Hening, W. A., Allen, R., Walters, A. S., & Chokroverty, S. (1999). Motor functions and dysfunctions of sleep. In S. Chokroverty (Ed.), *Sleep disorders medicine: Basic science, technical considerations, and clinical aspects* (pp. 441-507). Boston: Butterworth-Heinemann.

Herings, R.M.C., Stricker, B.H.Ch., deBoer, A., Bakker, A., & Sturmans, F. (1995). Benzodiazepines and the risk of falling leading to femur fractures. *Archives of Internal Medicine, 155*, 1801-1807.

Hohagen, F., Montero, R. F., Weiss, E., Lis, S., Schonbrunn, E., Dressing, H., Riemann, D., & Berger, M. (1994). Treatment of primary insomnia with trimipramine: An alternative to benzodiazepine hypnotics? *European Archives of Psychiatry and Clinical Neuroscience, 244*(2), 65-72.

Hughes, R. J., Sack, R. L., & Lewy, A. J. (1998). The role of melatonin and circadian phase in age-related sleep-maintenance insomnia: Assessment in a clinical trial of melatonin replacement. *Sleep, 21*, 52-68.

Jacobsen, F. M. (1990). Low-dose trazodone as a hypnotic in patients treated with MAOIs and other psychotropics: A pilot study. *Journal of Clinical Psychiatry, 51*(7), 298-302.

James, S. P., Mendelson, W. B., Sack, D. A., Rosenthal, N. E., & Wehr, T. A. (1987). The effect of melatonin on normal sleep. *Neuropsychopharmacology, 1,* 41-44.

James, S. P., Sack, D. A., Rosenthal, N. E., & Mendelson, W. B. (1989). Melatonin administration in insomnia. *Neuropsychopharmacology, 3*(1), 19-23.

Kales, A., Kales, J. D., Bixler, E. O., Scharf, M. B., & Russek, E. (1976). Hypnotic efficacy of triazolam: Sleep laboratory evaluation of intermediate-term effectiveness. *Journal of Clinical Pharmacology, 16*(8-9), 399-406.

Koski, K., Luukinen, H., Laippala, P., & Kivelä, S. L. (1998). Risk factors for major injurious falls among the home-dwelling elderly by functional abilities. *Gerontology, 44,* 232-238.

Kripke, D. F., Klauber, M. R., Wingard, D. L., Fell, R. L., Assmus, J. D., & Garfinkel, L. (1998). Mortality hazard associated with prescription hypnotics. *Biological Psychiatry, 43,* 687-693.

Kummer, J., Guendel, L., Linden, J., Eich, F. X., Attali, P., Coquelin, J. P., & Kyrein, H. J. (1993). Long-term polysomnographic study of the efficacy and safety of zolpidem in elderly psychiatric in-patients with insomnia. *Journal of International Medical Research, 21*(4), 171-184.

Kupfer, D. J., Perel, J. M., Pollock, B. G., Nathan, R. S., Grochocinski, V. J., Wilson, M. J., & McEachran, A. B. (1991). Fluvoxamine versus desipramine: Comparative polysomnographic effects. *Biological Psychiatry, 29,* 23-40.

Kuppermann, M., Lubeck, D. P., Mazonson, P. D., Patrick, D. L., Stewart, A. L., Buesching, D. P., & Fifer, S. K. (1995). Sleep problems and their correlates in a working population. *Journal of General Internal Medicine, 10*(1), 25-32.

Lader, M. (1994). Anxiety or depression during withdrawal of hypnotic treatments. *Journal of Psychosomatic Research, 38,* 113-123.

Leger, D., Quera-Salva, M. A., & Philip, P. (1996). Health-related quality of life in patients with insomnia treated with zopiclone. *Pharmacoeconomics, 10*(1), 39-44.

Leveille, S. G., Buchner, D. M., Koepsell, T. D., McCloskey, L. W., Wolf, M. E., & Wagner, E. H. (1994). Psychoactive medications and injurious motor vehicle collisions involving older drivers. *Epidemiology, 5,* 591-598.

Lewy, A. J., Ahmed, S., Jackson, J. M., & Sack, R. L. (1992). Melatonin shifts human circadian rhythms according to a phase-response curve. *Chronobiology International, 9*(5), 380-392.

Maarek, L., Cramer, P., Attali, P., Coquelin, J. P., & Morselli, P. L. (1992). The safety and efficacy of zolpidem in insomniac patients: A long-term open study in general practice. *Journal of International Medical Research, 20*(2), 162-170.

MacFarlane, J. G., Cleghorn, J. M., Brown, G. M., & Streiner, D. L. (1991). The effects of exogenous melatonin on the total sleep time and daytime alertness of chronic insomniacs: A preliminary study. *Biological Psychiatry, 30*(4), 371-376.

Maksoud, A., Moore, C. A., & Harshkowitz, M. (1997). The effect of melatonin administration on patients with sleep apnea. *Sleep Research, 26,* 114.

Mamelak, M., Csima, A., Buck, L., & Price, V. (1989). A comparative study on the effects of brotizolam and flurazepam on sleep and performance in the elderly. *Journal of Clinical Psychopharmacology, 9*(4), 260-267.

Martinez, H. T., & Serna, C. T. (1982). Short-term treatment with quazepam of insomnia in geriatric patients. *Clinical Therapeutics, 5*(2), 174-178.

Mellinger, G. D., Balter, M. B., & Uhlenhuth, E. H. (1985). Insomnia and its treatment: Prevalence and correlates. *Archives of General Psychiatry, 42,* 225-232.

Mendelson, W. B. (1997). A critical evaluation of the hypnotic efficacy of melatonin. *Sleep, 20*(10), 916-919.

Metz, A., & Shader, R. I. (1990). Adverse interactions encountered when using trazodone to treat insomnia associated with fluoxetine. *International Clinical Psychopharmacology, 5,* 191-194.

Meuleman, J. R., Nelson, R. C., & Clark, R. L., Jr. (1987). Evaluation of temazepam and diphenhydramine as hypnotics in a nursing-home population. *Drug Intelligence and Clinical Pharmacy, 21*(9), 716-720.

Middelkoop, H.A.M., Smilde-van den Doel, D. A., Neven, A. K., Kamphuisen, H.A.C., & Springer, C. P. (1996). Subjective sleep characteristics of 1,485 males and females aged 50-93: Effects of sex and age, and factors related to self-evaluated quality of sleep. *Journal of Gerontology, 51A*(3), M108-M115.

Middleton, B. A., Stone, B. M., & Arendt, J. (1996). Melatonin and fragmented sleep patterns. *Lancet, 348,* 551-552.

Mitler, M. M., Seidel, W. F., Van Den Hoed, J., Greenblatt, D. J., & Dement, W. C. (1984). Comparative hypnotic effects of flurazepam, triazolam, and placebo: A long-term simultaneous nighttime and daytime study. *Journal of Clinical Psychopharmacology, 4*(1), 2-13.

Montgomery, I., Oswald, I., Morgan, K., & Adam, K. (1983). Trazodone enhances sleep in subjective quality but not in objective duration. *British Journal of Clinical Pharmacology, 16,* 139-144.

Morgan, K., & Clarke, D. (1997). Longitudinal trends in late-life insomnia: Implications for prescribing. *Age and Ageing, 26,* 179-184.

Morin, C. M., Colecchi, C. A., Ling, W. D., & Sood, R. K. (1995). Cognitive behavior therapy to facilitate benzodiazepine discontinuation among hypnotic-dependent patients with insomnia. *Behavior Therapy, 26,* 733-745.

Mouret, J., Ruel, D., Maillard, F., & Bianchi, M. (1990). Zopiclone versus triazolam in insomniac geriatric patients: A specific increase in delta sleep with zopiclone. *International Clinical Psychopharmacology, 5*(Suppl. 2), 47-55.

Mustard, C. A., & Mayer, T. (1997). Case-control study of exposure to medication and the risk of injurious falls requiring hospitalization among nursing home residents. *American Journal of Epidemiology, 145,* 738-745.

Neutel, C. I., Hirdes, J. P., Maxwell, C. J., & Patten, S. B. (1996). New evidence on benzodiazepine use and falls: The time factor. *Age and Ageing, 25,* 273-278.

Nierenberg, A. A., Adler, L. A., Peselow, E., Zornberg, G., & Rosenthal, M. (1994). Trazodone for antidepressant-associated insomnia. *American Journal of Psychiatry, 151*(7), 1069-1072.

Nierenberg, A. A., Cole, J. O., & Glass, L. (1992). Possible trazodone potentiation of fluoxetine: A case series. *Journal of Clinical Psychiatry, 53*(3), 83-85.

Nolen, W. A., Haffmans, P.M.J., Bouvy, P. F., & Duivenvoorden, H. J. (1993). Hypnotics as concurrent medication in depression: A placebo-controlled, double-blind comparison of flunitrazepam and lormetazepam in patients with major depression, treated with a (tri)cyclic antidepressant. *Journal of Affective Disorders, 28,* 179-188.

Nowell, P. D., Mazumdar, S., Buysse, D. J., Dew, M. A., Reynolds, C. F., & Kupfer, D. J. (1997). Benzodiazepines and zolpidem for chronic insomnia: A meta-analysis of treatment efficacy. *Journal of the American Medical Association, 278*(24), 2170-2177.

Nowell, P. D., Reynolds, C. F., Buysse, D. J., Dew, M. A., & Kupfer, D. J. (1999). Paroxetine in the treatment of primary insomnia: Preliminary clinical and EEG sleep data. *Journal of Clinical Psychiatry, 60*(2), 89-95.

Noyes, R., Garvey, M. J., Cook, B., & Suelzer, M. (1991). Controlled discontinuation of benzodiazepine treatment for patients with panic disorder. *American Journal of Psychiatry, 148,* 517-523.

Ohayon, M. M. (1996). Epidemiological study on insomnia in a general population. *Sleep*, *19*(3), S7-S15.

Ohayon, M. M. (1997). Prevalence of DSM-IV diagnostic criteria of insomnia: Distinguishing insomnia related to mental disorders from sleep disorders. *Journal of Psychiatric Research*, *31*(3), 333-346.

Ohayon, M. M., & Caulet, M. (1996). Psychotropic medication and insomnia complaints in two epidemiological studies. *Canadian Journal of Psychiatry*, *41*, 457-464.

Olfson, M., & Pincus, H. A. (1994). Use of benzodiazepines in the community. *Archives of Internal Medicine*, *154*, 1235-1240.

Oswald, I., French, C., Adam, K., & Gilham, J. (1982). Benzodiazepine hypnotics remain effective for 24 weeks. *British Medical Journal*, *284*, 860-863.

Parrino, L., Spaggiari, M. C., Boselli, M., Di Giovanni, G., & Terzano, M. G. (1994). Clinical and polysomnographic effects of trazodone CR in chronic insomnia associated with dysthymia. *Psychopharmacology*, *116*, 389-395.

Parrino, L., & Terzano, M. G. (1996). Polysomnographic effects of hypnotic drugs: A review. *Psychopharmacology*, *126*, 1-16.

Perlis, M. L., Giles, D. E., Mendelson, W. B., Bootzin, R. R., & Wyatt, J. K. (1997). Psychophysiological insomnia: The behavioural model and a neurocognitive perspective [Review]. *Journal of Sleep Research*, *6*(3), 179-188.

Petrie, K., Conaglen, J. V., Thompson, L., & Chamberlain, K. (1989). Effect of melatonin on jet lag after long haul flights. *British Medical Journal*, *298*, 705-707.

Piccione, P., Zorick, F., Lutz, T., Grissom, T., Kramer, M., & Roth, T. (1980). The efficacy of triazolam and chloral hydrate in geriatric insomniacs. *Journal of International Medical Research*, *8*(5), 361-367.

Quera-Salva, M. A., McCann, C., & Boudet, J. (1994). Effects of zolpidem on sleep architecture, night time ventilation, daytime vigilance and performance in heavy snorers. *British Journal of Clinical Pharmacology*, *37*(6), 539-543.

Rascati, K. (1995). Drug utilization review of concomitant use of specific serotonin reuptake inhibitors or clomipramine with antianxiety/sleep medications. *Clinical Therapeutics*, *17*(4), 786-790.

Ray, W. A., Griffin, M. R., & Downey, W. (1989). Benzodiazepines of long and short elimination half-life and the risk of hip fracture. *Journal of the American Medical Association*, *262*, 3303-3307.

Reiter, R. J. (1995). The pineal gland and melatonin in relation to aging: A summary of the theories and of the data. *Experimental Gerontology*, *30*, 199-212.

Reynolds, C. F., Regestein, Q. R., Nowell, P. D., & Neylan, T. C. (1998). Treatment of insomnia in the Elderly. In C. Salzman (Ed.), *Clinical Geriatric Psychopharmacology* (3rd ed., pp. 395-416). Baltimore: Williams & Wilkins.

Richelson, E. (1996). Synaptic effects of antidepressants. *Journal of Clinical Psychopharmacology*, *16*(3, Suppl. 2), 1S-9S.

Rickels, K. (1988). Long-term treatment of anxiety and risk of withdrawal: Prospective comparison of clorazepate and buspirone. *Archives of General Psychiatry*, *45*, 444-450.

Rickels, K., Case, W. G., Schweizer, E., Garcia-Espana, F., & Fridman, R. (1991). Long-term benzodiazepine users 3 years after participation in a discontinuation program. *American Journal of Psychiatry*, *148*, 757-761.

Rickels, K., Morris, R. J., Newman, H., Rosenfeld, H., Schiller, H., & Weinstock, R. (1983). Diphenhydramine in insomniac family practice patients: A double-blind study. *Journal of Clinical Pharmacology*, *23*(5-6), 234-242.

Riemann, D., Hohagen, F., Krieger, S., Gann, H., Muller, W. E., Olbrich, R., Wark, H. J., Bohus, M., Low, H., & Berger, M. (1994). Cholinergic REM induction test: Muscarinic supersensitivity underlies polysomnographic findings in both depression and schizophrenia. *Journal of Psychiatric Research, 28*(3), 195-210.

Roehrs, T. A., Tietz, E. L., Zorick, F. J., & Roth, T. (1984). Daytime sleepiness and antihistamines. *Sleep, 7*(2), 137-141.

Roehrs, T. A., Zorick, F., Wittig, R., & Roth, T. (1985). Efficacy of a reduced triazolam dose in elderly insomniacs. *Neurobiology of Aging, 6*(4), 293-296.

Roger, M., Attali, P., & Coquelin, J. P. (1993). Multicenter, double-blind, controlled comparison of zolpidem and triazolam in elderly patients with insomnia. *Clinical Therapeutics, 15*(1), 127-136.

Rogers, N. L., Phan, O., Kennaway, D., & Dawson, D. (1997). Effect of oral daytime melatonin administration on cognitive psychomotor performance in humans. *Sleep Research, 26,* 212.

Romach, M., Busto, U., Somer, G., Kaplan, H. L., & Sellers, E. (1995). Clinical aspects of chronic use of alprazolam and lorazepam. *American Journal of Psychiatry, 152,* 1161-1167.

Roth, T. G., Roehrs, T. A., Koshorek, G. L., Greenblatt, D. J., & Rosenthal, L. D. (1997). Hypnotic effects of low doses of quazepam in older insomniacs. *Journal of Clinical Psychopharmacology, 17,* 401-406.

Roth, T., Roehrs, T., Koshorek, G., Sicklesteel, J., & Zorick, F. (1987). Sedative effects of antihistamines. *Clinical Immunology, 80,* 94-98.

Roth, T., Roehrs, R., Wittig, R., & Zorick, F. (1984). Benzodiazepines and memory. *British Journal of Clinical Pharmacology, 18,* 45S-49S.

Rush, A. J., Armitage, R., Gillin, J. C., Yonkers, K., Winokur, A., Moldofsky, H., Vogel, G. W., Kaplita, S. B., Fleming, J. B., Montplaisir, J., Erman, M. K., Albala, B. J., & McQuade, R. D. (1998). Comparative effects of nefazodone and fluoxetine on sleep in outpatients with major depressive disorder. *Biological Psychiatry, 44*(3), 14.

Sack, R. L., Hughes, R. J., Edgar, D. M., & Lewy, A. J. (1997). Sleep-promoting effects of melatonin: At what dose, in whom, under what conditions, and by what mechanisms? *Sleep, 20*(10), 908-915.

Sack, R. L., Lewy, A. J., Blood, M. L., Stevenson, J., & Keith, L. D. (1991). Melatonin administration to blind people: Phase advances and entrainment. *Journal of Biological Rhythms, 6*(3), 249-261.

Saletu, B., Saletu-Zyhlarz, G., Anderer, P., Brandstatter, N., Frey, R., Gruber, G., Klosch, G., Mandl, M., Grunberger, J., & Linzmayer, L. (1997). Nonorganic insomnia in generalized anxiety disorder. *Neuropsychobiology, 36*(3), 130-152.

Salzman, C., Fisher, J., Nobel, K., Glassman, R., Wolfson, A., & Kelley, M. (1992). Cognitive improvement following benzodiazepine discontinuation in elderly nursing home residents. *International Journal of Geriatric Psychiatry, 7,* 89-93.

Satterlee, W. G., & Faries, D. (1995). The effects of fluoxetine on symptoms of insomnia in depressed patients. *Psychopharmacology Bulletin, 31*(2), 227-237.

Scharf, M. B., Hirschowitz, J., Zemlan, F. P., Lichstein, M., & Woods, M. (1986). Comparative effects of limbitrol and amitriptyline on sleep efficiency and architecture. *Journal of Clinical Psychiatry, 47,* 587-591.

Scharf, M. B., Roth, T., Vogel, G. W., & Walsh, J. K. (1994). A multicenter, placebo-controlled study evaluating zolpidem in the treatment of chronic insomnia. *Journal of Clinical Psychiatry, 55*(5), 192-199.

Scharf, M. B., & Sachais, B. A. (1990). Sleep laboratory evaluation of the effects and efficacy of trazodone in depressed insomniac patients. *Journal of Clinical Psychiatry, 51,* 13-17.

Schlich, D., L'Heritier, C., Coquelin, J. P., Attali, P., & Kryrein, H. J. (1991). Long-term treatment of insomnia with zolpidem: A multicentre general practitioner study of 107 patients. *Journal of International Medical Research, 19*(3), 271-279. [Published erratum appears in *Journal of International Medical Research, 21*(6), 346]

Seppälä, M., Hyyppä, M. T., Impivaara, O., Knuts, L. R., & Sourander, L. (1997). Subjective quality of sleep and use of hypnotics in an elderly urban population. *Aging: Clinical and Experimental Research, 9*, 327-334.

Sharpley, A. L., & Cowen, P. J. (1995). Effect of pharmacologic treatments on the sleep of depressed patients. *Biological Psychiatry, 37*(2), 85-98.

Shaw, S. H., Curson, H., & Coquelin, J. P. (1992). A double-blind, comparative study of zolpidem and placebo in the treatment of insomnia in elderly psychiatric in-patients. *Journal of International Medical Research, 20*(2), 150-161. [Published erratum appears in *Journal of International Medical Research, 20*(6), following 494]

Sherin, J. E., Shiromani, P. J., McCarley, R. W., & Saper, C. B. (1996). Activation of ventrolateral preoptic neurons during sleep. *Science, 271*, 216-219.

Shipley, J. E., Kupfer, D. J., Griffin, S. J., Dealy, R. S., Coble, P. A., McEachran, A. B., Grochocinski, V. J., Ulrich, R., & Perel, J. M. (1985). Comparison of effects of desipramine and amitriptyline on EEG sleep of depressed patients. *Psychopharmacology, 85*, 14-22.

Simon, G. E., & VonKorff, M. (1997). Prevalence, burden, and treatment of insomnia in primary care. *American Journal of Psychiatry, 154*(10), 1417-1423.

Simon, G. E., VonKorff, M., Barlow, W., Pabiniak, C., & Wagner, E. (1996). Predictors of chronic benzodiazepine use in a health maintenance organization sample. *Journal of Clinical Epidemiology, 49*(9), 1067-1073.

Smith, R. B., Divoll, M., Gillespie, W. R., & Greenblatt, D. J. (1983). Effect of subject age and gender on the pharmacokinetics of oral triazolam and temazepam. *Journal of Clinical Psychopharmacology, 3*(3), 172-176.

Swartz, M., Landerman, R., George, L., Melville, M., Blazer, D., & Smith, K. (1991). Benzodiazepine anti-anxiety agents: Prevalence and correlates of use in a southern community. *American Journal of Public Health, 81*, 592-596.

Tallman, J. F., Paul, S. M., Skolnick, P., & Gallagher, D. W. (1980). Receptors for the age of anxiety: Pharmacology of the benzodiazepines. *Science, 207*, 274-281.

Tata, P. R., Rollings, J., Collins, M., Pickering, A., & Jacobson, R. R. (1994). Lack of cognitive recovery following withdrawal from long-term benzodiazepine use. *Psychological Medicine, 24*, 203-213.

Thase, M. E. (1998). Depression, sleep, and antidepressants. *Journal of Clinical Psychiatry, 59*(4), 55-65.

Tönne, U., Hiltunen, A. J., Vikander, B., Ngelbrektsson, K., Ergman, H., Ergman, I., Eifman, H., & Org, S. (1995). Neuropsychological changes during steady-state drug use, withdrawal and abstinence in primary benzodiazepine-dependent patients. *Acta Psychiatrica Scandinavica, 91*, 299-304.

Tzischinsky, O., & Lavie, P. (1994). Melatonin possesses time-dependent hypnotic effects. *Sleep, 17*, 638-645.

vanBemmel, A. L. (1997). The link between sleep and depression: The effects of antidepressants on EEG sleep. *Journal of Psychosomatic Research, 42*(6), 555-564.

Vgontzas, A. N., Kales, A., Bixler, E. O., & Myers, D. C. (1994). Temazepam 7.5 mg: Effects on sleep in elderly insomniacs. *European Journal of Clinical Pharmacology, 46*(3), 209-213.

Viukari, M., & Miettinen, P. (1984). Diazepam, promethazine and propiomazine as hypnotics in elderly inpatients. *Neuropsychobiology, 12*(2-3), 134-137.

Waldhauser, F., Saletu, B., & Trinchard-Lugan, I. (1990). Sleep laboratory investigations on hypnotic properties of melatonin. *Psychopharmacology, 100*(2), 222-226.

Walsh, J. K., & Engelhardt, C. L. (1992). Trends in the pharmacologic treatment of insomnia. *Journal of Clinical Psychiatry, 53*(12, Suppl.), 10-17; discussion, 18.

Walsh, J. K., & Schweitzer, P. K. (1999). Ten-year trends in the pharmacological treatment of insomnia. *Sleep, 22*(3), 371-375.

Ware, J. C., Brown, F. W., Moorad, P. J., Pittard, J. T., & Cobert, B. (1989). Effects on sleep: A double-blind study comparing trimipramine to imipramine in depressed insomniac patients. *Sleep, 12,* 537-549.

Weissman, M. M., Greenwald, S., Nino-Murcia, G., & Dement, W. C. (1997). The morbidity of insomnia uncomplicated by psychiatric disorders. *General Hospital Psychiatry, 19*(4), 245-250.

Woods, J. H., & Winger, G. (1995). Current benzodiazepine issues [Review]. *Psychopharmacology, 118*(2), 107-115; discussion, 118.

Wurtman, R. J., & Zhdanova, I. (1995). Improvement of sleep quality by melatonin. *Lancet, 346,* 1491.

Zhdanova, I. V., Wurtman, R. J., Morabito, C., Piotrovska, V. R., & Lynch, H. J. (1996). Effects of low oral doses of melatonin, given 2-4 hours before habitual bedtime, on sleep in normal young humans. *Sleep, 19*(5), 423-431.

PART III

Special
Treatment Topics

11

Discontinuation
of Sleep Medications

CHARLES M. MORIN
LUCIE BAILLARGEON
CÉLYNE BASTIEN

Pharmacotherapy is the most frequently used approach to the management of insomnia across all age groups, and particularly in late life (Mant, Mattick, Burgh, Donnelly, & Hall, 1995). Although sleep medications may be indicated for situational insomnia, prolonged usage usually is not recommended, especially in older persons, because of the associated risk of tolerance and dependence (National Institutes of Health [NIH], 1984, 1991). Discontinuation of sleep medications often poses a significant challenge to clinicians and patients alike, particularly after prolonged usage. This chapter describes treatment guidelines to facilitate tapering of such medications among older adults. After reviewing some epidemiological data on usage of sleep medications, a conceptual model of hypnotic-dependent insomnia is presented, and a typical withdrawal protocol is

AUTHORS' NOTE: Preparation of this chapter was supported in part by grant #MH52790 from the National Institute of Mental Health and by a grant from Health Canada (National Health Research and Development Program).

271

outlined. We conclude with a brief review of selected studies evaluating the efficacy of hypnotic/anxiolytic withdrawal programs and outline some practical strategies to guide practitioners in this challenging task. Although most of the evidence available is based on studies of benzodiazepine discontinuation, the more generic term of hypnotic medications (i.e., any prescribed or over-the-counter drugs used to promote sleep) will be used in this chapter.

Nature and Scope of Hypnotic-Dependent Insomnia

Epidemiology of Hypnotic Use

Approximately 7.4% of the adult population uses a hypnotic medication, including both prescribed and over-the-counter sleep aids, during the course of a year (Mellinger, Balter, & Uhlenhuth, 1985). The prescription and usage of sleep-promoting agents increase significantly with aging. For instance, the utilization rate is twice as high (14%) among those in the 65 to 79-year-old range as in the adult population as a whole. This rate is even higher among elderly patients attending medical practices, with 26% of women and 6% of men using sleep medications (Hohagen et al., 1994). Overall, it is estimated that nearly 40% of all prescriptions for hypnotics are written for persons over 60 years of age, although this age group represents only about 15% of the population.

Prescribed sleep-promoting agents include benzodiazepine-hypnotics (e.g., temazepam, flurazepam) and anxiolytics (e.g., lorazepam, clonazepam), non-benzodiazepine hypnotics (e.g., zolpidem, zopiclone), and sedating antidepressants (e.g., trazodone, amitryptyline, doxepin). Some elderly persons may still be using older hypnotic drugs (e.g., chloral hydrate, meprobamate, nembutal), although those medications have been replaced almost completely by safer agents (Walsh & Engelhardt, 1992). Many people also rely on over-the-counter medicines (e.g., Sominex, Unisom, Nytol), all of which contain an antihistamine, but these agents seem less popular among older adults. Alcohol is probably used more frequently as a sleep aid among older adults than by younger people. The risks, benefits, and limitations of hypnotic medications for older adults have been described in Chapter 10 of this volume and will not be discussed here.

The majority of those who use a sleep medication use it only for a limited period of time; however, some people continue using it for prolonged periods, often much longer than was intended initially. Long-term users (> 3 months) of hypnotic medications are mostly older adults. One study found that 71% of long-term users surveyed were aged 50 or older, and one-third were over 65 years of age (Mellinger et al., 1985). In a sample of British community-dwelling residents over 65, 11% reported using hypnotic drugs regularly for more than a year and an additional 4% for more than 10 years (Morgan, Dallosso, Ebrahim, Arie, & Fentem, 1988). These estimates nearly triple among institutionalized elders (Morgan & Clarke, 1997). In general, long-term users are older adults who report greater sleep dissatisfaction, more chronic medical illnesses, and higher psychological distress (Englert & Linden, 1998; Mellinger et al., 1985).

The Natural History of Hypnotic Dependency

Treatment of insomnia with hypnotic medications typically is initiated during periods of acute stress, medical illness, or hospitalization, or simply when a person can no longer cope with the daytime sequelae of chronic sleep disturbance (e.g., fatigue, attention and concentration problems). Despite the initial intent to limit their use to a few nights, some people continue using hypnotics for prolonged periods of time. The onset of this pattern of prolonged usage is often insidious, with both psychological and physiological factors contributing to its maintenance. Some individuals continue using medications because of chronic insomnia, but others may do so even after their sleep difficulties have subsided. For those people, sleep medications are used simply on a prophylactic basis, to prevent the recurrence of insomnia. The distress experienced during the first episode of insomnia and the fear of not sleeping maintain the pill-taking behavior. Sometimes, prescriptions of hypnotic drugs are renewed without adequate evaluations of continued need or sustained efficacy of the medication. With nightly use, tolerance may develop and increased dosage is sometimes necessary to maintain efficacy (Barnas, Whithworth, & Fleischhacker, 1993). When the maximum safe dosage is reached, the person is caught in a vicious cycle (see Figure 11.1). Although the medication may have lost its sleep-inducing effects, any attempt to stop it is followed by some withdrawal symptoms

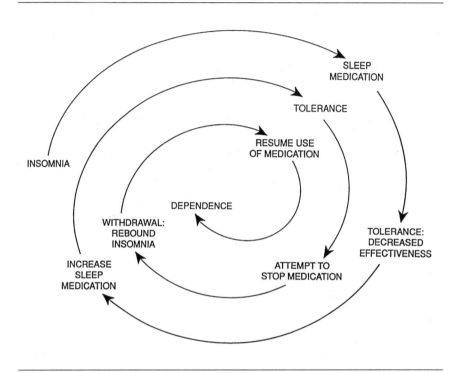

Figure 11.1. The Cycle of Hypnotic-Dependent Insomnia
SOURCE: From *Insomnia: Psychological Assessment and Management* (p. 164), Morin. © Copyright 1993 by Guilford Press. Reprinted with permission.

and a worsening of sleep difficulties. This rebound insomnia, which is typically transient in nature, heightens the patient's anticipatory anxiety and reinforces the belief that he or she cannot sleep without medication. Naturally, this chain reaction is powerful in prompting the patient to resume usage of sleeping pills and, hence, the cycle of hypnotic-dependent insomnia (Morin, 1993).

Conditioning principles also play an important role in perpetuating drug use for insomnia. For example, the hypnotic (and anxiolytic) properties of most benzodiazepines alleviate an aversive state (i.e., sleeplessness); as such, the drug-taking behavior itself is negatively reinforced. Although sleeping pills usually are recommended on an "as needed" basis to prevent tolerance, such an intermittent schedule of administration is very powerful in perpetuating a habitual pattern of drug use. Another factor that may contribute to prolonged hypnotic usage is the reversed sleep state misperception while under the influence of benzodiazepines. It is well recognized that unmedicated insomniacs overestimate the time required to fall asleep and underestimate total sleep time. Conversely, medicated insomniacs tend to have impaired recollection of wakefulness (i.e., they underestimate the amount of time spent awake) while on benzodiazepines and to perceive their sleep as of better quality than is actually recorded by EEG measures. This phenomenon has been attributed to the amnesic properties of most benzodiazepines (Schneider-Helmert, 1988). Upon drug withdrawal, patients become acutely aware of their sleep disturbances, often prompting the quick return to hypnotic drugs.

In summary, several risk factors (e.g., stressful life events, medical illness, poor coping skills), besides insomnia, may contribute to the initial use of hypnotic medications, and several additional factors may perpetuate their continued usage over time. The latter include the lack of standard monitoring and follow-up procedures, failure to educate patients about the transient rebound insomnia, the conditioning/reinforcing effect of intermittent hypnotic use, and the reversed sleep state misperception when under the influence of benzodiazepines. It is quite plausible that other factors (e.g., chronic stress/anxiety, dependent personality traits) are also involved in this pattern of prolonged usage.

Distinction Between Abuse and Misuse of Hypnotic Medications and Dependency

Before describing methods for discontinuation of sleep medications, it is important to distinguish several patterns of drug-taking behaviors among hypnotic users. First, very few people abuse hypnotic drugs in the same manner as some abuse narcotics or stimulants. Instead, most people tend to misuse their sleep medications not even in terms of exceeding the recommended therapeutic dosage but more in using them for prolonged periods. Patients may have gradually increased the amount and frequency of medications, but it is only in rare instances that dosage is higher than the upper recommended limit. Nevertheless, this self-contained pattern of habitual and prolonged use typically will lead to hypnotic-dependent insomnia. Although this type of dependency has been documented primarily for benzodiazepines, it may also develop with other prescribed or even with over-the-counter agents used as sleep aids. As such, dependency on hypnotic medications is often more psychological than physical in nature (Morin, 1993).

The formal diagnosis of hypnotic-dependent insomnia involves a complaint of poor sleep with nearly daily use of a hypnotic agent for at least 3 weeks (American Sleep Disorders Association [ASDA], 1990). By definition, it also implies tolerance to hypnotics and withdrawal effects following discontinuation. This type of physical dependence is more likely to occur with high doses of benzodiazepines or with older hypnotic drugs (e.g., barbiturates). Because most people remain on therapeutic doses without escalation for extensive periods of time, it is not entirely clear what proportion of long-term users meet criteria for hypnotic-dependent insomnia.

Clinical Guidelines for Discontinuation of Hypnotics

A step-by-step withdrawal protocol to discontinue hypnotic medications is described in this section. The procedures outlined here, or some variations of them, have been evaluated in several studies of benzodiazepines discontinuation with anxiety disorders patients and a few more with insomnia patients. The latter included two controlled clinical trials conducted by our team with more than 100 older patients who had used benzodiazepines as hypnotics for prolonged periods. The general principles of this medication tapering program also can be used with patients of any age and those using other classes of hypnotic medications.

Evaluate Patient's Readiness and Motivation

Before initiating drug tapering, it is essential to evaluate the patient's readiness and motivation concerning the undertaking of this program. If a person is still in a pre-contemplation phase, it may not be indicated to even attempt this program. It is also preferable to postpone it if the patient is under severe stress (e.g., impending surgery, hospitalization). Tapering a hypnotic drug is more likely to be successful if motivation is intrinsic (e.g., desire to achieve greater self-control) rather than extrinsic (e.g., pressure from the family). If the patient is reluctant to undertake a withdrawal program, it is important to determine whether lack of motivation or anticipatory anxiety is the main barrier. Providing information about the risks and adverse effects associated with benzodiazepine use (e.g., motor vehicle accidents, falls and hip fractures, memory impairment) may be useful, but ultimately the patient should make the decision on his or her own. Some patients are apprehensive about withdrawal symptoms and rebound insomnia. Information about the gradual tapering schedule and about the transient nature of most withdrawal symptoms should alleviate some of those concerns. Other patients may have very low self-confidence regarding their ability to discontinue medication; they should be encouraged to view this program as an opportunity to achieve greater self-control over their sleep and their life in general. The clinician needs to convey a high level of confidence about the process of discontinuation while remaining realistic about the outcome.

Self-Monitoring and Goal Setting

Keeping a daily sleep/medication diary should be an integral component of any insomnia treatment. A typical diary includes entries for quantitative and qualitative sleep parameters and for the type, frequency, and dosage of all sleep aids (prescribed or over-the-counter drugs, and alcohol). It is completed for a 2-week baseline period and throughout the tapering regimen. In addition to establishing baseline levels, the diary is very helpful for monitoring progress, severity of symptoms, and compliance with the tapering regimen.

Another useful procedure is to have the patient set a weekly goal for target reductions in dosage and number of medicated nights for any given week. Typically, we ask patients to indicate verbally their self-efficacy level in achieving that goal. When this rating is too low, it may be necessary to keep the patient on the same schedule for an additional week to have him or her gain a greater sense of mastery before proceeding to a lower dosage. For example, if a patient expresses only a 50% self-efficacy rating to reduce his lorazepam (Ativan) from 2.0 mg to 1.5 mg per night, this goal should be revised and made more attainable, or simply postponed until the following week. To keep the patient focused and goal-oriented, it is also helpful to keep a summary data form

TABLE 11.1 A Sample Medication Withdrawal Schedule

Week	Type	Dosage (mg)	Number of Nights	Total Amount (mg)	% Dosage Reduction	Self-Efficacy (0-100%)
Baseline	Ativan	2	7	14	—	—
Week 1	Ativan	1.5	7	10.5	25	—
Week 2	Ativan	1.5	4	9	36	—
		1.0	3			
Week 3	Ativan	1	7	7	50	80
Week 4	Ativan	1	4	5.5	61	65
		0.5	3			
Week 5	Ativan	0.5	7	3.5	75	75
Week 6	Ativan	0.5	5	2.5	82	80
Week 7	Ativan	0.5	5	2.5	82	75
Week 8	Ativan	0.5	3	1.5	89	60
Week 9	Ativan	0.5	1	0.5	96	80
Week 10	Ativan	0	0	0	100	75

(see Table 11.1) to compute the weekly amount of medication used, the number of medicated/drug-free nights, and the self-efficacy level in reaching one's goal for each week.

Stabilization Period

When two or more hypnotic drugs are used, either concomitantly or in alternation, the first task is to stabilize the patient on a single agent. This scenario is not infrequent among older adults. For example, if a patient alternates between clonazepam and triazolam, possibly to minimize tolerance, the task would be to get the patient stable on a single drug, in this case clonazepam. It may be necessary initially to increase the dosage of the drug retained. When two benzodiazepines are used, it is preferable to retain the drug with the longest half-life because of its built-in tapering properties. Switching from a short- to a long-acting compound may minimize rebound effects. Table 11.2 provides information on equivalent benzodiazepine dosages. This stabilization period should be 1 to 2 weeks. At the end of this period, the patient should take only one drug at

---

TABLE 11.2 Equivalent Dosages of Benzodiazepines

Benzodiazepines	Equivalent Dosage	Usual Dosage (mg)	Half-Life[a] (hours)
Alprazolam (Xanax®)	0.5 mg	0.25-1	12-19
Bromazepam (Lectopam®)	3 mg	1.5-6	8-19
Chlordiazepoxide (Librium®)	10 mg	5-25	5-30
Clonazepam (Klonopin®)	0.25-0.5 mg	0.5-2	20-60
Clorazepate (Tranxene®)	7.5 mg	3.75-15	
Diazepam (Valium®)	5 mg	5-10	20-60
Flurazepam (Dalmane®)	15 mg	15-30	48-100
Lorazepam (Ativan®)	1 mg	0.5-2	10-20
Nitrazepam (Mogadon®)	10 mg	5-10	16-18
Oxazepam (Serax®)	15 mg	10-30	5-10
Quazepam (Doral®)	15 mg	7.5-30	40-120
Temazepam (Restoril®)	15 mg	7.5-30	9-17
Triazolam (Halcion®)	0.25 mg	0.125-0.25	2-4

a. May be longer in older adults.

---

the same dosage every night and have ceased all other sleep aids (e.g., alcohol, over-the-counter).

Gradual Tapering Schedule

Use of a gradual withdrawal schedule is always preferable to abrupt discontinuation in order to minimize rebound effects (Greenblatt,

Harmatz, Zinny, & Shader, 1987). This principle is particularly true for an older person who has used a hypnotic drug for a prolonged period of time. Depending on the initial dosage, drug potency, and duration of use, the length of the tapering schedule may vary between 4 and 16 weeks in outpatient settings (DuPont, 1990; Lader, 1986; Murphy & Tyrer, 1991; Rickels, Case, Schweizer, Garcia-Espana, & Fridman, 1990). In our experience with older adults, a period of 8-10 weeks has proved adequate for the large majority of patients using hypnotics at dosages that remained within therapeutic range (Baillargeon et al., 1998; Morin et al., 1997; Morin, Colecchi, Ling, & Sood, 1995). The dosage is usually reduced by 25% at intervals of 1-2 weeks. This interval may vary as a function of initial dosage and drug potency, as well as withdrawal symptoms and patient's tolerance of those symptoms. When withdrawal symptoms are pronounced, it is best to slow the tapering schedule. Intervals of less than 1 week between dosage reduction usually are not recommended because of the associated risk of rebound insomnia, which can interfere with the tapering process and perpetuate the use of sleeping pills.

Once the lowest available dosage is reached, it is time to introduce "drug holidays." Medication is allowed only on a number of predetermined nights. This will entail skipping 1 or 2 nights the first week, 2 or 3 nights the next week, and so on. To minimize apprehension about impairments of daytime functioning, it is best to skip medication initially on nights when there are no significant obligations the next day, usually on weekends. The next step is to schedule additional drug-free nights even when there is a full agenda on the next day. When medication intake is reduced to only a few nights per week, the patient is instructed to use it on a fixed schedule rather than on an as-needed basis. This means he or she will use sleep medication on preselected nights (e.g., Sunday, Tuesday, and Thursday) and at a fixed time (i.e., 30 minutes before bedtime), regardless of whether or not sleep difficulties are experienced. With this time-contingent schedule, the patient may not be allowed to use medication on some nights when, indeed, he or she has sleep difficulties; conversely, he or she may be obligated to use it on some other nights when he or she would not need it. This "time-contingent" method is helpful to dissociate or weaken the association between sleeplessness and the drug-taking behavior.

The final step is to completely stop the medication. This step is difficult for some patients who become anxious, or even obsessed, with the idea of giving up the last few milligrams of their pills and about the expected consequences this will have on their sleep. This is often difficult for an older person who may have been using a sleeping pill for 20 years or more. It may be reassuring to simply remind him or her that such a small quantity of medication may have very little therapeutic effect on sleep.

The tapering principles outlined here are fairly similar for younger and older adults. The only exception may be for those using very high dosages of sleep medications. Because of greater risk of toxicity and withdrawal effects among older adults, it is particularly important to proceed gradually and under close supervision by a physician.

Concurrent Psychological Interventions

Although a systematic and supervised drug tapering program may be sufficient for some individuals, it is likely that most long-term users will benefit from the addition of some forms of nonpharmacological interventions (e.g., support, education, psychological treatment). These interventions are likely to help patients cope with the sleep disturbances that may arise or worsen during the tapering period as well as with some of the other withdrawal symptoms (e.g., anxiety). The nature and extent of this concurrent intervention will vary according to the patient's needs and severity of withdrawal symptoms and sleep difficulties. For some, simple encouragement, support, and education about the transient nature of withdrawal symptoms and rebound effects may be sufficient to get them through the discontinuation process. Information about age-appropriate sleep norms is very useful for older adults with unrealistic sleep requirement expectations. Others who are anxious even before withdrawal will benefit from relaxation training. Patients who engaged in maladaptive sleep habits and endorsed dysfunctional sleep cognitions may require formal cognitive-behavioral therapy involving sleep restriction, stimulus control, and cognitive restructuring. These procedures may be particularly needed if sleep deteriorates during the tapering program. For example, sleep restriction is very useful to minimize rebound insomnia during the tapering period. Cognitive therapy is especially helpful in controlling apprehensions about discontinuation of hypnotic medications and for reappraisal of withdrawal symptoms as temporary and manageable (Morin, 1993; Morin et al., 1995).

Relapse Prevention

Insomnia is often a recurrent problem (Vollrath, Wicki, & Angst, 1989), and even after successful treatment, it is not uncommon for patients to have occasional sleep problems. It is particularly important to address this issue of insomnia recurrence before the end of formal treatment. Patients should be guided to identify high-risk situations, both for insomnia and for use of sleeping pills. Once those situations are identified, the patient may be in a better position to either prevent major sleep difficulties (by restricting time in bed) or plan a strategy to cope with the occasional, but inevitable, poor night's sleep. For example, the occasional poor night's sleep should be seen as natural or resulting from identifiable causes (e.g., stress) rather than as evidence that chronic insomnia has returned. The patient should be encouraged to develop greater tolerance to these few bad nights. He or she also should be reminded that he or she could always return to newly learned behavioral strategies to cope with insomnia. In spite of all these precautions, some patients will be unable to remain completely drug free. It will be important to distinguish lapses from relapses and not to catastrophize if the patient should have to use a sleep medication for a very brief period. On the other hand, patients also should be encouraged to limit their usage to the occasional use of the smallest dosage available to avoid returning to the old pattern of drug dependency. To prevent relapse and foster maintenance of therapeutic benefits, it may be necessary for some patients to plan a maintenance phase involving periodic phone calls or follow-up therapy sessions. For some patients, simply having a few hypnotics available at home to face an emergency situation may be enough to reduce anticipatory anxiety and actually prevent further insomnia and the use of hypnotic medications.

Nature and Course of Withdrawal Symptoms

Three different syndromes may be associated with benzodiazepine discontinuation (DuPont, 1990; Noyes, Garvey, Cook, & Perry, 1988).

Withdrawal symptoms are new symptoms not present before discontinuation. *Rebound* symptoms refer to a worsening of the original symptoms beyond their baseline levels. In *relapse*, there is a recurrence of the same old symptoms, which persist throughout the drug-free period until some other form of treatment is initiated. Typical withdrawal symptoms associated with benzodiazepine discontinuation include insomnia, anxiety, restlessness, increased perceptual acuity, and impaired concentration (Gillin, Spinweber, & Johnson, 1989; Kales et al., 1986; Roehrs, Vogel, & Roth, 1990). More severe symptoms (e.g., seizures, persistent tinnitus) may follow abrupt discontinuation of high doses of benzodiazepines. Although rare, those symptoms are more likely to affect elders (Lader, 1990; Noyes et al., 1988; Petursson & Lader, 1981).

With short-acting benzodiazepines, withdrawal symptoms usually start at a very low dosage or within 24 hours of discontinuation; they peak within the next 3-4 days and return close to baseline by the second or third week (Fontaine, Chouinard, & Annable, 1984; Rickels, Schweizer, Case, & Greenblatt, 1990). With long-acting benzodiazepines, those symptoms start later, usually after 2 to 3 days, with a peak at approximately 6 to 7 days. Perceptual symptoms may last longer (Rickels, Case, et al., 1990). Withdrawal symptoms are minimal during the initial phase of a gradual taper; most symptoms occur in the latter part of tapering and disappear in most patients after several weeks without using benzodiazepines.

Some withdrawal symptoms may occur in about 50% of short-term users (less than 1 month), and their incidence may range from 40% to 100% among chronic users (Rickels, Schweizer, et al., 1990; Rickels, Schweizer, Csanalosi, Case, & Chung, 1988; Schweizer, Rickels, Case, & Greenblatt, 1990). Although the majority of long-term users will be free of any residual symptoms a few weeks after benzodiazepine discontinuation, 10%-15% of patients develop a postwithdrawal syndrome that may linger for months. It is sometimes difficult to distinguish between persisting withdrawal symptoms and reemergence of premorbid insomnia and anxiety symptoms.

Several drug- and patient-related factors influence the incidence and severity of withdrawal symptoms. The most important are dosage, half-life, and duration of drug use. Withdrawal symptoms are more severe and more immediate with higher dosages and with short half-life (triazolam) than with long half-life (flurazepam) benzodiazepines (Busto et al., 1986; Schweizer, Case, & Rickels, 1989; Schweizer et al., 1990). When treatment duration is less than 2 weeks, there is minimal rebound insomnia upon hypnotic discontinuation (Lingjaerde, Bratlid, Westby, & Gordeladze, 1983; Vogel & Vogel, 1983). Abrupt discontinuation leads to more severe and more rapid withdrawal symptoms relative to gradual cessation, particularly with short half-life benzodiazepines (Greenblatt et al., 1987; Rickels, Case, et al., 1990; Rickels et al., 1988). Sociodemographics and psychological factors may also influence the incidence of withdrawal symptoms. Those symptoms are more frequent among younger patients, women, and patients under chronic stress and those with preexisting anxiety, depression, and dependent personality (Rickels, Case, et al., 1990; Schweizer et al., 1989; Tyrer, Owen, & Dawling, 1983).

Clinical and Practical Issues

Treatment Implementation

Ideally, the patient should be seen once a week during the withdrawal period. During each visit, the clinician reviews the daily diary for hypnotic usage and changes in sleep and inquires about withdrawal symptoms during the previous week. After reviewing this material with the patient, objectives for target dosage are set for the next week. The clinician verifies the patient's level of confidence about successfully reducing his or her medication. When the self-efficacy rating is too low, the weekly goal is revised to be made more attainable. Brief consultations of 15-20 minutes each may be sufficient for implementing the medication tapering program alone. When psychological treatment is implemented concurrently with the tapering program, enough time should be allowed to review behavioral and cognitive procedures. Whether or not formal psychological treatment is implemented, patients' fears, apprehensions, and unrealistic beliefs should be carefully examined and dealt with during therapy sessions. When patients display high levels of anxiety, it is helpful to give them the opportunity to call the clinician between scheduled visits. In our experience, patients seldom call, but they are reassured by having this opportunity available in case of an emergency. Sometimes, it is also helpful to give patients the permission to use a small extra dose if an emergency situation arises or withdrawal symptoms become too severe. To foster a sense of mastery, patients should be given as much control as possible over the implementation of their drug tapering regimen. They should be involved in deciding when to initiate the withdrawal program, by how much the medication should be reduced on any given week, and when to introduce nights without medication.

Preparing Medications

Practical problems may arise in cutting down medication when the lowest available dosage has been reached. For example, it may be difficult to cut in half the smallest available dose (0.5 mg) of lorazepam (Ativan) or to reduce by 25% a capsule of 15 mg of temazepam (Restoril). Because older patients may have more dexterity problems, it may be necessary to ask them to buy a pill-cutter at the pharmacy or have the pharmacist prepare the small dosages (the physician has to write this on the prescription). A temazepam capsule could be dissolved in 100 ml of water or juice, and the patient could drink the quantity corresponding to the desired dose (e.g., 75 ml if the desired reduction is 25% of 15 mg). Temazepam and clorazepate (Tranxene) are tasteless in water, but flurazepam (Dalmane) is bitter and should be dissolved in juice.

Drug Substitution

Drug substitution is sometimes useful to minimize withdrawal symptoms. Because long-acting benzodiazepines produce less severe withdrawal symptoms, some authors recommend substituting long-acting for short-acting benzodiazepines before initiating withdrawal (American Psychiatric Association [APA] Task Force on Benzodiazepine Dependency, 1990; Ashton, 1994). Diazepam, chlordiazepoxide, and clonazepam have been used with patients suffering from insomnia and/or anxiety (Ashton, 1994; Closser & Brower, 1994; Herman, Rosenbaum, & Brotman, 1987). Equivalent dosages are shown in Table 11.2. After a stabilization period of 1-2 weeks, a gradual tapering of the long half-life benzodiazepine is done as described above. Long half-life benzodiazepines may facilitate the reduction of medication initially, but withdrawal symptoms are not completely eliminated with longer-acting agents; they are simply delayed.

Switching from a benzodiazepine to zopiclone, which is a cyclopyrrolone with more specific hypnotic actions without anxiolytic effects, may reduce withdrawal symptoms. Rebound insomnia can occur with abrupt cessation of zopiclone, but withdrawal symptoms are less frequent and less severe than those observed with benzodiazepines (Lader, 1997). Shapiro, Sherman, and Peck (1995) compared three methods of drug substitution with 134 insomniacs who had used benzodiazepines for at least 3 months. The abuttal method (i.e., change to zopiclone the same day the benzodiazepine was stopped) was better than the overlap and gap methods. Most patients remained on zopiclone for 1 month before it was discontinued. There was an increase of side effects (mostly dry mouth and a bitter taste) when subjects began to take zopiclone. Unfortunately, this study did not document withdrawal symptoms after cessation of zopiclone.

The substitution of phenobarbital may be useful for hospitalized patients with mixed chemical dependency (benzodiazepine with alcohol or other drugs) (APA Task Force, 1990; Ravi, Maany, Burke, Dhopesh, & Woody, 1990). Phenobarbital is a long-acting barbiturate with stable blood levels between doses, allowing the safe use of a progressively smaller daily dose. The patient's average daily dose of benzodiazepine is converted to phenobarbital equivalent. Patients are maintained on their initial dose of phenobarbital for 2 days, then the tapering begins on the third day. The rapidity of tapering depends on the half-life of the benzodiazepine that was used. If it is a long-acting one, the phenobarbital taper should be done over 14-20 days. Short- to intermediate-acting benzodiazepine dependence can be treated by reducing phenobarbital by 10% per day, resulting in a 10-day detoxification program.

Several other drugs have been used to facilitate benzodiazepine discontinuation among anxiety disorders patients. Beta-blockers, such as propanolol (Inderal), and other agents such as clonidine attenuate symptoms of autonomic hyperactivity associated with benzodiazepine withdrawal. Carbamazepine has also been used for alleviating withdrawal symptoms, but the results have been mixed (Johansson, Berglund, & Frank, 1997). An important point to remember for the clinician is that most patients have developed a drug dependency that is often more psychological than pharmacological in nature. For this reason, it may be difficult to have the patient switch from one pill, of a particular shape and color, to another format. In our experience, attempts at substituting a long-acting for a short-acting benzodiazepine have not always been successful. In most cases, it is simply easier to implement the drug tapering regimen with the actual medication the patient has been using for months or even years.

Ambulatory vs. Inpatient Withdrawal

The majority of older patients who are dependent on benzodiazepines as hypnotics can be managed on an outpatient basis. Drug tapering may need to be supervised on an inpatient basis, however, for patients who are using more than twice the highest recommended dosages (e.g., 60 mg of flurazepam or temazepam). An inpatient program will provide a safer environment to reduce the medication and respond promptly to severe withdrawal symptoms (e.g., seizures). Although few patients are actually abusing hypnotic medications, those who do should be referred to a detoxification program. An outpatient detoxification program is appropriate for highly motivated individuals with minimal coexisting medical or psychiatric illness and strong support from their family. Regular visits should be scheduled, and no more than 1 week's supply of benzodiazepine should be given. Patients with coexisting substance or alcohol abuse problems should be referred to a specialized detoxification program. The American Society of Addiction Medicine (1991) has published guidelines to help clinicians in determining the most appropriate level of care as a function of the patient's clinical profile.

Individual, Group, and Self-Help Treatment Formats

Individual therapy is often preferred to group therapy in the management of benzodiazepine discontinuation. Some patients are reluctant to discuss in a group format personal problems associated with their anxiety or insomnia, and others may feel embarrassed if they are unsuccessful in reducing their medications. Although it may be easier to implement a drug tapering program on an individual basis, group treatment offers several advantages. It is a powerful source of support and motivation for patients to work on a common treatment goal. The group format may also serve as a social inhibitor for some patients who bring materials that are not entirely relevant to the drug tapering program. Also, group treatment is more economical and may be more accessible and affordable to some older persons. Self-help treatment in the form of bibliotherapy is very beneficial for some patients (Mimeault & Morin, 1999; Morawetz, 1989; Riedel, Lichstein, & Dwyer, 1995), but professional guidance is often needed for long-term hypnotic users. Self-help organizations run by former benzodiazepine users can also provide excellent support for patients (Tattersall & Hallstrom, 1992); however, because of the possible withdrawal symptoms associated with the reduction/cessation of hypnotic medication, it is essential to enlist the collaboration of a physician (ideally the prescribing physician) and/or a pharmacist when implementing a withdrawal program.

Relative Contraindications to Drug Tapering

Although the use of hypnotics should be time-limited for most patients, long-term use may be necessary for some individuals. For example, drug therapy may be necessary when persistent insomnia is associated with chronic psychiatric (e.g., severe anxiety, major depression, schizophrenia) or medical conditions (e.g., chronic pain), particularly when treatment of the underlying condition does not alleviate the associated sleep disturbances. Behavioral interventions can still be a useful adjunct, but there is currently limited evidence on the efficacy of those interventions for secondary insomnia. Hypnotic medications may also be indicated when insomnia is associated with other sleep disorders such as restless legs syndrome and periodic leg movements, two conditions particularly prevalent among older adults (APA Task Force, 1990; NIH, 1984, 1991). The risk-benefit ratio of hypnotic withdrawal should be carefully evaluated for patients who have had seizures in the past, especially if those were associated with hypnotic discontinuation.

Review of Selected Studies of Hypnotic/Anxiolytic Discontinuation Programs

Several studies have examined the efficacy of different withdrawal protocols to assist patients in benzodiazepine discontinuation. The majority of those studies have been conducted with anxiety patients using benzodiazepines as anxiolytics (e.g., Fraser, Peterkin, Gamsu, & Baldwin, 1990; Otto et al., 1993; Schweizer et al., 1989), and a few more have focused on insomnia patients using either benzodiazepines or other agents as hypnotic medications (e.g., Baillargeon et al., 1998; Espie, Lindsay, & Brooks, 1988; Kirmil-Gray, Eagleston, Thorensen, & Zarcone, 1985; Lichstein & Johnson, 1993; Lichstein et al., 1999; Morin et al., 1997; Morin et al., 1995). Of those studies, only a handful have been conducted with older adults. In this section, we will summarize the evidence regarding the short- and long-term efficacy of different interventions in the management of benzodiazepine/hypnotic discontinuation.

In a pilot study with five older adults (aged 55 to 69 years), a medication taper combined with cognitive-behavior therapy (CBT), and implemented in a group format, was effective in reducing usage of benzodiazepines as hypnotics (Morin et al., 1995). Four of five patients discontinued medications completely within a period of 6 to 8 weeks, and one patient decreased drug intake by 90%. Sleep was slightly disrupted during the initial tapering period but improved at the 3-month follow-up assessment. There was significant variability across patients in the impact of benzodiazepine discontinuation on sleep during and after tapering.

A recent randomized clinical trial conducted with 65 elderly insomniacs using benzodiazepines showed that a supervised withdrawal program, combined with CBT for insomnia, was more effective than a medication taper alone (Baillargeon et al., 1998). The medication tapering was supervised by a physician in the context of eight weekly, brief consultation sessions. CBT included stimulus control and sleep restriction, cognitive restructuring, and sleep hygiene education (Morin, 1993). It was provided by a psychologist in eight weekly group therapy sessions. Posttreatment evaluation revealed that 77% of participants in the combined treatment condition withdrew completely from medications compared to 38% in the taper alone group. This difference was maintained at 3- and 12-month follow-ups. Sleep measures were improved at posttreatment for the combined treatment group but not for the medication taper alone condition.

In an ongoing study of late-life insomnia (Morin et al., 1997), we are currently comparing three treatment conditions (taper alone, CBT alone, and combined taper plus CBT) for benzodiazepine discontinuation; all treatments last 10 weeks, and polysomnographic evaluations of sleep are obtained at baseline, at posttreatment, and at a 1-year follow-up. Preliminary data from the first 61 patients enrolled in this protocol indicate that all three conditions produced significant reductions (> 90%) in both the quantity and frequency of benzodiazepine usage at the end of the 10-week intervention; there is currently no significant difference on those two dependent measures across the three conditions. The typical patient enrolled in this protocol is 65 years old and has used a benzodiazepine for sleep on a regular basis for more than 13 years. Average nightly dosage used before treatment is the equivalent of 2 mg of lorazepam

(Ativan) or 10 mg of diazepam (Valium). For the three conditions combined, 72% of the patients were drug-free at posttreatment, and this proportion was higher in the combined condition (82%) compared to the medication taper (71%) or CBT (61%) alone conditions. Treatment gains were well maintained at 3- and 12-month follow-ups in terms of the quantity and frequency of medication used; however, the proportion of patients who were still drug-free went down from an overall posttreatment rate of 72%, to 68% at 3-month follow-up, and 50% at the 12-month follow-up. Although sleep was improved only slightly, the absence of sleep deterioration following discontinuation of hypnotic drugs is, in itself, a positive outcome.

In a series of studies, Lichstein and his colleagues have examined the impact of relaxation training and stimulus control with medicated insomniacs. In their first study (Lichstein & Johnson, 1993), elderly community-dwelling women (mean age of 66 years) were provided with a brief relaxation intervention consisting of three training sessions over a 2-week period. Although there were no specific tapering instructions, a 47% reduction of hypnotic medications was obtained from baseline to a 6-week follow-up, without sleep deterioration. In another study that included a structured withdrawal program, Lichstein and his colleagues (1999) reported an 80% reduction of medication intake among the long-term hypnotic users treated with relaxation; once again, minimal rebound insomnia was reported during the tapering program. Post-tapering sleep remained either unchanged (number of awakenings) or improved (latency to sleep, total sleep time, and sleep efficiency) compared to baseline measures. Finally, in a study of medicated and unmedicated middle-aged adults (Riedel et al., 1998), stimulus control was found to produce significant sleep improvements after withdrawal (i.e., 8 weeks posttreatment). Those benefits, however, were generally smaller than those observed in the unmedicated group. For the medicated insomniacs, the addition of stimulus control to a supervised withdrawal program did not yield greater reduction of hypnotics relative to a supervised withdrawal program alone.

The relative efficacy of a medication withdrawal program implemented in the context of a brief consultation, or as part of a stress management program, was evaluated with 12 middle-aged women (mean age of 50 years) who were dependent on hypnotic medications

(Kirmil-Gray et al., 1985). The interventions were equally successful in eliminating medication use in all patients, in an average of 8 weeks. Sleep improvements were modest at posttreatment, possibly because of persisting rebound effects; however, patients receiving concurrent stress management showed more improvements on sleep and mood measures compared to those receiving treatment that focused exclusively on medication withdrawal. At 6- and 12-month follow-ups, half of the participants had resumed use of hypnotic drugs between one and four times per week, while the other half limited their use to no more than twice a month.

An important issue that often arises in clinical practice is whether drug tapering should be implemented before, during, or after behavioral treatment for insomnia. Espie and his colleagues (1988) compared two withdrawal protocols. Five chronic hypnotic users were withdrawn before and five after receiving behavioral therapies (i.e., relaxation training, stimulus control, and paradoxical intention). Patients who were withdrawn from medication early in treatment achieved a better outcome on sleep onset latency than those withdrawn after behavior therapy. Four patients (one in the early and three in the late withdrawal) had resumed usage of hypnotic medication at the 1-year follow-up. Consistent with other studies, the long-term results suggest that maintenance therapy (i.e., booster sessions, periodic phone calls) may be necessary to prevent relapse.

Additional studies of benzodiazepine discontinuation with anxious patients indicate that 65% of patients trying to taper their anxiolytic medications on their own will relapse 1 year later, compared to 45% of those who receive some information and support during the tapering program (Rickels, Case, et al., 1990). Other findings reveal that a gradual taper is equally as successful with patients older than 60 as with those younger than 55 years old, and the older group report less withdrawal symptoms relative to younger patients (Schweizer et al., 1989). Because rebound insomnia and anxiety are classic symptoms associated with abrupt benzodiazepine withdrawal, it is important to use a gradual discontinuation approach to minimize those difficulties. Even with a gradual approach, however, some people may still experience withdrawal symptoms that are severe enough to jeopardize the tapering process. The addition of psychological treatment to a drug tapering regimen may reduce the frequency and severity of reported withdrawal symptoms relative to a standard tapering alone in patients with anxiety disorders (Fraser et al., 1990; Otto et al., 1993).

In summary, the evidence currently available indicates that a supervised taper combined with psychological treatment produces significant reduction in the quantity and frequency of hypnotic medications used by insomnia patients. Between 70% and 80% of older adults who are long-term hypnotic users are drug-free after an average of 8 to 10 weeks. Although promising, these short-term benefits must be tempered against long-term outcomes because significant relapse rates occur at intermediate (6-month) and long-term (12-month) follow-ups. As for other forms of substance abuse/dependency, it seems essential to integrate formal relapse prevention training in order to maintain therapeutic gains.

In terms of treatment modality, the evidence indicates that a supervised tapering regimen is an essential therapeutic component to discontinue benzodiazepines among older adults. Brief consultations integrated into a structured, time-limited, and gradual tapering regimen are very important in keeping patients focused and goal-oriented. On the other hand, behavioral treatment of insomnia, without specific guidance in reducing hypnotic medications, may not be sufficient for long-term users who may have failed several previous attempts to discontinue medications on their own. The addition of psychological treatment to drug tapering enhances therapeutic benefits; it facilitates benzodiazepine discontinuation and reduces withdrawal symptoms. In addition, cognitive-behavior therapy specifically targeting insomnia improves sleep more than discontinuation of hypnotic medications alone. Sleep improvements, although modest initially, become more noticeable after patients have been off medication for several weeks or months.

Conclusions

The prevalence of insomnia increases with aging, and older adults are more likely than any other age group to be prescribed and to use sleep medications. Although hypnotic drugs may be indicated in the short-term management of late-life insomnia, their long-term use is still controversial. Many older adults continue using sleep medications much longer than was initially intended. This prolonged usage is often maintained by difficulties coming off the medication because of anticipatory anxiety, worsening of insomnia, and other withdrawal symptoms. Controlled studies of cognitive-behavioral interventions for late-life insomnia have yielded promising results for unmedicated patients. It is only recently, however, that the management of hypnotic-dependent insomnia has received some attention in the literature. The evidence available indicates that a supervised medication tapering is a necessary component to guide patients in discontinuing hypnotic medications. A structured medication taper may be sufficient for some patients, but the addition of formal cognitive-behavior therapy, specifically targeting insomnia and withdrawal symptoms (e.g., anxiety), appears to facilitate drug discontinuation by minimizing sleep disruptions during the withdrawal program. Treatment responses of older adults to structured medication tapering programs are comparable to if not better than those of younger adults. Additional research is needed to evaluate the long-term effects of various interventions and the benefits of relapse prevention training in maintaining a drug-free status over time. Longitudinal studies are also warranted to identify risk factors for prolonged usage of hypnotic medications and predictors of relapse/successful discontinuation. On a more clinical note, it would be important to examine carefully the indications for benzodiazepine discontinuation and to evaluate the broader impact of hypnotic discontinuation on sleep, cognitive functioning (memory), and quality of life.

References

American Psychiatric Association Task Force on Benzodiazepine Dependency. (1990). *Benzodiazepine: Dependence, toxicity and abuse.* Washington, DC: Author.

American Sleep Disorders Association. (1990). *The International Classification of Sleep Disorders: Diagnostic and coding manual.* Rochester, MN: Author.

American Society of Addiction Medicine. (1991). *Patient placement criteria for the treatment of psychoactive substance use disorders.* Washington, DC: Author.

Ashton, H. (1994). The treatment of benzodiazepine dependence. *Addiction, 89,* 1535-1541.

Baillargeon, L., Landreville, P., Verreault, R., Beauchemin, J.-P., Grégoire, J.-P., & Morin, C. M. (1998). *Réduction de la consommation de benzodiazépines chez les aîné-e-s souffrant d'insomnie: Effets d'une intervention cognitive et comportementale combinée avec un sevrage médicamenteux* [Reduction of benzodiazepine usage among older adults with insomnia: Effects of a cognitive-behavioral intervention combined with medication tapering]. Unpublished manuscript, Programme national de recherche et de développement en matière de santé, Ottawa, Ontario, Canada.

Barnas, C., Whithworth, A., & Fleischhacker, W. W. (1993). Are patterns of benzodiazepine use predictable? *Psychopharmacology, 111*, 301-305.

Busto, U. E., Sellers, E. M., Naranjo, C. A., Cappell, H., Sanchez-Craig, M., & Sykora, K. (1986). Withdrawal reactions after long-term therapeutic use of benzodiazepines. *New England Journal of Medicine, 315*, 854-859.

Closser, M. H., & Brower, K. J. (1994). Treatment of alprazolam withdrawal with chlordiazepoxide substitution and taper. *Journal of Substance Abuse Treatment, 11*, 319-323.

DuPont, R. L. (1990). A practical approach to benzodiazepine discontinuation. *Journal of Psychiatric Research, 24*, 81-90.

Englert, S., & Linden, M. (1998). Differences in self-reported sleep complaints in elderly persons living in the community who do or do not take sleep medication. *Journal of Clinical Psychiatry, 59*, 137-144.

Espie, C. A., Lindsay, W. R., & Brooks, N. (1988). Substituting behavioural treatment for drugs in the treatment of insomnia: An exploratory study. *Journal of Behavior Therapy and Experimental Psychiatry, 19*, 51-56.

Fontaine, R. G., Chouinard, L., & Annable, L. (1984). Rebound anxiety in anxious patients after abrupt withdrawal of benzodiazepine treatment. *American Journal of Psychiatry, 141*, 848-852.

Fraser, D., Peterkin, G. S., Gamsu, C. V., & Baldwin, P. J. (1990). Benzodiazepine withdrawal: A pilot comparison of three methods. *British Journal of Clinical Psychology, 29*, 231-233.

Gillin, J. C., Spinweber, C. L., & Johnson, L. C. (1989). Rebound insomnia: A critical review. *Journal of Clinical Psychopharmacology, 9*, 161-172.

Greenblatt, D. J., Harmatz, B. A., Zinny, M. A., & Shader, R. I. (1987). Effects of gradual withdrawal on the rebound sleep disorder after discontinuation of triazolam. *New England Journal of Medicine, 317*, 722-728.

Herman, J. B., Rosenbaum, J. F., & Brotman, A. W. (1987). The alprazolam to clonazepam switch for the treatment of panic disorder. *Journal of Clinical Psychopharmacology, 7*, 175-178.

Hohagen, F., Käppler, C., Schramm, E., Rink, K., Weyerer, S., Riemann, D., & Berger, M. (1994). Prevalence of insomnia in elderly general practice attenders and the current treatment modalities. *Acta Psychiatrica Scandinavica, 90*, 102-108.

Johansson, B., Berglund, M., & Frank, A. (1997). Effects of gradual benzodiazepine taper during a fixed 10-day schedule: A pilot study. *Nordic Journal of Psychiatry, 51*, 281-286.

Kales, A., Bixler, E. O., Vela-Bueno, A., Soldatos, C. R., Niklaus, D. E., & Manfredi, R. L. (1986). Comparison of short and long half-life benzodiazepine hypnotics: Triazolam and quazepam. *Clinical Pharmacology Therapy, 40*, 378-386.

Kirmil-Gray, K., Eagleston, J. R., Thorensen, C. E., & Zarcone, V. P. (1985). Brief consultation and stress management treatments for drug-dependent insomnia: Effects on sleep quality, self-efficacy, and daytime stress. *Journal of Behavioral Medicine, 8*, 79-99.

Lader, M. H. (1986). Management of benzodiazepine dependence: Update 1986. *British Journal of Addiction, 81*, 7-10.

Lader, M. H. (1990). Benzodiazepine withdrawal. In R. Noyes, M. Roth, & G. D. Burrows (Eds.), *Handbook of anxiety* (pp. 57-71). Amsterdam: Elsevier.

Lader, M. H. (1997). Zopiclone: Is there any dependence and abuse potential? *Journal of Neurology, 244*(Suppl. 1), 18-22.

Lichstein, K. L., & Johnson, R. S. (1993). Relaxation for insomnia and hypnotic medication use in older women. *Psychology and Aging, 8*, 103-111.

Lichstein, K. L., Peterson, B. A., Riedel, B. W., Means, M. K., Epperson, M. T., & Aguillard, R. N. (1999). Relaxation to assist sleep medication withdrawal. *Behavior Modification, 23,* 379-402.

Lingjaerde, O., Bratlid, T., Westby, O. C., & Gordeladze, J. O. (1983). Effect of midazolam, flunitrazepam, and placebo against midwinter insomnia in northern Norway. *Acta Psychiatrica Scandinavica, 67,* 118-129.

Mant, A., Mattick, R. P., Burgh, S., Donnelly, N., & Hall, W. (1995). Benzodiazepine prescribing in general practice: Dispelling some myths. *Family Practice, 12,* 37-43.

Mellinger, G. D., Balter, M. B., & Uhlenhuth, E. H. (1985). Insomnia and its treatment: Prevalence and correlates. *Archives of General Psychiatry, 42,* 225-232.

Mimeault, V., & Morin, C. M. (1999). Self-help treatment for insomnia: Bibliotherapy with and without professional guidance. *Journal of Consulting and Clinical Psychology, 67,* 511-519.

Morawetz, D. (1989). Behavioral self-help treatment for insomnia: A controlled evaluation. *Behavior Therapy, 20,* 365-379.

Morgan, K., & Clarke, D. (1997). Longitudinal trends in late-life insomnia: Implications for prescribing. *Age and Ageing, 26,* 179-184.

Morgan, K., Dallosso, H., Ebrahim, S., Arie, T., & Fentem, P. H. (1988). Prevalence, frequency, and duration of hypnotic drug use among elderly living at home. *British Medical Journal, 296,* 601-602.

Morin, C. M. (1993). *Insomnia: Psychological assessment and management.* New York: Guilford.

Morin, C. M., Bastien, C. H., Radouco-Thomas, M., Guay, B., Leblanc, J., & Gagné, A. (1997, November). *Treatment of insomnia and benzodiazepine dependance in late-life.* Paper presented at the annual meeting of the Association for Advancement of Behavior Therapy, Miami, FL.

Morin, C. M., Colecchi, C. A., Ling, W. D., & Sood, R. K. (1995). Cognitive behavior therapy to facilitate benzodiazepine discontinuation among hypnotic-dependent patients with insomnia. *Behavior Therapy, 26,* 733-745.

Murphy, S. M., & Tyrer, P. (1991). Double-blind comparison of the effects of gradual withdrawal of lorazepam, diazepam and bromazepam in benzodiazepine dependence. *British Journal of Psychiatry, 158,* 511-516.

National Institutes of Health. (1984). Drugs and insomnia: The use of medications to promote sleep. *Journal of the American Medical Association, 18,* 2410-2414.

National Institutes of Health. (1991). Consensus development conference statement: The treatment of sleep disorders of older people. *Sleep, 14,* 169-177.

Noyes, R., Garvey, M. J., Cook, B. L., & Perry, P. L. (1988). Benzodiazepine withdrawal: A review of the evidence. *Journal of Clinical Psychiatry, 49,* 382-389.

Otto, M. W., Pollack, M. H., Sachs, G. S., Reiter, S. R., Meltzer-Brody, S., & Rosenbaum, J. F. (1993). Discontinuation of benzodiazepine treatment: Efficacy of cognitive-behavioral therapy for patients with panic disorder. *American Journal of Psychiatry, 150,* 1485-1490.

Petursson, H., & Lader, M. H. (1981). Withdrawal from long-term benzodiazepine treatment. *British Medical Journal, 283,* 643-645.

Ravi, N. V., Maany, I., Burke, W. M., Dhopesh, V., & Woody, G. E. (1990). Detoxification with phenobarbital of alprazolam-dependent polysubstance abusers. *Journal of Substance Abuse Treatment, 7,* 55-58.

Rickels, K., Case, W. G., Schweizer, E., Garcia-Espana, F., & Fridman, R. (1990). Benzodiazepine dependence: Management of discontinuation. *Psychopharmacology Bulletin, 26,* 63-68.

Rickels, K., Schweizer, E., Case, W. G., & Greenblatt, D. J. (1990). Long-term therapeutic use
of benzodiazepines: I. Effects of abrupt discontinuation. *Archives of General Psychiatry,*
47, 899-907.
Rickels, K., Schweizer, E., Csanalosi, I., Case, W. G., & Chung, H. (1988). Long-term treatment of anxiety and risk of withdrawal: Prospective comparison of clorazepate and
buspirone. *Archives of General Psychiatry, 45,* 444-450.
Riedel, B. W., Lichstein, K. L., & Dwyer, W. O. (1995). Sleep compression and sleep education for older insomniacs: Self-help versus therapist guidance. *Psychology and Aging, 10,*
54-63.
Riedel, B. W., Lichstein, K. L., Peterson, B. A., Epperson, M. T., Means, M., & Aguillard,
R. N. (1998). A comparison of the efficacy of stimulus control for medicated and
nonmedicated insomniacs. *Behavior Modification, 22,* 3-28.
Roehrs, T., Vogel, G., & Roth, T. (1990). Rebound insomnia: Its determinants and significance. *The American Journal of Medicine, 88*(Suppl. 3A), 39-42.
Schneider-Helmert, D. (1988). Why low-dose benzodiazepine-dependent insomniacs can't
escape their sleeping pills. *Acta Psychiatrica Scandinavica, 78,* 706-711.
Schweizer, E., Case, W. G., & Rickels, K. (1989). Benzodiazepine dependence and withdrawal in elderly patients. *American Journal of Psychiatry, 146,* 529-531.
Schweizer, E., Rickels, K., Case, W. G., & Greenblatt, D. J. (1990). Long-term therapeutic use
of benzodiazepines: II. Effects of gradual taper. *Archives of General Psychiatry, 47,*
908-915.
Shapiro, C. M., Sherman, D., & Peck, D. F. (1995). Withdrawal from benzodiazepines by initially switching to zopiclone. *European Psychiatry, 10*(Suppl. 3), 145-151.
Tattersall, M. L., & Hallstrom, C. (1992). Self-help and benzodiazepine withdrawal. *Journal*
of Affective Disorders, 24, 193-198.
Tyrer, P., Owen, R., & Dawling, S. (1983). Gradual withdrawal of diazepam after long-term
therapy. *Lancet, 1,* 1402-1406.
Vogel, G. W., & Vogel, F. (1983). Effect of midazolam on sleep of insomniacs. *British Journal*
of Clinical Pharmacology, 16(Suppl. 1), 103-108.
Vollrath, M., Wicki, W., & Angst, J. (1989). The Zurich Study: VIII. Insomnia: Association
with depression, anxiety, somatic syndromes, and course of insomnia. *European Ar-*
chives of Psychiatry and Clinical Neuroscience, 239, 113-124.
Walsh, J. K., & Engelhardt, C. L. (1992). Trends in the pharmacological treatment of insomnia. *Journal of Clinical Psychiatry, 53*(Suppl.), 10-17.

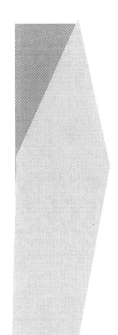

12

Secondary Insomnia

KENNETH L. LICHSTEIN

One can distinguish between primary insomnia (PI) and secondary insomnia (SI). PI is thought to derive from a combination of three sources: (a) psychological tension, as exemplified by bedtime worry; (b) conditioned sleep inhibition associated with the bedroom resulting from past associations of this setting with activities, thoughts, and/or emotions that are sleep obstructing; and (c) cognitive and/or physiological arousal stemming from the above (American Psychiatric Association, 1994). In brief, PI arises from bio-psycho-social mechanisms unrelated to a defined disease. A large body of research has demonstrated good responsivity of PI to psychological interventions with younger (Lichstein & Riedel, 1994) and older (Lichstein, Riedel, & Means, 1999) samples. If the insomnia is precipitated or aggravated by another disease, disorder, or substance, then the other disorder is termed primary and the insomnia secondary. The pres-

AUTHOR'S NOTE: Preparation of this chapter was supported in part by grant AG12136 from the National Institute on Aging, by a grant from the H. W. Durham Foundation, by Methodist Healthcare, and by the Department of Psychology's Center for Applied Psychological Research, part of the state of Tennessee's Center of Excellence Grant program.

ent chapter will investigate SI with a focus on its occurrence among older adults.

The traditional reluctance to treat SI stems from the widespread beliefs among health professionals that direct treatment of the sleep disturbance would be fruitless as long as the primary condition provoking the insomnia persists, and that sleep improvement will follow amelioration of the primary condition (Mendelson & Jain, 1995; National Institutes of Health, 1991; Walsh & Sugerman, 1989). The scarcity of published accounts of direct treatment of SI evinces the ubiquity of this opinion.

Three assumptions are implicit in common conceptualizations of SI. These serve to bolster the aversion to treating this disorder but may be unjustified.

> *Assumption 1:* SI can be properly diagnosed.
> *Assumption 2:* SI and PI are mutually exclusive conditions, precluding the possibility of partial SI.
> *Assumption 3:* SI, which may arise from a highly varied array of primary conditions, is uniformly unresponsive to direct treatment.

The remainder of this chapter will examine the nature and treatment of SI and, in so doing, will challenge the validity of these discouraging assumptions.

Demography of SI

Diagnosis

DSM-IV and *ICSD*

The *DSM-IV* (American Psychiatric Association, 1994) recognizes three kinds of SI: (a) arising from a primary mental disorder, termed insomnia related to another mental disorder; (b) arising from a medical condition, termed sleep disorder due to a general medical condition, insomnia type; and (c) substance-induced sleep disorder, insomnia type. To qualify for the first type, the insomnia must be "temporally and causally" (p. 592) related to the mental disorder, but the *DSM-IV* gives little advice on how to establish these criteria. More detail is provided for the second type. There should be an association between the "onset, exacerbation, or remission of the general medical condition and that of the sleep disturbance" (p. 598). Further, the presence of atypical characteristics of the insomnia and a rationale for the mechanism of action of the primary condition on sleep strengthen the diagnosis. The third type may be due to drugs of abuse or medications.

The International Classification of Sleep Disorders (*ICSD*) (American Sleep Disorders Association, 1990) takes a similar approach to SI. It lists 19 psychiatric and medical conditions and substances that may induce SI. Here too, a temporal relationship between the insomnia and the primary condition and a rationale for the connection are the main criteria, though few details are given on the mechanics of establishing the diagnosis.

Diagnostic Complexity in SI

In conformity with the *DSM* and the *ICSD*, there is general agreement that the following two conditions must be met. First, one must be able to specify the mechanism by which the primary condition produces insomnia. This standard will minimize misdiagnoses resulting from serendipitous joint occurrence. Second, there must be a correlated history between the primary disorder and insomnia, including a temporal sequence compatible with causality. This standard will minimize misdiagnoses resulting from misattributions of insomnia to conditions that sometimes do cause insomnia. The presence of comorbidity does not by itself reduce PI to SI. Also, determining that there was a plausible temporal sequence (i.e., the primary condition precedes the insomnia) is critical, because insomnia will sometimes act as the primary condition and provoke another disorder (see discussion below).

By correlated history, we mean that the origin of the insomnia shortly followed that of the primary condition and/or that variations in severity of the primary condition over time are followed shortly by comparable variations in insomnia. This latter criterion recognizes that there may have been a preexisting PI that was worsened by a primary condition. Thus, we wish to introduce the concept of partial SI, in that SI may not be entirely under the control of a primary condition. Two versions of partial SI are possible. A preexisting PI may be exacerbated by a primary condition, or insomnia created by a primary condition may acquire some degree of functional independence over time.

In brief, the diagnosis of SI requires the determination that a comorbid condition owns a causal influence over reported insomnia, and such a judgment may be difficult, even for experienced clinicians. The only study that measured the reliability of this diagnosis highlighted the difficulty inherent in this process (Buysse, Reynolds, Hauri, et al., 1994). Sleep specialists and general clinicians rendered independent diagnoses on a series of individuals reporting insomnia complaints. Agreement between them in conferring the diagnosis of insomnia secondary to a mental disorder was at the lower boundary of the moderately good range, median kappa = 0.42.

We now recognize two varieties of SI: *absolute SI*, which requires that the origin *and* the variation in severity of the insomnia mirror the course of the primary condition, and *partial SI*, in which only one of these constraints holds. Further, we wish to introduce a third type that we shall call *specious SI*, in which appearances satisfy the definition of absolute or partial SI but in truth no causal link exists. Specious SI arises when comorbidity is mistaken for causality.

In most cases of SI, we cannot rule out specious SI for two reasons. First, the data on which the diagnosis of SI rests often are shaky. Typically, the patient's historical accounting of the course of the primary condition and of the insomnia is the main basis for the diagnosis. The reliability of this source of data will vary greatly. Second, even when high-quality data are obtained, the diagnosis of SI usually constitutes an educated guess. Only under the uncommon circumstance of a naturally occurring single-subject experimental design (i.e., ABAB, wherein the primary condition is absent-present-absent-present and fluctuations in the insomnia closely track this sequence) do we have the opportunity to elevate our confidence in the hypothesized causal link. By this reasoning, only absolute SI under uncommon circumstances holds even the potential of definitive diagnosis.

To illustrate the several forms of SI, consider an individual suffering arthritic pain. Absolute SI would be inferred if insomnia onset shortly followed the beginning of the pain and if the severity of the insomnia varied over the years in conformity with increases and decreases in pain. Presumably, the insomnia is under control of the pain, and sleep treatment would be futile as long as the pain persisted. Normal sleep would be expected to return if the pain ceased. Partial SI would appear to be an appropriate diagnosis if the insomnia preceded pain onset but the insomnia grew worse after the pain began. Similarly, the diagnosis of partial SI might be conferred if the insomnia followed pain onset but variations in pain did not instigate like change in the insomnia. It is critical to note that in all three of the above examples, the causal link between pain and insomnia is inferred from a correlated history. The stronger the correlation, the more confident the diagnosis. Nevertheless, rarely is the causal link unequivocally established.

The matter of specious SI is a bit more circuitous. Had the provider not believed a causal link existed, the insomnia and the pain would simply be said to be comorbid. Thus, the diagnosis of specious SI is not given when causality is thought to be absent; rather, specious SI is a diagnosis held in reserve when a diagnosis of either absolute or partial SI is conferred. Unfortunately, in nearly all cases of absolute and partial SI, we cannot dismiss the possibility that this is really specious SI. When in fact we have partial or specious SI, successful treatment of the "primary" condition can be expected to yield partial or no insomnia relief. Alternatively, partial and specious SI can be expected to be responsive to direct sleep treatment.

It should be obvious that the differential diagnosis of the three types of SI is rarely clear-cut. Rendering a diagnosis of SI is more inferential than definitive. Some unknown proportion of absolute and partial SI cases are misdiagnoses of specious SI, but by definition, it would be difficult to distinguish specious SI from alternative diagnoses.

The diagnosis of SI should also consider the dimension of the primary disorder that is responsible for the insomnia. Disturbed sleep may arise directly from the physiological mechanisms of the primary disorder (particularly in the case of neurological disorders), from secondary symptoms associated with the disease (such as pain or nocturia), from alerting medications treating the primary disorder, and/or from associated stress (Aldrich, 1993; Hu & Silberfarb, 1991). The treatment responsivity of the insomnia may be dependent on the dimension of the primary disorder disrupting sleep.

A thorough understanding of the complexity of the diagnosis of SI is important because it softens barriers to psychological treatment in this domain. Even were it true that psychological treatment of some types of absolute SI holds little promise, we usually do not know if we are treating absolute, partial, or specious SI; therefore, what may pass for the treatment of SI may in fact be treatment of PI or some mixture of PI and SI. In the latter case, it can be expected that at least some portion of the insomnia will be responsive to psychological intervention.

Common Causes of SI

SI may derive from a variety of sources. For example, insomnia is routinely encountered among individuals suffering a broad range of psychiatric disorders (Walsh & Sugerman, 1989). Dozens of medical conditions may instigate insomnia. Examples are asthma, fibromyalgia, chronic fatigue syndrome, alcohol abuse, pulmonary disease, gastroesophageal reflux, renal failure, headaches, heart disease, arthritis, and a variety of neurological diseases, such as Parkinson's, Alzheimer's, and Huntington's diseases and seizures (Mitler, Poceta, Menn, & Erman, 1991; Williams, 1988; Wooten, 1989). Although the diagnosis of SI usually relies on self-report of sleep complaints, a number of studies have employed all-night sleep studies (polysomnography) to objectively document SI, as exemplified by studies of depression (Kupfer & Reynolds, 1992), pain (Wittig, Zorick, Blumer, Heilbronn, & Roth, 1982), and Huntington's disease (Wiegand et al., 1991).

A number of specific mechanisms exist by which a primary disorder causes insomnia. A particular mechanism may operate across numerous disorders, and a single disorder may operate through several mechanisms. Pain is a high-frequency instigator of insomnia (Haythornthwaite, Hegel, & Kerns, 1991; Morin, Gibson, & Wade, 1998) and is the likely SI mechanism in a substantial proportion of cases of cancer (Hu & Silberfarb, 1991; Strang & Qvarner, 1990; World Health Organization, 1986, p. 20), back pain (Currie, Wilson, & Gauthier, 1995), and headache (Spierings & van Hoof, 1997). Stress associated with the primary condition may be the SI mechanism in cases of cancer (Hu & Silberfarb, 1991). Muscle tremors and stiffness may disturb sleep and are found in many of the neurological diseases (Aldrich, 1993).

Several studies are discussed in detail below because they were done carefully and illuminate important dimensions of SI. Some of the issues they explore are the types of sleep disturbance that can manifest in SI, the diversity of causal mechanisms operating in SI, and the complex interaction between the primary disorder and the sleep disturbance.

A small amount of data alerts us to the possibility that the type of insomnia associated with different primary conditions may vary. Kaye,

Kaye, and Madow (1983) collected self-report sleep data from 30 outpatients suffering from several types of inoperable cancer, 28 outpatients with differing types of chronic cardiac disease, and 24 matched, healthy controls. Cancer patients were distinguished by their high rate of maintenance insomnia (main difficulty is awakenings during the night), and cardiac patients primarily reported onset (difficulty falling asleep initially) or terminal (final awakening early in the morning) insomnia. Such contrasts in the type of insomnia may help guide treatment selection. For example, meta-analytic data suggest that relaxation therapy is more effective for onset than maintenance insomnia (Morin, Culbert, & Schwartz, 1994).

Sleep is a fragile, vulnerable biologic function. Any condition that instigates physiological arousal, psychological distress, or pain is likely to provoke SI. A recent study of Parkinson's disease (PD) exemplifies a multifactorial model of SI (Smith, Ellgring, & Oertel, 1997). Sleep disturbance may arise in PD following the direct physical effects of the disease (tremor, rigidity, excessive sweating), physical by-products of the disease (nocturia, pain), alerting medications taken for PD (levodopa, selegiline), and/or emergent psychiatric distress (depression). To evaluate these factors, self-report data were collected from 153 PD patients and their spouses and from 103 healthy, age-matched controls. The rate of insomnia among the PD patients and their spouses about doubled that found in the control group. Indeed, insomnia was slightly *more common in the spouses than in the patients themselves*, underscoring the burden attendant to being a caregiver of someone with chronic illness. For both patients and caregivers, depression was rated the most important factor in their insomnia. Although most PD studies report elevated rates of insomnia, at least one study found only a small increment in insomnia among PD patients compared to the level reported in age-matched controls (Factor, McAlarney, Sanchez-Ramos, & Weiner, 1990).

A study of nocturnal and morning headaches revealed insomnia may play reactive, instigative, or reciprocal roles in relation to the "primary" disorder (Paiva, Batista, Martins, & Martins, 1995). Twenty-five headache patients submitted to polysomnography, and seven of these individuals complained of insomnia. In many cases, other sleep disorders—sleep apnea and periodic limb movements—were discovered and found to be causing the headaches. There were numerous instances, however, of headache causing insomnia (reactive), insomnia causing headache (instigative), and insomnia and headache exacerbating each other (reciprocal). One case of SI was particularly interesting. Insomnia was induced by anticipatory worry that headache may appear during sleep. Consistent with the findings of this basic research, clinical studies have shown that successful treatment of the insomnia may elicit improvement in the primary condition as well (Morin, Kowatch, & O'Shanick, 1990; Morin, Kowatch, & Wade, 1989).

Pain is among the most common sources of medical SI but is reactive to insomnia as well, thus instigating a process of reciprocal escalation of symptoms. Studies of osteoarthritis may serve as a model for this syndrome (Moldofsky, 1989). Osteoarthritis pain may provoke insomnia, but two operative sleep factors may initiate or aggravate daytime pain. Sleep posture may strain joints and give rise to pain, and the sleep deprivation occasioned by insomnia will lower pain threshold.

Sleep is reactive to a broad range of substances. Some common nonprescription substances may disrupt sleep: caffeine, nicotine, and alcohol (Mendelson & Jain, 1995; Moran & Stoudemire, 1992). Over-the-counter medications, such as nasal decongestants and pain medications that contain caffeine (e.g., Anacin, Excedrin), may also adversely affect sleep. In addition, many prescribed medications may cause insomnia, dependent on the dosage level, time of administration, age of the patient, and idiosyncratic response (Becker & Jamieson, 1992; Mitler et al., 1991; Monane, 1992). The main classes of drugs that can induce insomnia are energizing antidepressants, antihypertensives, bronchodilators, diuretics, beta-blockers, and corticosteroids. It should be noted that drugs differ with respect to their mechanism of action, and not all drugs within a class will cause insomnia in most people. Table 12.1 lists examples of the many prescription drugs known to cause insomnia, though this list is not exhaustive.

Prevalence

Numerous epidemiological studies (see Chapter 1, this volume) have estimated the prevalence of insomnia in the general population and among older adults, but such data are less common for SI specifically and are more difficult to interpret. For example, large surveys may have collected data on comorbid psychiatric and medical conditions with insomnia and found increased insomnia prevalence when such comorbidity

TABLE 12.1 Examples of Medications That May Induce Insomnia

Generic Name	Target Disorder
Clonidine	Hypertension
Fluoxetine	Depression
Imipramine	Depression
Levodopa	Parkinson's disease
Methyldopa	Hypertension
Phenelzine	Depression
Phenytoin	Seizures
Propranolol	Hypertension
Protriptyline	Depression
Quinidine	Arrhythmia
Steroids	Inflammation
Theophylline	Asthma
Thyroid hormone	Thyroid dysfunction
Triamterene	Edema

exists, but these may lack the detailed inquiry to assert a causal link establishing the diagnosis of SI (Foley et al., 1995; Mellinger, Balter, & Uhlenhuth, 1985). We can nevertheless infer a rough estimate of its occurrence by reports of varying levels of sophistication and by analyses of small samples of people with insomnia (PWI).

Numerous studies have estimated the prevalence of insomnia associated with particular disorders. These studies are characterized by inference of SI by the presence of comorbidity, and most did little to determine if the primary condition owned a causal relationship to the sleep disturbance. The following prevalence rates may overstate sleep disturbance rightfully owing to the primary condition. Studies of patients experiencing pain from varied sources report that 50% to 70% of these individuals suffer insomnia (Atkinson, Ancoli-Israel, Slater, Garfin, & Gillin, 1988; Morin et al., 1998; Pilowsky, Crettenden, & Townley, 1985). Morin et al. (1998) did take the additional diagnostic step of determining that 90% of the PWI reported that their poor sleep coincided with or followed the onset of their pain problem, consistent with the diagnosis of SI. Cordoba et al. (1998) found that 47.7% of cirrhotic and 38.6% of chronic renal failure patients complained of unsatisfactory sleep, compared to 4.5% of healthy controls. This study also monitored participants with wrist actigraphy to corroborate sleep complaints. Older adults experiencing stroke or heart disease have about twice the likelihood of developing insomnia over the next 3 years than others without these conditions (Monjan & Foley, 1996). Studying more than 3,000 individuals with chronic illness, Katz and McHorney (1998) found significantly elevated rates of severe insomnia among individuals with depression, congestive heart failure, obstructive airway disease, back problems, hip impairment, and peptic ulcer. An epidemiological survey (Mellinger et al., 1985) found that 47% of people reporting severe insomnia also admitted high psychiatric distress. Symptoms comparable to major depression were found in 21% of the insomnia sample, and symptoms comparable to generalized anxiety were found in 13%. Further, 53% of those complaining of severe insomnia also reported having at least two medical health problems, implying that medical factors were also contributory.

A small amount of data is specific to prevalence rates among older adults with SI (OASI). In a Gallup poll (Gallup Organization, 1995), when PWI were asked if medical problems were the basis of their sleep disturbance, affirmative responses were given by about 5% of PWI who were below the age of 55 and by about 15% of PWI 55 or older. A survey of 100 healthy older adults found high rates of reported sleep disruption: 59% complained of nocturia disturbing their sleep on a regular basis, 16% cited coughing or difficulty breathing, 12% pain, 10% feeling cold, 8% feeling hot, 6% leg cramps, and 3% dreams (Hoch, Buysse, Monk, & Reynolds, 1992).

Ohayon (1997) conducted the most carefully done epidemiological survey to evaluate SI. Representative sampling techniques produced telephone interviews with 5,622 people in France. The interviewers were not mental health professionals but were given $2\frac{1}{2}$ days of training specific to this interview task. Employing conservative criteria for insomnia, they found that 5.6% of the sample had clinically significant insomnia. Among these individuals, when comorbid psychiatric or medical conditions were present, an attempt was made to determine if the insomnia arose from this other condition, thus providing a reasonable effort to verify the diagnosis of SI. This study found that 51.8% of insomnia was secondary to psychiatric disorder (evenly split between a primary condition of anxiety or depression), 8.9% was secondary to medical disorder, and 3.6% was secondary to substance use. Of those with insomnia, 23.2% were judged to have PI. Nearly all the medical SI occurred in older adults, where its prevalence was nine times that of younger adults. Somewhat surprisingly, insomnia secondary to psychiatric disorder was 1½ times more common in younger adults.

Ford and Kamerow (1989) conducted one of the most important and enlightening epidemiologic studies of insomnia and psychiatric illness. They presented the most persuasive evidence of reciprocity between insomnia and depression. They reported the results of two interviews conducted 1 year apart on 7,954 people. At the first interview, 40.4% of PWI had a psychiatric disorder compared to 16.4% of those not complaining of insomnia. Anxiety and depression were the main diagnoses associated with insomnia. At the time of the second interview, incident anxiety and depression (meaning new cases) were significantly more common to individuals who reported insomnia at both the first and second interview compared either to individuals who reported insomnia at the first interview only (the sleep disturbance having resolved by the second interview) or to individuals who reported no insomnia at either interview. This study established insomnia as a risk factor for psychiatric disturbance. Further, it challenges the automatic diagnosis of presumed SI when insomnia and psychiatric disturbance jointly occur.

Several sleep disorders centers have broken down their patient pools to reveal insomnia subtypes. In all cases, these proportions reflect the normal patient flow at these centers, not recruited or sampled patients. Table 12.2 reports the proportion of all insomnia cases diagnosed as PI and SI. The percentages of PI and SI cases do not accumulate to 100% because many of the "insomnia" patients ultimately were diagnosed as having other sleep disorders such as sleep apnea, periodic limb movements, and delayed sleep phase syndrome. When the initial insomnia was later diagnosed as another sleep disorder, this case no longer fell within the categories of PI or SI.

Several of these studies have distinctive features that merit recognition or require explanation. Two of the studies combined data across several centers. The Buysse, Reynolds, Kupfer, et al. (1994) study combined data from five independent centers and employed the *ICSD, DSM-IV,* and *ICD-10* diagnostic systems. The present results are for the *ICSD* data only. A later report by this same group (Nowell et al., 1997) analyzed the factors contributing to diagnostic decisions. The presence of negative

TABLE 12.2 Prevalence of Primary and Secondary Insomnia at Sleep Disorders Centers

Study	N	% Primary	% Psychiatric	% Medical	% Substance	Largest Single Category (%)
			Main Categories of Secondary Insomnia			
Buysse, Reynolds, Kupfer, et al. (1994)	216	12.5	40.1	2.8	3.1	Mood (32.3)
Coleman et al. (1982)	1,214	15.3	34.9	3.8	12.4	Depression (17.5)
Edinger et al. (1989)	100	16	44	0	6	
Jacobs et al. (1988)	123	18.7	30.9	14	7.3	Depression (29.3)
Mendelson (1997)	312	16	20	6		Depression (13.0)
Roehrs et al. (1983): 20 to 40 years	68	9	24	3	3	
Roehrs et al. (1983): 41 to 60 years	84	19	19	6	5	
Roehrs et al. (1983): 61 years and older	48	15	6	10	15	
Zorick et al. (1981)	84	6	14	7	12	
Unweighted average across studies		14.2	25.9	5.8	8.0	

conditioning and poor sleep hygiene contributed most to the diagnosis of PI, and depression weighed most heavily in the diagnosis of insomnia secondary to psychiatric disorder. Coleman et al. (1982) combined data from 11 centers. One distinction in their data was the high rate of insomnia associated with personality disorders. Nearly half of the psychiatric cases (45%) were so classified.

Roehrs, Zorick, Sicklesteel, Wittig, and Roth (1983) reported their results for the full sample that spanned all ages, and they also broke their data down by age groups. Table 12.2 reports their data for each age group.

The interpretation of the data presented in Table 12.2 is subject to some qualifications. First, most of these studies did not carefully distinguish between SI versus PI with a comorbid psychiatric or medical condition; therefore, the rates of SI reported in Table 12.2 are probably inflated by some unknown amount. The most extreme example of prima facie inferring SI from the presence of other factors was a study omitted from Table 12.2 because its data were so deviant (Tan, Kales, Kales, Soldatos, & Bixler, 1984). This group evaluated 100 PWI and found 95 cases of psychiatric disturbance and 5 cases of medical disturbance responsible for the insomnia. Second, these are not random samples drawn from the population of PWI. These data describe self-referred individuals seeking clinical services at sleep disorders centers and individuals referred by their primary care physician. These data therefore fairly reflect treatment-seeking PWI but do not inform us about others who do not seek treatment because of insurance/financial barriers, lack of motivation or diminished expectations of successful treatment, lack of knowledge about the availability of services, or for other reasons.

Some summary conclusions can be drawn from the sleep center data. Of all those diagnosed with PI or SI, 73.7% were labeled SI. There is general agreement among centers that the prevalences of PI and insomnia secondary to medical factors are low and that of psychiatric SI is high. This does not necessarily mean that medical causes are rare. It may be that these individuals do not report to sleep disorders centers.

SI and Older Adults

SI is most likely more common and more severe in older adults. A number of factors can be identified that cause the prevalence of SI to be preponderant in older adults compared to younger age groups.

1. Older adults have lighter sleep (see Chapter 1, this volume), and this makes their sleep more sensitive to medical and psychiatric irritants.

2. Higher rates of medical illness in older adults produce greater exposure to potential sources of SI, including secondary symptoms of illness and polypharmacy effects. The higher rate of medical SI in older adults is striking (see above discussion of Ohayon, 1997). Many neurological diseases, such as Parkinson's disease, Huntington's disease, and Alzheimer's disease, are most prevalent among older adults and are high-risk factors for SI (Aldrich, 1993). Nocturnal confusion and wandering, termed sundowning, is a peculiar form of SI associated with Alzheimer's disease (Bliwise, 1993). Oftentimes, dementia patients are sustained by a spouse or child caregiver, who may themselves be an older adult. The patient's insomnia may very well be disruptive to the caregiver's sleep as well (McCurry, Logsdon, & Teri, 1996).

3. The impact of illness may be greater in older adults. For example, Guerrero and Crocq (1994) studied two groups of depressed individuals matched for severity of mood disturbance, a group under age 55 and a group older than 65. Insomnia was more frequent and more severe in the older group.

4. Normal physiologic changes associated with aging retard drug absorption, distribution, metabolism, and elimination, and elevate target site sensitivity (Gottlieb, 1990; Monane, 1992). The net effect of these changes is increased drug exposure and greater risk of insomnia secondary to medication.

5. A number of factors that may spawn psychiatric threats to sleep are more likely to occur in older adults. Death of a spouse, other loved one, or close friend will occur more often among older adults, and bereavement is a risk factor for insomnia (Hall et al., 1997; Hoch et al., 1992; Monjan & Foley, 1996). Retirement, social isolation, and restricted movement resulting from disability may provoke anxiety or depression and thereby affect sleep (De Berry, 1981-1982).

6. Other sleep disorders, such as sleep apnea and periodic limb movements, occur at higher rates among older adults, will produce insomnia-like symptoms, and will sometimes give rise to the incorrect diagnosis of insomnia (Hoch et al., 1992).

Treatment of SI

SI and its primary condition may evolve into a reciprocal relationship over time, wherein each is both an instigator and a reactor to the other. For example, insomnia may result from cancer, but the emergence of poor sleep diminishes the patient's physical and emotional resources to cope with the disease (Hu & Silberfarb, 1991). This cautionary note is to

remind the reader that we usually are not certain if we are treating absolute SI, partial SI, or specious SI, and that SI trials should monitor the primary condition as well document "side" benefits that may arise.

A variety of insomnia treatments have been tested with SI, as noted
below. The present chapter will identify, but not describe in detail, the
psychological treatments enlisted for this disorder; such descriptions are
provided in the collective chapters of this book or are well documented
in the literature.

SI Interventions With Varied Age Groups

Five case studies relate insomnia improvement associated with psychological treatment when the insomnia was secondary to chronic pain
(French & Tupin, 1974), cancer (Stam & Bultz, 1986), depression and
pain (Morin et al., 1990), multiple medical problems (Kolko, 1984), or he-
mophilia (Varni, 1980). Treatments were relaxation (French & Tupin,
1974; Kolko, 1984; Stam & Bultz, 1986; Varni, 1980); slow, deep breathing
(Varni, 1980); sleep restriction (Morin et al., 1990); stimulus control
(Varni, 1980); and imagery (French & Tupin, 1974; Stam & Bultz, 1986;
Varni, 1980).

One study evaluated a single group of 20 severe PWI (Tan et al., 1987).
These individuals were treated on an inpatient psychiatry unit for an average of 5 weeks, after outpatient insomnia treatment failed. All these
patients experienced a significant stressful life event at the time of insomnia onset. Nineteen patients had an Axis I diagnosis, and all 20 had
Axis II diagnoses according to the *DSM-III-R*. Insomnia was judged to be
secondary to the Axis I diagnosis in 9 cases and secondary to the Axis II
diagnosis in the remaining 11 cases. Treatment was intense, multimodal,
and individualized. The main treatment options were individual psychotherapy, group psychotherapy, marital therapy, occupational therapy, sleep medication, progressive relaxation, stimulus control, and biofeedback. Employing global quality of sleep ratings that ranged from 0 to
8, significant improvement was achieved from pretreatment ($M = 1.6$,
$SD = 0.2$) to posttreatment ($M = 6.0$, $SD = 0.4$), and gains were well maintained to 6-month follow-up ($M = 6.9$, $SD = 0.4$).

Morin et al. (1989) presented a carefully done multiple baseline design
evaluating the treatment of insomnia secondary to chronic pain in three

individuals. Treatment comprised six weekly sessions of stimulus control and sleep restriction. All patients simultaneously continued in their usual care for their particular pain problem, which included physical therapy, nerve blocks, and other treatments. This single-subject experimental design demonstrated close association between the introduction of treatment and self-reported sleep gains on a number of measures: latency to sleep, wake time during the night, and number of awakenings. Six-month follow-up revealed good maintenance of gains. All-night sleep studies (polysomnography) conducted pre- and posttreatment generally corroborated the self-report data. Further, two of three patients showed substantial improvement over the course of treatment on measures of depression and anxiety.

The only randomized group study of SI in a mixed-age sample tested progressive relaxation (PR) with patients diagnosed with various cancers (Cannici, Malcolm, & Peek, 1983). Thirty patients with mean age of 56 years were randomly assigned to usual medical care for their cancer or usual care plus three sessions of PR. Treatment sessions were conducted on 3 consecutive days, and pre-post self-report sleep assessments lasted only 3 days. Thus, this study was conducted over a 9-day period. In addition, 3-month follow-up data were collected.

Latency to sleep was significantly improved in the PR group, going from 124 minutes at pretreatment to 29 minutes post. This variable was unchanged in the comparison group. At 3-month follow-up, the PR group reported latency to sleep of 33 minutes, and the comparison group was unchanged. The changes observed in this measure were large and clinically meaningful. Unfortunately, this is the only measure that registered statistically significant treatment gains. Changes in most of the other sleep measures (e.g., total sleep time, number of awakenings during the night, rated sleep satisfaction) and pain ratings favored the PR group, but the differences did not reach statistical significance, a possible consequence of low power resulting from small sample size.

In summary, relatively few data are available on the treatment of SI, reflecting the prevailing opinion of the clinical community that this disorder is not suited for psychological intervention. The most convincing data are those by Morin et al. (1989), but there is little by way of replication or extension of these findings. There is, however, enough suggestive data available to conclude that this domain may be more amenable to psychological treatment than formerly believed, and more active research in this area is justified.

SI Interventions With Older Adults

We recently completed one of the few randomized studies on SI and the only study to focus on older adults (Lichstein, Wilson, & Johnson, in press). Forty-four volunteers met our screening criteria: age 58 or older, exhibiting insomnia by self-report for at least 6 months, and free of sleep medication. Further, to qualify as SI, the following conditions were satisfied as well: there was a plausible rationale establishing the causal link of the psychiatric or medical disorder to the insomnia, the onset of the insomnia closely followed the onset of the primary disorder, and/or variations in the severity of the insomnia closely tracked variations in the course of the primary disorder.

Our sample was evenly divided between insomnia secondary to psychiatric and to medical disorders. The most common primary disorders were depression and chronic pain associated with a variety of conditions. Other primary conditions represented in descending order of frequency were anxiety, prostate disease, neurologic disorders, and chronic respiratory disease.

Participants were randomized to two groups: a treatment group given four sessions combining hybrid passive relaxation, stimulus control, and sleep hygiene instructions, and a no treatment control group. Self-report sleep assessments were conducted at pretreatment, posttreatment, and 3-month follow-up.

There was significantly greater improvement at posttreatment and follow-up for the treated group on three sleep measures: wake time during the night, sleep efficiency percent (the ratio of time slept to time in bed × 100), and rated quality of sleep (from 1 = *very poor* to 5 = *excellent*). From baseline to follow-up for the treated group, wake time went from 87.3 minutes to 56.4, sleep efficiency went from 66.7% to 77.7%, and rated quality of sleep went from 2.7 to 3.2. Participants with medical and psychiatric SI were comparably responsive. Given the small number of treatment sessions we used with this difficult-to-treat population, we found these results highly encouraging.

Consistent with the discussion earlier in this chapter, in most cases we could not be certain if we were treating absolute SI, partial SI, or specious SI because individuals' memories of the course of their insomnia and primary disorder often were indefinite. It is clear, however, that this sample typified the population of people that are usually labeled SI and who have in the past been denied psychological treatment for their insomnia.

Conclusions

This chapter began by identifying three assumptions that militate against psychological treatment of SI: assumptions of satisfactory diagnoses, of expectation of absolute SI, and of uniform lack of responsiveness to treatment. Thoughtful consideration of the data suggests that these assumptions are false, or at least that there are commonly encountered circumstances in which they do not hold. Obstructing assumptions have been dismissed, and preliminary clinical data have provided encouraging results. The clinical environment is ripe for active exploration of psychological management of SI.

Simplistic conceptions of SI will lead to overdiagnosis of this condition and missed opportunities for effective insomnia treatment. When considering the SI diagnosis, the clinician/researcher is obliged to scrutinize relationships and processes between the "primary" condition and the sleep disturbance. Although some investigators conclude that the co-occurrence of poor sleep and a psychiatric/medical disorder evinces SI, others have questioned this assumption. There may evolve an upward spiraling, reciprocal relationship between the insomnia and the primary disorder, whereby each aggravates the other and each subsequently suffers as the other worsens (Paiva et al., 1995; Pilowsky et al., 1985). A downward spiraling, beneficial version of this reciprocity has been reported (Morin et al., 1990; Morin et al., 1989), and we have seen this phenomenon in our own research with pain patients experiencing SI (Lichstein et al., in press). Several of our participants commented that as their treated insomnia improved, daytime pain discomfort lessened and pain tolerance increased. At other times, the insomnia may precede and instigate the "primary" disorder (Ford & Kamerow, 1989; Paiva et al., 1995).

There is surprising agreement between two independent and divergent sources of information on the prevalence of PI and SI. Data from the sleep centers (Table 12.2) and the large survey conducted by Ohayon (1997) both find that PI occurs in less than 25% of insomnia cases, and SI may be three times more common than PI. These data may not fairly represent population distributions, but they are the best data available. The nearly exclusive focus of psychological treatments on PI stands in sharp contrast to the high frequency of occurrence of SI. The misfit of effort and prevalence should alert health care professionals that SI is highly deserving of their attention.

There seems to be some consistency in the data from varied sources that insomnia secondary to depression is the most common type of insomnia. Arguably, the commonality of this syndrome should command a fair amount of clinical/research attention, but it has not. No study has concurrently treated depression and insomnia in such individuals, nor has any study incorporated any special procedures to tailor insomnia interventions for this group. For example, perhaps cognitive therapy for insomnia popularized by Morin (1993) would fit this subtype of SI well in that it could also be adapted easily to address associated depressive cognitions. Depression SI deserves more attention in the future.

At this point, the study of psychological treatment of SI is in its infancy. Indeed, it was not more than a decade ago that the same statement could be made about psychological treatment of insomnia in older adults. The great progress made in treating older adults with insomnia should buoy advances in treating SI, particularly because SI is in large part a disorder of older adults.

There are enough data by now to strongly encourage further study, but not enough to draw definitive conclusions. Major questions remain regarding the clinical strategies to be used and the resulting therapeutic process. For example, it may be unjustified to assume that the same treatments found useful with PI among older adults will fare equally well with OASI. Similarly, we expect an uneven therapeutic response among the varieties of SI, but there are insufficient data to indicate if psychiatric or medical SI is more responsive to psychological intervention, and further, which subtypes within these two categories are the best therapy candidates.

Age and gender may also be associated with SI outcome. Within the older adult range, some have used the cutoff of 75 years to designate young-old and old-old groups. Are psychological interventions equally effective for both these groups, and do men and women respond equally?

Perhaps the near future will see an accelerating level of research in this area to clarify these important questions and bring sleep relief to a very needy group. At the very least, clinicians must begin to challenge the prevailing conviction that individuals with SI should receive little consideration for psychological treatment of their sleep disturbance.

References

Aldrich, M. S. (1993). Insomnia in neurological diseases. *Journal of Psychosomatic Research, 37*(Suppl. 1), 3-11.

American Psychiatric Association. (1994). *Diagnostic and statistical manual of mental disorders* (4th ed.). Washington, DC: Author.

American Sleep Disorders Association. (1990). *The International Classification of Sleep Disorders: Diagnostic and coding manual.* Rochester, MN: Author.

Atkinson, J. H., Ancoli-Israel, S., Slater, M. A., Garfin, S. R., & Gillin, J. C. (1988). Subjective sleep disturbance in chronic back pain. *Clinical Journal of Pain, 4,* 225-232.

Becker, P. M., & Jamieson, A. O. (1992). Common sleep disorders in the elderly: Diagnosis and treatment. *Geriatrics, 47*(3), 41-42, 45-48, 51-52.

Bliwise, D. L. (1993). Sleep in normal aging and dementia. *Sleep, 16,* 40-81.

Buysse, D. J., Reynolds, C. F., III, Hauri, P. J., Roth, T., Stepanski, E. J., Thorpy, M. J., Bixler, E. O., Kales, A., Manfredi, R. L., Vgontzas, A. N., Stapf, D. M., Houck, P. R., & Kupfer, D. J. (1994). Diagnostic concordance for DSM-IV sleep disorders: A report from the APA/NIMH DSM-IV field trial. *American Journal of Psychiatry, 151,* 1351-1360.

Buysse, D. J., Reynolds, C. F., III, Kupfer, D. J., Thorpy, M. J., Bixler, E., Manfredi, R., Kales, A., Vgontzas, A., Stepanski, E., Roth, T., Hauri, P., & Mesiano, D. (1994). Clinical diagnoses in 216 insomnia patients using the International Classification of Sleep Disorders (ICSD), DSM-IV and ICD-10 categories: A report form the APA/NIMH DSM-IV field trial. *Sleep, 17,* 630-637.

Cannici, J., Malcolm, R., & Peek, L. A. (1983). Treatment of insomnia in cancer patients using muscle relaxation training. *Journal of Behavior Therapy and Experimental Psychiatry, 14,* 251-256.

Coleman, R. M., Roffwarg, H. P., Kennedy, S. J., Guilleminault, C., Cinque, J., Cohn, M. A., Karacan, I., Kupfer, D. J., Lemmi, H., Miles, L. E., Orr, W. C., Phillips, E. R., Roth, T., Sassin, J. F., Schmidt, H. S., Weitzman, E. D., & Dement, W. C. (1982). Sleep-wake disorders based on polysomnographic diagnosis: A national cooperative study. *Journal of the American Medical Association, 247,* 997-1003.

Cordoba, J., Cabrera, J., Lataif, L., Penev, P., Zee, P., & Blei, A. T. (1998). High prevalence of sleep disturbance in cirrhosis. *Hepatology, 27,* 339-345.

Currie, S. R., Wilson, K. G., & Gauthier, S. T. (1995). Caffeine and chronic low back pain. *Clinical Journal of Pain, 11,* 214-219.

De Berry, S. (1981-1982). An evaluation of progressive muscle relaxation on stress related symptoms in a geriatric population. *International Journal of Aging and Human Development, 14,* 255-269.

Edinger, J. D., Hoelscher, T. J., Webb, M. D., Marsh, G. R., Radtke, R. A., & Erwin, C. W. (1989). Polysomnographic assessment of DIMS: Empirical evaluation of its diagnostic value. *Sleep, 12,* 315-322.

Factor, S. A., McAlarney, T., Sanchez-Ramos, J. R., & Weiner, W. J. (1990). Sleep disorders and sleep effect in Parkinson's disease. *Movement Disorders, 5,* 280-285.

Foley, D. J., Monjan, A. A., Brown, S. L., Simonsick, E. M., Wallace, R. B., & Blazer, D. G. (1995). Sleep complaints among elderly persons: An epidemiologic study of three communities. *Sleep, 18,* 425-432.

Ford, D. E., & Kamerow, D. B. (1989). Epidemiologic study of sleep disturbances and psychiatric disorders: An opportunity for prevention? *Journal of the American Medical Association, 262,* 1479-1484.

French, A. P., & Tupin, J. P. (1974). Therapeutic application of a simple relaxation method. *American Journal of Psychotherapy, 28,* 282-287.

Gallup Organization. (1995). *Sleep in America: 1995.* Princeton, NJ: Author.

Gottlieb, G. L. (1990). Sleep disorders and their management: Special considerations in the elderly. *American Journal of Medicine, 88*(Suppl. 3A), 29S-33S.

Guerrero, J., & Crocq, M. A. (1994). Sleep disorders in the elderly: Depression and post-traumatic stress disorder. *Journal of Psychosomatic Research, 38*(Suppl. 1), 141-150.

Hall, M., Buysse, D. J., Dew, M. A., Prigerson, H. G., Kupfer, D. J., & Reynolds, C. F., III. (1997). Intrusive thoughts and avoidance behaviors are associated with sleep disturbances in bereavement-related depression. *Depression and Anxiety, 6,* 106-112.

Haythornthwaite, J. A., Hegel, M. T., & Kerns, R. D. (1991). Development of a sleep diary for chronic pain patients. *Journal of Pain and Symptom Management, 6,* 65-72.

Hoch, C. C., Buysse, D. J., Monk, T. H., & Reynolds, C. F., III. (1992). Sleep disorders and aging. In J. E. Birren, R. B. Sloane, & G. D. Cohen (Eds.), *Handbook of mental health and aging* (2nd ed., pp. 557-581). San Diego, CA: Academic Press.

Hu, D. S., & Silberfarb, P. M. (1991). Management of sleep problems in cancer patients. *Oncology, 5*(9), 23-27.

Jacobs, E. A., Reynolds, C. F., III, Kupfer, D. J., Lovin, P. A., & Ehrenpreis, A. B. (1988). The role of polysomnography in the differential diagnosis of chronic insomnia. *American Journal of Psychiatry, 145,* 346-349.

Katz, D. A., & McHorney, C. A. (1998). Clinical correlates of insomnia in patients with chronic illness. *Archives of Internal Medicine, 158,* 1099-1107.

Kaye, J., Kaye, K., & Madow, L. (1983). Sleep patterns in patients with cancer and patients with cardiac disease. *Journal of Psychology, 114,* 107-113.

Kolko, D. J. (1984). Behavioral treatment of excessive daytime sleepiness in an elderly woman with multiple medical problems. *Journal of Behavior Therapy and Experimental Psychiatry, 15,* 341-345.

Kupfer, D. J., & Reynolds, C. F., III. (1992). Sleep and affective disorders. In E. S. Paykel (Ed.), *Handbook of affective disorders* (pp. 311-323). New York: Guilford.

Lichstein, K. L., & Riedel, B. W. (1994). Behavioral assessment and treatment of insomnia: A review with an emphasis on clinical application. *Behavior Therapy, 25,* 659-688.

Lichstein, K. L., Riedel, B. W., & Means, M. K. (1999). Psychological treatment of late-life insomnia. In R. Schulz, G. Maddox, & M. P. Lawton (Eds.), *Annual Review of Gerontology and Geriatrics: Vol. 18. Focus on interventions research with older adults* (pp. 74-110). New York: Springer.

Lichstein, K. L., Wilson, N. M., & Johnson, C. T. (in press). Psychological treatment of secondary insomnia. *Psychology and Aging.*

McCurry, S. M., Logsdon, R. G., & Teri, L. (1996). Behavioral treatment of sleep disturbance in elderly dementia caregivers. *Clinical Gerontologist, 17*(2), 35-50.

Mellinger, G. D., Balter, M. B., & Uhlenhuth, E. H. (1985). Insomnia and its treatment. *Archives of General Psychiatry, 42,* 225-232.

Mendelson, W. B. (1997). Experiences of a sleep disorders center: 1700 patients later. *Cleveland Clinic Journal of Medicine, 64,* 46-51.

Mendelson, W. B., & Jain, B. (1995). An assessment of short-acting hypnotics. *Drug Safety, 13,* 257-270.

Mitler, M. M., Poceta, S., Menn, S. J., & Erman, M. K. (1991). Insomnia in the chronically ill. In P. J. Hauri (Ed.), *Case studies in insomnia* (pp. 223-236). New York: Plenum.

Moldofsky, H. (1989). Sleep influences on regional and diffuse pain syndromes associated with osteoarthritis. *Seminars in Arthritis and Rheumatism, 18*(4, Suppl. 2), 18-21.

Monane, M. (1992). Insomnia in the elderly. *Journal of Clinical Psychiatry, 53*(Suppl.), 23-28.

Monjan, A., & Foley, D. (1996, June). *Incidence of chronic insomnia associated with medical and psychosocial factors: An epidemiological study among older persons.* Paper presented at the meeting of the Association of Professional Sleep Societies, Washington, DC.

Moran, M. G., & Stoudemire, A. (1992). Sleep disorders in the medically ill patient. *Journal of Clinical Psychiatry, 53*(Suppl.), 29-36.

Morin, C. M. (1993). *Insomnia: Psychological assessment and management.* New York: Guilford.

Morin, C. M., Culbert, J. P., & Schwartz, S. M. (1994). Nonpharmacological interventions for insomnia: A meta-analysis of treatment efficacy. *American Journal of Psychiatry, 151,* 1172-1180.

Morin, C. M., Gibson, D., & Wade, J. (1998). Self-reported sleep and mood disturbance in chronic pain patients. *The Clinical Journal of Pain, 14,* 311-314.

Morin, C. M., Kowatch, R. A., & O'Shanick, G. (1990). Sleep restriction for the inpatient treatment of insomnia. *Sleep, 13,* 183-186.

Morin, C. M., Kowatch, R. A., & Wade, J. B. (1989). Behavioral management of sleep disturbances secondary to chronic pain. *Journal of Behavior Therapy and Experimental Psychiatry, 20,* 295-302.

National Institutes of Health. (1991). The treatment of sleep disorders of older people, March 26-28, 1990. *Sleep, 14,* 169-177.

Nowell, P. D., Buysse, D. J., Reynolds, C. F., III, Hauri, P. J., Roth, T., Stepanski, E. J., Thorpy, M. J., Bixler, E., Kales, A., Manfredi, R. L., Vgontzas, A. N., Stapf, D. M., Houck, P. R., & Kupfer, D. J. (1997). Clinical factors contributing to the differential diagnosis of primary insomnia and insomnia related to mental disorders. *American Journal of Psychiatry, 154,* 1412-1416.

Ohayon, M. M. (1997). Prevalence of DSM-IV diagnostic criteria of insomnia: Distinguishing insomnia related to mental disorders from sleep disorders. *Journal of Psychiatric Research, 31,* 333-346.

Paiva, T., Batista, A., Martins, P., & Martins, A. (1995). The relationship between headaches and sleep disturbances. *Headache, 35,* 590-596.

Pilowsky, I., Crettenden, I., & Townley, M. (1985). Sleep disturbance in pain clinic patients. *Pain, 23,* 27-33.

Roehrs, T., Zorick, F., Sicklesteel, J., Wittig, R., & Roth, T. (1983). Age-related sleep-wake disorders at a sleep disorder center. *Journal of the American Geriatrics Society, 31,* 364-370.

Smith, M. C., Ellgring, H., & Oertel, W. H. (1997). Sleep disturbances in Parkinson's disease patients and spouses. *Journal of the American Geriatrics Society, 45,* 194-199.

Spierings, E.L.H., & van Hoof, M. J. (1997). Fatigue and sleep in chronic headache sufferers: An age- and sex-controlled questionnaire study. *Headache, 37,* 549-552.

Stam, H. J., & Bultz, B. D. (1986). The treatment of severe insomnia in a cancer patient. *Journal of Behavior Therapy and Experimental Psychiatry, 17,* 33-37.

Strang, P., & Qvarner, H. (1990). Cancer-related pain and its influence on quality of life. *Anticancer Research, 10,* 109-112.

Tan, T. L., Kales, J. D., Kales, A., Martin, E. D., Mann, L. D., & Soldatos, C. R. (1987). Inpatient multidimensional management of treatment-resistant insomnia. *Psychosomatics, 28,* 266-272.

Tan, T. L., Kales, J. D., Kales, A., Soldatos, C. R., & Bixler, E. O. (1984). Biopsychobehavioral correlates of insomnia, IV: Diagnosis based on DSM-III. *American Journal of Psychiatry, 141,* 357-362.

Varni, J. W. (1980). Behavioral treatment of disease-related chronic insomnia in a hemophiliac. *Journal of Behavior Therapy and Experimental Psychiatry, 11,* 143-145.

Walsh, J. K., & Sugerman, J. L. (1989). Disorder of initiating and maintaining sleep in adult psychiatric disorders. In M. H. Kryger, T. Roth, & W. C. Dement (Eds.), *Principles and practice of sleep medicine* (pp. 448-455). Philadelphia: Saunders.

Wiegand, M., Moller, A. A., Lauer, C. J., Stolz, S., Schreiber, W., Dose, M., & Krieg, J. C. (1991). Nocturnal sleep in Huntington's disease. *Journal of Neurology, 238*, 203-208.

Williams, R. L. (1988). Sleep disturbances in various medical and surgical conditions. In R. L. Williams, I. Karacan, & C. A. Moore (Eds.), *Sleep disorders: Diagnosis and treatment* (2nd ed., pp. 265-291). New York: Wiley.

Wittig, R. M., Zorick, F. J., Blumer, D., Heilbronn, M., & Roth, T. (1982). Disturbed sleep in patients complaining of chronic pain. *Journal of Nervous and Mental Disease, 170*, 429-431.

Wooten, V. (1989). Medical causes of insomnia. In M. H. Kryger, T. Roth, & W. C. Dement (Eds.), *Principles and practice of sleep medicine* (pp. 456-475). Philadelphia: Saunders.

World Health Organization. (1986). *Cancer pain relief.* Geneva: Author.

Zorick, F. J., Roth, T., Hartze, K. M., Piccione, P. M., & Stepanski, E. J. (1981). Evaluation and diagnosis of persistent insomnia. *American Journal of Psychiatry, 138*, 769-773.

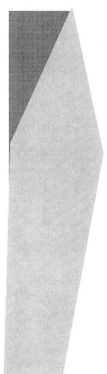

13

Insomnia in Dementia and in Residential Care

DONALD L. BLIWISE
MICHAEL J. BREUS

Institutional settings provide a unique challenge to psychologists and other health care professionals dealing with disturbed sleep. As the population continues to age, working with individuals residing in such environments is likely to assume increased importance. At present, 2.5 million individuals in the United States reside in nursing home or assisted living environments. With the number of persons over the age of 65 increasing from about 30 million to 70 million by the year 2030, these numbers will only grow. In this chapter, we will focus largely on the data derived from skilled nursing facilities because among those few studies that have examined sleep and wakefulness in institutionalized adults, most have been conducted in these settings. We should stress that even within the general category of skilled nursing care, however, the specifics of care in these environments vary widely. For example, some nursing homes offer environments specifically devoted to patients with dementia (i.e., Alzheimer's disease special

AUTHORS' NOTE: This research was supported by a grant from the National Institute of Aging (AG-10643).

care units), whereas others include patients with only medical disease and yet others may include both kinds of patients. It is thus important to note that although we will be discussing institutions as though they are uniform environments, this is a gross simplification. Put simply, there is no single nursing home environment.

Nursing homes are complex in a number of respects. First, the residents represent a wide variety of medical, neurologic, and psychological conditions, many of which, even when studied in the outpatient setting (i.e., independent living situation), have been shown to disrupt nocturnal sleep and cause daytime sleepiness. Second, the environments themselves are often unwieldy because of the social and architectural constraints that exist at every site. For example, the scheduling of staff on different shifts, varying staff-to-patient ratios, the level of training of various aides and personnel, and the physical adequacy of the facility itself may play major roles in affecting how the residents sleep. Finally, last, but certainly not least, the impact of economic reality, as brought to bear by the standards for care specified by Medicare/Medicaid guidelines for nursing home care, almost certainly have a direct bearing on the practices in a given nursing home, not only in terms of reduction of antipsychotic medication but also in terms of nighttime care. In this chapter we will discuss these issues and how they may affect how residents sleep. After describing what is known about person-related and environmental factors affecting sleep/wakefulness, we will discuss current pharmacologic and nonpharmacologic approaches that may be relevant to residents living in such settings.

A final point relevant for discussing disturbed sleep in institutional settings involves the notion of a "successful" outcome. Gauging improvement is a particularly complex issue for such individuals. Even more so than for individuals living independently, knowing what constitutes a desired outcome, particularly when the individuals in question are too mentally and cognitively impaired to report improvement or have electroencephalograms too abnormal to define conventional sleep stages, is challenging at one level and, ultimately, frustrating at another level. The psychologist and other health care professionals working with elderly residents in institutional settings may come to define improvement using criteria that may seem unconventional or even trivial to some, yet the biologic capacities of the aged, infirm human accompanied by social and economic constraints may leave no other options. In fact, a "success" might be defined, in some cases, by removal of a noxious stimulus (e.g., reduction of high-dose neuroleptic medication, fewer nocturnal bed checks) rather than increases in sleep efficiency or total sleep time.

Person-Related Factors

Numerous person-related factors affect the sleep of the older individual living in an institutional environment. Many of these are similar to factors that affect sleep for the older individual living independently. Thus, for example, increased sleep fragmentation, decreased slow-wave sleep, and susceptibility to external arousal affect the sleep of ambulatory older persons and certainly would be expected to affect sleep in long-term care as well (see Chapter 1, this volume, for a review of these effects). The prevalence of specific sleep disorders such as sleep apnea has been shown to be particularly high in nursing home patients (Ancoli-Israel, Klauber, Kripke, Parker, & Cobarrubies, 1989), although specific sleep-wake symptoms may not always accompany sleep-disordered breathing. This problem is particularly salient for periodic leg movements during sleep, which may have an even higher prevalence than sleep-disordered breathing (Bliwise, in press-b) but may have fewer symptomatic correlates. To the extent that older individuals in long-term care are no longer able to self-care because of infirmity, one would expect the impact and severity of all diseases to be greater in such patients relative to individuals living outside such institutions. Such conditions can be broadly categorized as involving medical disease, neurologic conditions, and psychological/behavioral factors.

Among *medical* diseases, congestive heart failure is a particularly disruptive condition for sleep. Sleep is often severely fragmented by rhythmic oscillations in breathing (referred to as Cheyne-Stokes respiration), and such patients typically have highly disturbed sleep consisting of frequent alternations among wakefulness and Stage 1 and Stage 2 sleep. Patients with chronic obstructive pulmonary disease (COPD), a condition characterized by reduced lung volumes, retention of carbon dioxide, and dyspnea upon exertion, also have highly fragmented sleep and may show marked oxygen desaturation in REM sleep. Curiously, COPD patients may not be overtly sleepy during the daytime (Orr,

Shamma-Othman, Levin, Othman, & Rundell, 1990). Conversely, end stage renal disease patients are often markedly hypersomnolent (Parker, Bliwise, & Rye, in press), particularly if dialysis occurs early in the morning or late in the afternoon. Renal patients may also have higher rates of sleep apnea and restless legs syndrome. Perhaps the most common medical cause of sleep disturbance in older individuals living in institutions is chronic pain. Pain not only fragments sleep and changes conventional sleep architecture but also often is associated with a specific polysomnographic feature referred to as "alpha-delta sleep," in which alpha waves, typically characteristic of wakefulness, are present throughout nREM sleep. Rheumatoid arthritis patients, for example, have both alpha-delta sleep as well as excessively large numbers of periodic leg movements.

Perhaps the most widely recognized *neurologic* condition afflicting nursing home patients and affecting their sleep is dementia. Dementia is a global description that refers to a wide array of neurodegenerative and cerebrovascular conditions in which the primary symptom is cognitive deterioration and insidious loss of mental faculties. Typical diagnoses of dementia include Alzheimer's disease (probably the most common, in about 70% of dementia cases) as well as conditions such as vascular (multi-infarct) dementia, Parkinson's disease, Shy-Drager syndrome, progressive supranuclear palsy, frontal lobe dementia, Lewy body dementia, and a host of other less common, but no less devastating, progressive neurologic conditions. Important differences in sleep patterns among these various conditions exist and are reviewed elsewhere (Bliwise, 1994a, in press-a) and have implications for understanding mechanisms involved in the control of sleep and circadian rhythms. Other than for diseases primarily involving the motor system, however, such as Parkinson's disease, the issues insofar as treatment of the underlying sleep disturbance may not be all that different. Certain basic principles (e.g., exposure to relevant zeitgebers such as light and physical activity) may still operate within the context of a deteriorating central nervous system and are worthy of consideration (see the section on intervention, below). It is worth noting, however, that a small proportion of dementias in the elderly are reversible (Bliwise, 1996; Clarfield, 1988). Although a thorough differential diagnosis is beyond the ken of a psychologist and most other health care professionals working in a nursing home and it is unlikely that a reversible dementia would be unrecognized for such an extended time so as to result in unjustified institutionalization, cognizance of such factors is important.

Given the large number of diseases that are likely to affect the sleep/wake cycle in the institutionalized elderly, it is easy to disregard *psychological* factors that may be relevant. Many older persons who undergo a change in living situation from a private dwelling to an institutional setting may have considerable psychological difficulty with such a relocation. Whether such a change is merely an adjustment reaction or represents development of a diagnosable affective disorder is an important distinction that may hold implications for treatment. Although some aged patients in long-term care may develop a primary psychiatric diagnosis for the first time in their lives, it is far more likely that depression in such individuals may represent any number of late-life personal losses of family and friends. Some data have suggested that such bereavement results in polysomnographic changes (lower sleep efficiency, altered sleep architecture, decreased sleep continuity) that may be virtually indistinguishable from those alterations seen in primary affective disorder in the absence of such conditions (Reynolds et al., 1992). Epidemiologic data suggest the importance of active treatment of such adjustment reactions in the elderly so as to prevent the development of primary affective disorder. Late-life emergence of posttraumatic stress disorder has also been described, with ruminations, at least in the group described, involving Holocaust trauma (Rosen, Reynolds, Yeager, Houck, & Hurwitz, 1991). This may be prototypical for the manifestation of war-related trauma in late life for other historical periods as well. Finally, the emergence of full-fledged dream enactment behavior, also referred to as REM behavior disorder (Schenck, Bundlie, Ettinger, & Mahowald, 1986), may also be suggestive of long-term psychological distress particular to any specific patient's history. Although in some sense "psychiatric" in nature, converging evidence suggests that such nocturnal behavior may be more reflective of functional disinhibition of striatal dopaminergic centers controlling brainstem systems responsible for REM atonia than of purely psychological issues (Rye & Bliwise, 1997; Schenck, Bundlie, & Mahowald, 1996).

All these conditions may affect sleep, but in many cases their associated treatments also disturb sleep. Polypharmacy is associated with a wide variety of adverse reactions in the aged (Stewart & Hale, 1992). One study reported that the average nursing home patient received a total of

8.1 medications (Gurwitz, Soumerai, & Avorn, 1990). Morgan, Dallosso, Ebrahim, Arie, & Fentem (1988) have shown that the number of medications an elderly person receives (not necessarily psychoactive medication) was correlated with the overall quality of that person's sleep. Although this observation was made in community-residing elderly, there is a high likelihood that such a result would occur in institutionalized elderly as well, given the higher number of medications used in a more infirm population. Typical medications seeing common use in geriatric patients, such as beta-blockers, diuretics, respiratory stimulants, and nonsteroidal anti-inflammatories, have all been shown to disrupt sleep (Murphy, Badia, Myers, Boecker, & Wright, 1994; Rosen & Kostis, 1985). In some cases these are direct effects on sleep architecture (e.g., lipophilic beta-blockers), whereas in other cases the effects are indirect (nocturia induced by diuretics). Even psychoactive medications can disrupt sleep. Based on his review, Morgan (1987) reported that as many as 50% of elderly in institutions received psychoactive medications. Although this may have changed in the United States in recent years owing to the new practice guidelines (see the section on interventions, below), undoubtedly there are examples of such medications causing as many problems as they are intended to treat. Little, Satlin, Sunderland, and Volicer (1995), for example, have presented some evidence that use of psychoactive medications may be associated with "sundowning" phenomena in dementia. Additionally, although now seeing widespread use within nursing homes because of their safety and relative success, selective serotonin reuptake inhibitors (e.g., sertraline, paroxetine, fluoxetine) are associated with high rates of treatment emergent insomnia with incidence rates as high as 20% (*Physicians' Desk Reference*, 1999). Use of such medications is often counterbalanced in practice by simultaneous administration of more sedating antidepressant medication, thus compounding the problem of polypharmacy.

Environmental Factors

Few studies have specifically examined the effects of institutionalization per se on the sleep of elderly individuals residing within such facilities. Ideally, individuals' 24-hour sleep/wake cycle would be well characterized for some time prior to institutionalization and then, subsequent to adaptation to the new environment (e.g., 3 to 4 weeks), sleep could be re-evaluated to determine what changes might have occurred in 24-hour sleep/wake function. No such studies currently exist. Because decisions to enter institutions typically are made under duress following a precipitating medical (e.g., stroke, hip fracture) or psychosocial (e.g., death of a spouse) event, such prospective studies are unlikely to occur. Instead, some knowledge of the effects of institutionalization on sleep can be inferred from other types of data, including (a) studies of young adults that have experimentally manipulated variables relevant to the long-term care environment such as physical activity and bed rest, (b) retrospective data from elderly persons who are capable of verbally describing changes in their sleep subsequent to institutionalization, and (c) careful descriptive studies that examine the variability of sleep across different institutional settings, thereby allowing some appreciation of how varying environmental characteristics and routines may affect sleep. We will review research in each of these areas below.

The sheer act of spending excessive time in bed is disruptive to the sleep/wake cycle. In an early study sponsored by the National Aeronautics and Space Administration, Winget et al. (1972) noted that a period of prolonged bed rest (56 days) resulted in a less robust body temperature cycle, which would be expected to undermine the integrity of the sleep/wake cycle. About a decade later, Campbell (1984) found that young adults who were forced to spend 60 consecutive hours in bed displayed considerable sleep fragmentation as assessed polysomnographically. In an early study of exercise deprivation, Baekeland (1970) noted that if healthy young adults who customarily exercised were asked to refrain from exercising on a given day, their sleep the subsequent night was characterized by greater levels of nocturnal wakefulness and decreased Stage 4 sleep. More recently Edgar and Dement (1991) showed that, in rodents, the mere locking of a running wheel can lead to disruption of the sleep/wake cycle. Taken together, these results suggest that the prolonged bed rest and generalized inactivity experienced by many institutionalized elderly individuals probably contributes substantially to the poor-quality sleep that they experience. Surprisingly, the role of physical activity interventions for such individuals has seldom been studied systematically (see the section on interventions, below).

Although several studies relying upon self-report (Cohen et al., 1983; Gentili, Weiner, Kuchibhatla, & Edinger, 1997), actigraphic (Ancoli-Israel et al., 1991; Ancoli-Israel, Parker, Sinaee, Fell, & Kripke, 1989;

Jacobs, Ancoli-Israel, Parker, & Kripke, 1989), and behavioral observations (Bliwise, Bevier, Bliwise, Edgar, & Dement, 1990; Bliwise, Carroll, & Dement, 1990) of nursing home patients have been reported, few of these studies have made any attempt to retrospectively determine how residents slept *before* entering the facility. Even if these studies had reported such findings, much of such data, of course, would have to be considered unreliable because of the confusion and presumed dementia of many of the residents, apart from the obvious issue of recall bias, which would be expected to affect even cognitively normal individuals. Nevertheless, one study did report some such data in institutionalized, (presumably) non–grossly demented patients after at least 2 months in long-term care. Clapin-French (1986) reported that increased napping during the day, earlier nocturnal bedtimes and more difficulty falling asleep, and more frequent awakenings during the night were all more commonly reported by these elderly subjects after moving to a nursing home environment.

In a more recent study comparing institutionalized patients (mean duration in facility about 3 years) and noninstitutionalized elderly controls, Middelkoop, Kerkhof, Smilde-van den Doel, Ligthart, and Kamphuisen (1994) reported that elderly individuals living independently had significantly later bedtimes and wake-up times and fewer daytime naps than individuals residing in a nursing home setting or a "service home," which appeared to be roughly equivalent to an intermediate-level care facility. The total time spent in bed per 24 hours was also significantly greater in the two institutionalized populations, with the nursing home group spending, on average, 12.5 per 24 hours in bed. Of interest was that for all three groups, nocturia was the most common cause of nighttime awakenings. Although there were no age differences across groups, the overall level of infirmity (as indexed by the number of medications prescribed) showed a predictable relationship with level of incapacity. Perhaps most surprising in this study was that, in a small subanalysis comparing independently living individuals and individuals residing in the service home (who had significantly more sleep complaints), polysomnographic measures showed no significant differences in any measures. The meaning of the latter result remains uncertain; however, given the other evidence of environmental effects on sleep discussed below, this lack of differences may reflect either the small sample size or the fact that only those individuals not receiving any sedative/hypnotic medication were selected for participation in the polysomnographic portion of the study. In one of the few other studies that attempted to examine the effects of institutionalization (in a nongeriatric population), Espie and Tweedie (1991) examined sleep in mentally handicapped individuals by examining an institutionalized population and a community-dwelling population with a similar diagnosis. The latter was somewhat younger than the former (mean ages 41.6 vs. 31.1), and although a few statistically significant differences emerged (more frequent awakenings and longer sleep latencies in the community-residing residents), these results may have been more likely to reflect the age differences in the samples.

A final source of inference regarding the effects of institutionalization per se are studies that have compared elderly persons residing in different types of institutional environments. In one recent study of 230 residents residing across eight different nursing homes studied specifically because of incontinence, Schnelle et al. (1998) reported substantial differences across sites for critical variables such as time in bed during the day, total time observed asleep, and the amount of sleep observed out of bed. By way of example, in some facilities residents were observed to spend as little as 19% of the daytime hours in bed (i.e., the percentage of daytime observations in which the resident was in bed), whereas in other facilities this figure was 51%. The mean across sites was 35.8%. Conversely, the percentage of observations where sleep was observed in bed varied from about 10% to 26%. Curiously, on a site-by-site basis, the correlation between the percentage of time spent in bed and the amount of daytime sleep appeared unrelated, though this study cannot be considered definitive because the observations were intermittent rather than continuous and the data were presented only at a site-by-site level rather than at the level of the individual nursing home resident. Despite these interpretative limitations, this study is important in demonstrating that environmental factors play a large role in opportunities for daytime sleep, a factor that may be critically important in understanding sleep disturbance in the institutional environment.

Another recent paper, by Sloane et al. (1998), also serves to highlight differences across nursing homes. In this study, part of the efforts of the National Institute on Aging initiative to investigate Alzheimer's disease special care units, a total of 53 different institutions across four different states were examined in an attempt to determine environmental correlates of agitation across sites. Residents were observed using an identi-

cal, reliable rating scale at four different times of day. Perhaps most striking in these results were the huge differences across sites, with a range of
0% to 40% (median = 8%) of patients demonstrating agitation. Factors related to lower rates of observed agitation included staff involvement in
activities, low use of physical restraint use, fewer comorbid diseases,
lower levels of functional dependence, and "better" physical environments, including factors such as cleanliness of bathrooms and halls,
presence of a public kitchen, non-glare floors, and better activity room
lighting. A final factor, consisting of the routine practice of putting patients to bed for afternoon naps, was also shown to be predictive of *lower*
levels of agitation. These and other factors will be discussed more completely in the following section on interventions.

  In summary, there is considerable evidence that the nursing home environment itself exerts a major influence on the sleep of the elderly in
long-term care. The parameters of describing and quantifying the relevant environmental characteristics have only just begun to be understood and appreciated. Additionally, to what extent such factors interact
with the aforementioned patient-derived factors (i.e., a person × environment interaction) is unknown and unexplored in any study to date.
Undoubtedly individuals with particular types of diseases or disabilities
may be differentially affected by different components of nursing home
life insofar as their sleep is concerned. Novel attempts to try to model
such interactions in the nursing home have been attempted in the realm
of interpersonal behavior (Baltes, Kindermann, Reisenzein, & Schmid,
1987) but never for sleep.

Interventions

When discussing interventions in an institutionalized population, it is
important again to recall the heterogeneity of the populations and environments under consideration. For elderly persons residing in interme-
diate-care nursing facilities who remain largely independent in maintenance of activities of daily living, interventions to improve sleep will
resemble those described elsewhere in this volume (see Chapters 5-10).
In this section of our chapter, we will focus on issues that are more likely
to be relevant for aged individuals with greater levels of incapacity and
more significant medical and neurologic disease who reside in skilled

care nursing facilities and demonstrate more profound disturbance of sleep.

Many institutionalized elderly persons demonstrate agitated behavior during the nocturnal hours. Such behavior is often subsumed under the rubric of "sundowning" and has been the subject of numerous studies (Bliwise, 1994b; Bliwise, Carroll, Lee, Nekich, & Dement, 1993; Evans, 1987; Exum, Phelps, Nabers, & Osborne, 1993; Gallagher-Thompson, Brooks, Bliwise, Leader, & Yesavage, 1992). Some data suggest that the peak occurrence of such behavior may occur in the hours between 4 and 8 p.m. (Bliwise, 1994b), though the temporal delineation of the syndrome may be more difficult to ascertain, because many of these studies did not use 24-hour observations and instead relied on a window of daytime observations that ended at 8 or 9 p.m. In common parlance, usage of the term *sundowning* is not nearly so temporally specific and may refer to any increase in the frequency or intensity of agitated behaviors that occurs during the evening or nocturnal hours. Successful interventions for such behavioral disruption hold dramatic implications not only within but also outside the institutional environment. Several studies have reported that sleep disturbance represents a unique and independent risk factor predicting institutionalization (Pollak & Perlick, 1991; Pollak, Perlick, Linsner, Wenston, & Hsieh, 1990), and measures of caregiver stress are often correlated with such sleep disturbance (Gallagher-Thompson et al., 1992; Pollak, Stokes, & Wagner, 1997). Our focus in this section will be on interventions in the nursing home setting. Obviously, to the extent that it may be possible to implement such approaches, it may be possible to forestall eventual institutionalization, if indeed that is the desire of family and caregivers.

Pharmacologic Interventions

Polypharmacy in the nursing home environment is legion. The implications of such heavy use of often-overlapping medications and the emergence of toxic and delirious states related to such medication use are profound. For example, the risk of falling in the nursing home increases substantially as the number of medications increases (Granek et al., 1987). Additionally, several studies have suggested that residents' use of medication for sleep is only weakly associated with the quality of sleep (Monane, Glynn, & Avorn, 1996; Seppala, Rajala, & Sourander,

1993), and in an acute care hospital, use of sleep medication in selected elderly patients was associated with higher health care costs in those patients (Yuen, Zisselman, Louis, & Rovner, 1997).

As mentioned in the introduction to this chapter, usage of medications, particularly antipsychotic medications, in the typical long-term care environment in the United States has changed substantially over the last 10 years, following the Medicare guidelines adopted by Health Care Financing Administration (HCFA) rules, following passage of the 1987 Omnibus Budget and Reconciliation Act (OBRA-87). These guidelines stipulated that any such pharmacologic intervention be documented sufficiently so that the behavior(s) in question were documented to impair the resident's functional capacity, endanger the resident or others, or interfere with the staff's ability to provide care. Moreover, before instituting treatment with antipsychotic medication, a trial of nonpharmacologic management was required to be documented and, if such medication was employed, gradual dose reductions after 6 months of treatment were required. Shorr, Fought, and Ray (1994) have presented compelling data to suggest a decline in antipsychotic drug use in 172 Tennessee nursing homes in the 30-month period during the implementation of the OBRA-87 guidelines. Utilization of other psychoactive medications did not show parallel declines over the same period, suggesting that the specificity of the guidelines was not part of a more general trend for fewer prescriptions. Particularly relevant from the perspective of sleep disturbance, however, was the observation that third shift (nighttime) staffing was associated strongly with the extent of reduction of antipsychotic use. Specifically, nursing facilities that had the greatest number of night shift staff were better able to implement the OBRA guidelines. Short-staffed facilities showed far less of a reduction in such medication. These data imply that staffing is critical when considering how such medications are dispensed. The data also imply (but do not prove) that antipsychotic medication reduction probably can occur without untoward effects insofar as patient care is concerned. Although this latter point has been questioned because no behavioral data on residents were collected (Venable, 1994), the Shorr et al. (1994) study stands as a sobering reminder that antipsychotics probably have been overused in the past. Also of interest in this regard was a study by Gilbert, Innes, Owen, and Sansom (1993), who conducted a randomized clinical trial reducing usage of benzodiazepines in a nursing home environment without adverse effects on sleep. In a related observational, rather than interventional, study, Exum et al. (1993) noted that usage of all PRN psychoactive medications in the institutional environment peaked in the hours immediately prior to nursing staff shift changes. It is not hard to imagine busy and harried nurses "loading up" patients with psychoactive medication before leaving their shift for a variety of reasons related to institutional context and work environment rather than patient-related factors.

Taken together, these studies certainly raise the possibility that much usage of psychotropics in the nursing home is unnecessary. In fact, it is refreshing for psychologists and other health care professionals who employ behavioral interventions working in the setting of the nursing home that documented trials of nonpharmacologic interventions actually are required by law. Nevertheless, although the net outcome of the post-OBRA environment has been a dramatic decrease in the use of antipsychotic medications in nursing homes, clinical exigencies continue to occur that necessitate the use of such medications. The remainder of this section will highlight the spectrum of medications typically used for this purpose.

Elsewhere we have reviewed the diverse pharmacologic classes of medications that have been employed in the treatment of nocturnal agitation, including carbazepine, valproate, trazodone, lithium, L-deprenyl, pindolol, and propranolol (Bliwise, in press-a; McGaffigan & Bliwise, 1997). Benzodiazepines such as triazolam have not been shown to help dementia patients sleep (McCarten, Kovera, Maddox, & Cleary, 1995), though one report, which included about 60 demented patients, showed that a relatively high dose of zolpidem (20 mg), a site-specific benzodiazepine receptor agonist, improved sleep, as assessed with nurses' ratings (Shaw, Curson, & Coquelin, 1992). Adverse reactions at far more moderate dosages of zolpidem (10 mg) have been reported in younger patients, however, arguing for judicious use of this medication in dementia (Ansseau, Pitchot, Hansenne, & Moreno, 1992).

Traditionally, older antipsychotics such as haloperidol (0.5-1.0 mg) and thioridazine (25 mg) have been shown to improve sleep and reduce nocturnal agitation in dementia patients (McGaffigan & Bliwise, 1997), but both have adverse side effects. Currently, a newer generation of antipsychotic medications, including clozapine (typical initial dosage 12.5-25 mg), risperidone (typical initial dosage 2-4 mg), olanzapine (typical initial dosage 5-10 mg), and quetiapine (typical initial dosage 25-50 mg) are currently favored. Side effect profiles with these medications generally are more favorable than for the older generation of antipsychotics, though usage of clozapine requires frequent laboratory work to monitor white blood cell counts. The mechanisms of action of each of these medications differ; most are multiple receptor site antagonists, operating on dopaminergic, serotoninergic, and histaminergic neurotransmission (Bliwise, in press-a). In patients with advanced stage Parkinson's disease, whose nocturnal agitation may arise from awakenings from REM sleep (i.e., REM dyscontrol) and/or extensive use of levodopa (i.e., dopamimetic psychosis), medications with specific dopamine antagonist properties (clozaril, risperidone) are usually favored (Bliwise, in press-a; Rye & Bliwise, 1997).

Melatonin represents another possible avenue of treatment for nocturnal sleep disturbance and agitation in the demented, institutionalized patient; however, its potential role as a cardiac vasoconstrictor suggests extreme care in its use with frail elderly persons with possible cardiovascular or cerebrovascular disease. Several studies have suggested utility for melatonin at dosages of 2 mg in (apparently) nondemented individuals (Garfinkel, Laudon, Nof, & Zisapel, 1995; Haimov et al., 1995). These studies relied on actigraphy to assess outcome, and the lack of specificity regarding the nature of the aged populations under investigation leaves some doubt as to the value of the data. Singer et al. (1998) have presented preliminary data from a study examining the effects of melatonin in well-characterized, noninstitutionalized Alzheimer's disease patients that suggested only minimal effects at relatively high dosages (10 mg) and no effect at lower dosages. Finally, Hughes, Sack, and Lewy (1998) reported a double-blind, placebo-controlled, crossover polysomnographic study of melatonin in nondemented elderly insomniacs living independently that showed few effects on sleep. Although the scientific literature on the clinical utility of melatonin thus is expanding rapidly at this point, there is little conclusive evidence to support melatonin's widespread use in dementia at this time.

Nonpharmacologic Interventions

Nonpharmacologic interventions for disturbed sleep and nocturnal agitation in elderly persons in residential situations should always be considered as an alternative to pharmacologic treatment or as an adjunct to such treatment. Possible interventions include (a) exercise and physical activity, (b) light therapy, and (c) sleep hygiene, sleep restriction, and other adjustments to the sleep/wake cycle.

Lack of physical activity can be hypothesized as an important factor explaining much of the poor sleep of the infirm, institutionalized elderly. Unfortunately, there are no conclusive intervention studies in this area because of a number of methodologic difficulties. Although the studies of King, Oman, Brassington, Bliwise, and Haskell (1997) and Singh, Clements, and Fiatarone (1997) have shown that ambulatory, community-residing elderly individuals may report better sleep following aerobic or strength training, respectively, these results do not necessarily generalize to institutionalized populations. Vitiello, Prinz, and Schwartz (1994) also have examined the effects of aerobic activity on sleep with polysomnographic measurements and have shown increases in Stages 3 and 4 sleep with such exercise in an elderly, noninsomniac, ambulatory population. In the only study that appeared to apply such principles to a nursing home population, Alessi et al. (1995) examined the effects of an exercise routine involving sit-to-stand repetitions of wheelchair propulsions performed every 2 hours during the daytime, 5 days a week, for 9 weeks to a more conservative program of similar activity once a day, 3 times a week, for 9 weeks. Subjects included incontinent and physically restrained nursing home residents, and sleep was measured actigraphically. Results were equivocal. Neither intervention appeared to affect the poor sleep of these individuals. These results may have reflected the nature of the outcome measures (actigraphy) or the very modest intensity of the physical activity intervention used in these frail subjects. To what extent more intense physical activity could be employed in such a population to improve sleep remains uncertain. The mechanisms underlying the effects of exercise also remain unclear. Some have suggested that thermal stress may be the critical variable, and at least one study has reported improved sleep with passive body heating in elderly, independently living older women (Dorsey et al., 1996).

A role for light in the treatment of the insomnia of elderly persons was amply demonstrated in a well-controlled study by Campbell, Dawson, and Anderson (1993), who reported that in otherwise healthy, aged, ambulatory volunteers, early evening light exposure shifted the circadian rhythm of body temperature as well as improving polysomnographically defined measures of sleep quality, such as sleep efficiency.

There are a number of reasons to suspect that sleep in the institutional environment might be helped by increased illumination. First, several reports have documented the typically low levels of light exposure (often less than 300 lux) experienced by nursing home patients (Ancoli-Israel et al., 1991; Bliwise et al., 1993). Additionally, age-dependent visual impairments and optic neuropathy, common in aging and in neurodegenerative diseases such as Alzheimer's disease, may result in greatly reduced exogenous stimulation for the retinohypothalamic tract. The possible role of bright light in the treatment of sleep disturbance in dementia has been examined in several small-scale studies (Castor, Woods, Pigott, & Hemmes, 1991; Lovell, Ancoli-Israel, & Gevirtz, 1995; Meltzer-Brody, Mouton, Ge, Sanchez, & Zee, 1994; Mishima et al., 1994; Okawa et al., 1991; Satlin, Volicer, Ross, Herz, & Campbell, 1992). Although varying widely in the quality and type of outcomes assessed, these studies suggest some value of enhanced illumination, though the timing and duration of light exposure varied across studies and few included an adequate control intervention.

The foregoing studies of light all targeted their interventions at an individual, rather than a group, level, which would offer the greatest face validity as a pragmatic, group-based intervention. An important exception to this is the landmark study by the New York State Department of Health (1994), which established "light rooms" in two special care units for Alzheimer's disease patients in a New York City nursing home. Each room contained high-luminescence fixtures delivering 2,500 to 2,700 lux and parabolic reflectors to ensure even dispersion of light around the room. The intervention occurred between 2 p.m. and 4 p.m. over a period of 2 weeks. In this crossover design, a control group received "natural" light exposure of 400-500 lux during the same time period and then, after washout, both treatments were reversed. Outcomes consisted of nurses' ratings of affect, behavioral disruption, and sleep. (Attempts to use actigraphic measurements in this population were unsuccessful.) Results of the study showed few statistically significant treatment effects using strict, parametric MANOVA models with individual scales and instead noted considerable variability in ratings of agitation and other behavioral indicators over the 6 weeks of observation. Although employing 40 residents in the design, the authors felt that statistical power was insufficient to adequately appreciate predictors of individual response. Preliminary nonparametric analyses that were reported, however, suggested that among moderately to severely demented nursing home residents (mean Mattis Dementia Rating Scale [MDRS] = 61, mean Mini-Mental State Exam [MMSE] = 9), 11 of 20 showed improvement (shifts of greater than 0.5 standard deviations) on a cumulative index of at least two of five behavior rating scales after the light treatment. By contrast, among severely impaired nursing home residents (mean MDRS = 14, mean MMSE = 5), marked improvement was seen in only 2 of 24 residents. These results, although technically representing small effect sizes, continue to present some optimism regarding use of light treatment. As a final note to the issue of enhanced illumination, however, even if the positive effects of light therapy in the nursing home environment noted in this study could be replicated by others, the mechanistic basis for such effects (light serving as a zeitgeber to strengthen circadian rhythms vs. merely acting as a novel stimulus to prevent daytime napping) would continue to remain unclear. Nevertheless, the possibility of improving sleep for the millions of individuals residing in institutions by such a minimally invasive intervention appears promising.

The role of sleep hygiene in the treatment of insomnia in aged persons has been dealt with extensively elsewhere in this volume (Chapters 5-9). Although many of these principles may be relevant for the infirm, cognitively impaired elderly population in residential care, numerous issues arise in the latter population that make implementation of sleep hygiene far more difficult to achieve in this context. Additionally, some very recent data may even challenge the prevailing notions of conventional sleep restriction in the nursing home environment.

For the aged individual residing independently, initiating sleep hygiene may require some attention and effort but, at least in principle, maladaptive behavior is amenable to change. By contrast, elderly residents residing in long-term care environments often have little choice over matters that are critical factors in sleep hygiene. For example, the institutional environment typically offers residents little control as to when they are "put" to bed. Similarly, for those individuals who are wheelchair bound, transit within the facility (e.g., for physical or occupational therapy) may be impossible without staff assistance. Additionally, residents may be given caffeine with their supper and not only may be allowed to nap during the daytime but actually may be encouraged to do so, as this allows staff more time for charting and other duties. One study reported that individuals in the nursing home who napped during the

daytime hours were more likely to be those individuals awake the following night; similarly, those awake at night tended to be those asleep
the following day (Bliwise, Bevier, et al., 1990). Obviously, this establishes a vicious cycle in which such behaviors may be perpetuated. In
one of the few studies to attempt to affect institutional policy on this
problem, Edinger, Lipper, and Wheeler (1989) reported that, in an un-
blinded study performed on three sub-acute VA inpatient wards (average length of stay 30-40 days), elimination of daytime napping resulted
in increased sleep times, as derived from nursing observations. Whether
this finding might be replicable in the nursing home environment is unknown.

   Although prevention of daytime sleep would thus appear to be well
established as a guiding principle to improve nocturnal sleep, at least
one recent article inadvertently has raised a somewhat contrasting perspective. Sloane et al. (1998) reported a study of agitation performed in
53 Alzheimer's disease special care units. From among 40 different variables predicting differences in site-specific agitation rates, only a few
variables predicted agitation. These included somewhat expected variables such as lower numbers of comorbid diseases, lower rates of use of
physical restraints, and better physical environment ratings. Lower rates
of agitation also were detected, however, among facilities that routinely
placed residents in bed during the afternoon hours. Although this study
was correlational and the increased use of daytime bed rest might not
represent a consequence of lower agitated behavior rather than its cause,
the results are quite provocative. They also fit with a prevailing notion
among nursing home researchers that agitation is increased by fatigue
and that sleep ameliorates such fatigue (Cohen-Mansfield, Werner, &
Freedman, 1995). From a related perspective but in a much smaller intervention study, Creighton (1995) noted that "putting to bed" geriatric patients during the afternoon resulted in better cognitive performance and
increased sleepiness subsequent to the nap, perhaps suggesting a potential role for such midday sleep in decreasing agitation.

   In recent years the salience of not only daytime but also nighttime
sleep hygiene issues has been highlighted, most notably from the perspective of the standard of practice for the nocturnal care of bedridden
and/or incontinent patients. Development of pressure sores, which are
hastened by moisture, is a major cause of mortality in the nursing home
(Allman, 1989; Berlowitz & Wilking, 1990) and can be prevented by fre-

quent repositioning of patients while in bed. Because of this, conventional clinical practice guidelines endorsed by the United States Department of Health and Human Services for patients in nursing homes stipulate that such individuals be checked for wetness and immobility and, if necessary, have bedclothes changed and be repositioned every 2 hours during the night. Because of these guidelines and the economic reality entailed by potential loss of Medicare/Medicaid reimbursement, most nursing facilities have policies ensuring that such sleep disruption occurs on a routine, nightly basis. In fact, such interruptions are seen as part and parcel of high-quality nursing care.

Obviously, from the perspective of sleep hygiene, such practices leave much to be desired. Only recently, however, have researchers become interested in examining such issues systematically. The results to date may hold profound implications for future care of nursing home patients, specifically insofar as sleep is concerned. For example, nearly 66% of incontinent, bedridden patients demonstrated spontaneous mobility during the night, both at shoulder and hip, at rates in excess of one turn per hour (Schnelle, Ouslander, Simmons, Alessi, & Gravel, 1993b), thus possibly obviating the need for forced awakenings. In another study employing actigraphy, nearly half of all awakenings of nursing home patients could be attributed to forced nursing interruptions, sudden noise, or changes in room lighting (Cruise, Schnelle, Alessi, Simmons, & Ouslander, 1998). For example, nursing staff entering a patient's room for a wetness check or repositioning would typically speak and turn on overhead lights as well, thereby disrupting the sleep not only of the individual being checked but also that of any other room residents. Residents seldom appeared to sleep "through" such staff contact; 87% of all incontinence care practices were associated with episodes of waking at least 2 minutes in length (Schnelle, Ouslander, Simmons, Alessi, & Gravel, 1993a). They also had considerable difficulty returning to sleep; the mean length of awakening was 21 minutes (standard deviation = 38 minutes) (Schnelle et al., 1993a). Several other studies have also noted that episodes of agitation appeared more likely after staff interruptions during the night (Bliwise et al., 1993; Cohen-Mansfield, 1990). The impact of data such as these for care in the nursing home environment remains to be seen; however, it seems clear that to the extent that externally induced nocturnal sleep disturbance is considered to represent the sine qua non of optimal nursing care, attempts to modify staff behavior may be formidable and have legal and economic consequences. Perhaps, eventually, the relative importance of disrupted sleep and its impact on mortality, morbidity, and quality of life will be tested against other, better-established factors known to affect the welfare of the infirm, aged, institutionalized person.

Closing Comments

As mentioned in the introduction to our chapter, improving the sleep of aged individuals residing in long-term care environments may be exceptionally challenging. The psychologist or other health care professional working in this environment may be forced to deal with administrative issues involving staffing more customarily encountered in the province of organizational psychology, issues in medication usage more conventionally in the domain of geriatric medicine, and issues of lighting and sound abatement more typically falling in the fields of architecture and environmental engineering. As we have tried to stress, however, the need to gather more scientifically valid data about how residents of such facilities sleep and what can be done to improve their sleep and quality of life remains largely unexplored. Given the aging of the population and the fact that many of us will spend our final years living (and sleeping) in institutional environments, such effects would appear worthy of future study.

References

Alessi, C. A., Schnelle, J. F., MacRae, P. G., Ouslander, J. G., Al-Samarrai, N., Simmons, S. F., & Traub, S. (1995). Does physical activity improve sleep in impaired nursing home residents? *Journal of the American Geriatrics Society, 43*, 1098-1102.

Allman, R. M. (1989). Pressure ulcers among the elderly. *New England Journal of Medicine, 320*, 850-853.

Ancoli-Israel, S., Jones, D. W., Hanger, M. A., Parker, L., Klauber, M. R., & Kripke, D. F. (1991). Sleep in the nursing home. In S. Kuna, P. Suratt, & J. Remmers (Eds.), *Sleep and respiration in aging adults* (pp. 77-84). Amsterdam: Elsevier.

Ancoli-Israel, S., Klauber, M. R., Kripke, D. F., Parker, L., & Cobarrubies, M. (1989). Sleep apnea in female nursing home patients: Increased risk of mortality. *Chest, 96*, 1054-1058.

Ancoli-Israel, S., Parker, L., Sinaee, R., Fell, R. L., & Kripke, D. F. (1989). Sleep fragmentation in patients from a nursing home. *Journal of Gerontology: Medical Sciences, 44*, M18-M21.

Ansseau, M., Pitchot, W., Hansenne, M., & Moreno, A. G. (1992). Psychotic reactions to zolpidem. *Lancet, 339*, 809.

Baekeland, F. (1970). Exercise deprivation: Sleep and psychological reactions. *Archives of General Psychiatry, 22*, 365-369.

Baltes, M. M., Kindermann, T., Reisenzein, R., & Schmid, U. (1987). Further observational data on the behavioral and social world of institutions for the aged. *Psychology and Aging, 2*, 390-403.

Berlowitz, D. R., & Wilking, S.V.B. (1990). The short-term outcome of pressure sores. *Journal of the American Geriatrics Society, 38*, 748-752.

Bliwise, D. L. (1994a). Sleep in dementing illness. In J. M. Oldham & M. B. Riba (Eds.), *Review of psychiatry* (Vol. 13, pp. 757-776). Washington, DC: American Psychiatric Press.

Bliwise, D. L. (1994b). What is sundowning? *Journal of the American Geriatrics Society, 42*, 1009-1011.

Bliwise, D. L. (1996). Is sleep apnea a cause of reversible dementia in old age ? *Journal of the American Geriatrics Society, 44*, 1407-1409.

Bliwise, D. L. (in press-a). Dementia. In M. H. Kryger, T. Roth, & W. C. Dement (Eds.), *Principles and practice of sleep medicine* (3rd ed.). Philadelphia: W. B. Saunders.

Bliwise, D. L. (in press-b). Normal aging. In M. H. Kryger, T. Roth, & W. C. Dement (Eds.), *Principles and practice of sleep medicine* (3rd ed.). Philadelphia: W. B. Saunders.

Bliwise, D. L., Bevier, W. C., Bliwise, N. G., Edgar, D.M., & Dement, W. C. (1990). Systematic 24-hr behavioral observations of sleep wakefulness in a skilled care nursing facility. *Psychology of Aging, 5*, 16-24.

Bliwise, D. L., Carroll, J. S., & Dement, W. C. (1990). Predictors of observed sleep/wakefulness in residents in long term care. *Journal of Gerontology: Medical Sciences, 45*, M126-M130.

Bliwise, D. L., Carroll, J. S., Lee, K. A., Nekich, J. C., & Dement, W. C. (1993). Sleep and "sundowning" in nursing home patients with dementia. *Psychiatry Research, 48*, 277-292.

Campbell, S. (1984). Duration and placement of sleep in a "disentrained" environment. *Psychophysiology, 21*, 106-113.

Campbell, S. S., Dawson, D., & Anderson, M. W. (1993). Alleviation of sleep maintenance insomnia with timed exposure to bright light. *Journal of the American Geriatrics Society, 41*, 829-836.

Castor, D., Woods, D., Pigott, L., & Hemmes, R. (1991). Effect of sunlight on sleep patterns of the elderly. *Journal of the American Academy of Physician Assistants, 4*, 321-326.

Clapin-French, E. (1986). Sleep patterns of aged persons in long-term care facilities. *Journal of Advanced Nursing, 11*, 57-66.

Clarfield, A. M. (1988). The reversible dementias: Do they reverse? *Annals of Internal Medicine, 109*, 476-486.

Cohen, D., Eisdorfer, C., Prinz, P., Breen, A., Davis, M., & Gadsby, A. (1983). Sleep disturbances in the institutionalized aged. *Journal of the American Geriatrics Society, 31*, 79-82.

Cohen-Mansfield, J. (1990). The relationship between sleep disturbances and agitation in a nursing home. *International Journal of Aging and Health, 2*, 42-57.

Cohen-Mansfield, J., Werner, P., & Freedman, L. (1995). Sleep and agitation in agitated nursing home residents: An observational study. *Sleep, 18*, 674-680.

Creighton, C. (1995). Effects of afternoon rest on the performance of geriatric patients in a rehabilitation hospital: A pilot study. *The American Journal of Occupational Therapy, 49*, 775-779.

Cruise, P. A., Schnelle, J. F., Alessi, C. A., Simmons, S. F., & Ouslander, J. G. (1998). The nighttime environment and incontinence care practices in nursing homes. *Journal of the American Geriatrics Society, 46,* 181-186.

Dorsey, C. M., Lukas, S. E., Teicher, M. H., Harper, D., Winkelman, J. W., Cunningham, S. L., & Satlin, A. (1996). Effects of passive body heating on the sleep of older female insomniacs. *Journal of Geriatric Psychiatry & Neurology, 9,* 83-90.

Edgar, D. M., & Dement, W. C. (1991). Regularly scheduled voluntary exercise synchronizes the mouse circadian clock. *American Journal of Physiology, 261,* R928-R933.

Edinger, J. D., Lipper, S., & Wheeler, B. (1989). Hospital ward policy and patients' sleep patterns: A multiple baseline study. *Rehabilitation Psychology, 34,* 43-50.

Espie, C. A., & Tweedie, F. M. (1991). Sleep patterns and sleep problems amongst people with mental handicap. *Journal of Mental Deficiency Research, 35,* 25-36.

Evans, L. K. (1987). Sundown syndrome in institutionalized elderly. *Journal of the American Geriatrics Society, 35,* 101-108.

Exum, M. E., Phelps, B. J., Nabers, K. E., & Osborne, J. G. (1993). Sundown syndrome: Is it reflected in the use of PRN medications for nursing home residents? *Gerontologist, 33,* 756-761.

Gallagher-Thompson, D., Brooks, J. O., Bliwise, D., Leader, J., & Yesavage, J. A. (1992). The relations among caregiver stress, "sundowning" symptoms, and cognitive decline in Alzheimer's disease. *Journal of the American Geriatrics Society, 40,* 807-810.

Garfinkel, D., Laudon, M., Nof, D., & Zisapel, N. (1995). Improvement of sleep quality in elderly people by controlled-release melatonin. *Lancet, 346,* 541-544.

Gentili, A., Weiner, D. K., Kuchibhatla, M., & Edinger, J. D. (1997). Factors that disturb sleep in nursing home residents. *Aging: Clinical Experimental Research, 9,* 207-213.

Gilbert, A., Innes, J. M., Owen, N., & Sansom, L. (1993). Trial of an intervention to reduce chronic benzodiazepine use among residents of aged-care accommodation. *Australia and New Zealand Journal of Medicine, 23,* 343-347.

Granek, E., Baker, S. P., Abbey, H., Robinson, E., Myers, A. H., Samkoff, J. S., & Klein, L. E. (1987). Medications and diagnoses in relation to falls in a long-term care facility. *Journal of the American Geriatrics Society, 35,* 503-511.

Gurwitz, J. H., Soumerai, S. B., & Avorn, J. (1990). Improving medication prescribing utilization in the nursing home. *Journal of the American Geriatrics Society, 38,* 542-552.

Haimov, I., Lavie, P., Laudon, M., Herer, P., Vigder, C., & Zisapel, N. (1995). Melatonin replacement therapy in elderly insomniacs. *Sleep, 18,* 598-603.

Hughes, R. J., Sack, R. L., & Lewy, A. J. (1998). The role of melatonin and circadian phase in age-related sleep-maintenance insomnia: Assessment in a clinical trial of melatonin replacement. *Sleep, 21,* 52-68.

Jacobs, D., Ancoli-Israel, S., Parker, L., & Kripke, D. F. (1989). 24-hour sleep/wake patterns in a nursing home population. *Psychology and Aging, 4,* 352-356.

King, A. C., Oman, R. F., Brassington, G., Bliwise, D. L., & Haskell, W. L. (1997). Moderate-intensity exercise and self-rated quality of sleep in older adults. *Journal of the American Medical Association, 277,* 32-37.

Little, J. T., Satlin, A., Sunderland, T., & Volicer, L. (1995). Sundown syndrome in severely demented patients with probable Alzheimer's disease. *Journal of Geriatric Psychiatry and Neurology, 8,* 103-106.

Lovell, B. B., Ancoli-Israel, S., & Gevirtz, R. (1995). Effect of bright light treatment on agitated behavior in institutionalized elderly subjects. *Psychiatry Research, 57,* 7-12.

McCarten, J. R., Kovera, C., Maddox, M. K., & Cleary, J. P. (1995). Triazolam in Alzheimer's disease: Pilot study on sleep and memory effects. *Pharmacology, Biochemistry and Behavior, 52,* 447-452.

McGaffigan, S., & Bliwise, D. L. (1997). The treatment of sundowning: A selective review of pharmacological and nonpharmacological studies. *Drugs and Aging, 10*, 10-17.

Meltzer-Brody, S., Mouton, A., Ge, Y. R., Sanchez, R., & Zee, P. C. (1994). Effects of scheduled bright light exposure on subjective measurements of vigor in residents of an assisted living facility. *Sleep Research, 23*, 504.

Middelkoop, H.A.M., Kerkhof, G. A., Smilde-van den Doel, D. A., Ligthart, G. J., & Kamphuisen, H.A.C. (1994). Sleep and ageing: The effect of institutionalization on subjective and objective characteristics of sleep. *Age and Ageing, 23*, 411-417.

Mishima, K., Okawa, M., Hishikawa, Y., Hozumi, S., Hori, H., & Takahashi, K. (1994). Morning bright light therapy for sleep and behavior disorders in elderly patients with dementia. *Acta Psychiatrica Scandinavica, 89*, 1-7.

Monane, M., Glynn, R. J., & Avorn, J. (1996). The impact of sedative-hypnotic use on sleep symptoms in elderly nursing home residents. *Clinical Pharmacological Therapy, 59*, 83-92.

Morgan, K. (1987). *Sleep and aging: A research-based guide to sleep in later life.* Baltimore: The Johns Hopkins University Press.

Morgan, K., Dallosso, H., Ebrahim, S., Arie, T., & Fentem, P. H. (1988). Characteristics of subjective insomnia in the elderly living at home. *Age and Ageing, 17*, 1-7.

Murphy, P. J., Badia, P., Myers, B. L., Boecker, M. R., & Wright, K. P. (1994). Nonsteroidal anti-inflammatory drugs affect normal sleep patterns in humans. *Physiology and Behavior, 55*, 1063-1066.

New York State Department of Health. (1994). *Light therapy for residents of special care units: Final report.* Riverdale, NY: Hebrew Home for the Aged.

Okawa, M., Mishima, K., Hishikawa, T., Hozumi, S., Hori, H., & Takahashi, K. (1991). Circadian rhythm disorders in sleep-waking and body temperature in elderly patients with dementia and their treatment. *Sleep, 14*, 478-485.

Orr, W. C., Shamma-Othman, Z., Levin, D., Othman, J., & Rundell, O. H. (1990). Persistent hypoxemia and excessive daytime sleepiness in chronic obstructive pulmonary disease (COPD). *Chest, 97*, 583-585.

Parker, K. P., Bliwise, D. L., & Rye, D. B. (in press). Hemodialysis disrupts basic sleep regulatory mechanisms: Hypothesis building. *Nursing Research.*

Physicians' Desk Reference. (53rd ed.). (1999). Montvale, NJ: Medical Economics Company.

Pollak, C. P., & Perlick, D. (1991). Sleep problems and institutionalization of the elderly. *Journal of Geriatric Psychiatry and Neurology, 4*, 204-210.

Pollak, C. P., Perlick, D., Linsner, J. P., Wenston, J., & Hsieh, F. (1990). Sleep problems in the community elderly as predictors of death and nursing home placement. *Journal of Community Health, 15*, 123-135.

Pollak, C. P., Stokes, P. E., & Wagner, D. R. (1997). Nocturnal interactions between community elders and caregivers, as measured by cross-correlation of their motor activity. *Journal of Geriatric Psychiatry and Neurology, 10*, 168-173.

Reynolds, C. F., III, Hoch, C. C., Buysse, D. J., Houck, P. R., Schlernitzauer, M., & Frank, E. (1992). Electroencephalographic sleep in spousal bereavement and bereavement-related depression of late life. *Biological Psychiatry, 31*, 69-82.

Rosen, J., Reynolds, C. F., Yeager, A. L., Houck, P. R., & Hurwitz, L. F. (1991). Sleep disturbances in survivors of the Nazi Holocaust. *American Journal of Psychiatry, 148*, 62-66.

Rosen, R. C., & Kostis, J. B. (1985). Biobehavioral sequellae associated with adrenergic-inhibiting antihypertensive agents: A critical review. *Health Psychology, 4*, 579-604.

Rye, D. B., & Bliwise, D. L. (1997). Movement disorders specific to sleep and the nocturnal manifestations of waking movement disorders. In R. L. Watts & W. C. Koller (Eds.), *Movement disorders: Neurologic principles and practice* (pp. 687-713). New York: McGraw-Hill.

Satlin, A., Volicer, L., Ross, V., Herz, L., & Campbell, S. (1992). Bright light treatment of be-havioral and sleep disturbances in patients with Alzheimer's disease. *American Journal of Psychiatry, 149,* 1028-1032.

Schenck, C. H., Bundlie, S. R., Ettinger, M. G., & Mahowald, M. W. (1986). Chronic behav-ioral disorders of human REM sleep: A new category of parasomnia. *Sleep, 9,* 293-308.

Schenck, C. H., Bundlie, S. R., & Mahowald, M. W. (1996). Delayed emergence of a Parkinsonian disorder in 38% of 29 older men initially diagnosed with idiopathic rapid eye movement sleep behavior disorder. *Neurology, 46,* 388-393.

Schnelle, J. F., Cruise, P. A., Alessi, C. A., Ludlow, K., Al-Samarrai, N. R., & Ouslander, J. G. (1998). Sleep hygiene in physically dependent nursing home residents: Behavioral and environmental intervention implications. *Sleep, 21,* 515-523.

Schnelle, J. F., Ouslander, J. G., Simmons, S. F., Alessi, C. A., & Gravel, M. D. (1993a). The nighttime environment, incontinence care, and sleep disruption in nursing homes. *Jour-nal of the American Geriatrics Society, 41,* 910-914.

Schnelle, J. F., Ouslander, J. G., Simmons, S. F., Alessi, C. A., & Gravel, M. D. (1993b). Night-time sleep and bed mobility among incontinent nursing home residents. *Journal of the American Geriatrics Society, 41,* 903-909.

Seppala, M., Rajala, T., & Sourander, L. (1993). Subjective evaluation of sleep and the use of hypnotics in nursing homes. *Aging: Clinical and Experimental Research, 5,* 199-205.

Shaw, S. H., Curson, H., & Coquelin, J. P. (1992). A double-blind, comparative study of zolpidem and placebo in the treatment of insomnia in elderly psychiatric in-patients. *The Journal of International Medical Research, 20,* 150-161.

Shorr, R. I., Fought, R. L., & Ray, W. A. (1994). Changes in antipsychotic drug use in nursing home during implementation of the OBRA-87 regulations. *Journal of the American Medi-cal Association, 271,* 358-362.

Singer, C., Colling, E., Moffit, M., Cutler, N., Sack, R., & Lewy, A. (1998). Melatonin and sleep in patients with Alzheimer's disease. *Sleep, 21,* 248.

Singh, N. A., Clements, K. M., & Fiatarone, M. A. (1997). A randomized controlled trial of the effect of exercise on sleep. *Sleep, 20,* 95-101.

Sloane, P. D., Mitchell, C. M., Preisser, J. S., Phillips, C., Commander, C., & Burker, E. (1998). Environmental correlates of resident agitation in Alzheimer's disease special care units. *Journal of the American Geriatrics Society, 46,* 862-869.

Stewart, R. B., & Hale, W. E. (1992). Acute confusional states in older adults and the role of polypharmacy. *Annual Review of Health, 13,* 415-430.

Venable, R. J. (1994, July). Legislating drug prescribing practices [Letter to the editor]. *Jour-nal of the American Medical Association, 272,* 30.

Vitiello, M. V., Prinz, P. N., & Schwartz, R. S. (1994). Slow wave sleep but not overall sleep quality of healthy older men and women is improved by increased aerobic fitness. *Sleep Research, 23,* 149.

Winget, C. M., Vernikos-Danellis, J., Cronin, S. E., Leach, C. S., Rambout, P. C., & Mack, P. B. (1972). Circadian rhythm asynchrony in man during hypokinesis. *Journal of Applied Physiology, 33,* 640-643.

Yuen, E. J., Zisselman, M. H., Louis, D. Z., & Rovner, B. W. (1997). Sedative-hypnotic use by the elderly: Effects on hospital length of stay and costs. *The Journal of Mental Health Ad-ministration, 24,* 90-97.

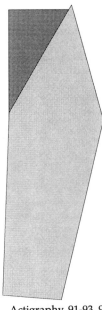

Index

345

About the Editors

Kenneth L. Lichstein is Professor of Psychology at The University of Memphis. He earned his doctoral degree in clinical psychology from the University of Tennessee in 1976. Most of his career has been devoted to investigating methodological and clinical aspects of behavioral medicine, with an emphasis on sleep disorders. He has published more than 75 journal articles and book chapters and one previous book. For most of the past 10 years, his research on insomnia in older adults has been supported by the National Institute on Aging. He has served on the editorial boards of several journals, including the *Journal of Consulting and Clinical Psychology* and *Behavior Therapy*, and he has served as a consultant to the National Institute of Health relating to behavioral medicine and sleep disorders.

Charles M. Morin is Professor of Psychology and Director of the Sleep Disorders Centre at the Université Laval in Quebec City. From 1986 to 1994, he was on the faculty of the Medical College of Virginia at Virginia Commonwealth University. He is a leading authority on insomnia treatment and has been conducting clinical sleep research and treating patients with insomnia for more than 15 years. He has published extensively and lectured internationally on the topic, and his research has been funded by the National Institute of Mental Health. A Diplomate of the American Board of Sleep Disorders Medicine, he received the Distinguished Scientific Award for an Early Career Contribution to Psychology from the American Psychological Association in 1995.

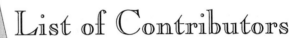

List of Contributors

Iris Alapin
Concordia University

Sally Bailes
Jewish General Hospital, Montreal

Lucie Baillargeon
Centre Hospitalier de l'Université Laval

Célyne Bastien
Université Laval

France C. Blais
Vancouver Hospital

Donald L. Bliwise
Emory University Medical School

Richard R. Bootzin
University of Arizona

Michael J. Breus
DeKalb Medical Center, Decatur

Daniel J. Buysse
University of Pittsburgh School of Medicine

Jack D. Edinger
VA Medical Center, Durham

Dana R. Epstein
Carl T. Hayden VA Medical Center, Phoenix

Colin A. Espie
University of Glasgow

Catherine S. Fichten
Dawson College

Eva Libman
Concordia University

Kenneth L. Lichstein
The University of Memphis

Kevin Morgan
Loughborough University, UK

Charles M. Morin
Université Laval

Charles F. Reynolds III
University of Pittsburgh School of Medicine

Brant W. Riedel
The University of Memphis

Josée Savard
Université Laval

William K. Wohlgemuth
Duke University Medical Center